ADOLESCENT PSYCHIATRY

DEVELOPMENTAL AND CLINICAL STUDIES

VOLUME 18

Annals of the American Society for Adolescent Psychiatry

ADOLESCENT PSYCHIATRY

DEVELOPMENTAL AND CLINICAL STUDIES

VOLUME 18

Edited by
SHERMAN C. FEINSTEIN
Editor in Chief

Senior Editors
AARON H. ESMAN
HARVEY A. HOROWITZ
JOHN G. LOONEY
GEORGE H. ORVIN
JOHN L. SCHIMEL
ALLAN Z. SCHWARTZBERG
ARTHUR D. SOROSKY
MAX SUGAR

The University of Chicago Press
Chicago and London

The University of Chicago Press, Chicago 60637
The University of Chicago Press, Ltd., London

© 1992 by The University of Chicago
All rights reserved. Published 1992
Printed in the United States of America

International Standard Book Number: 0-226-24064-9
Library of Congress Catalog Card Number: 70-147017

The paper used in this publication meets the minimum requirements of American National Standard for Information Sciences—Permanence of Paper for Printed Library Materials, ANSI Z39.48-1984. ∞ ™

CONTENTS

Special Section

STANLEY SCHNEIDER, Special Editor

PART V. ADOLESCENT SUBSTANCE ABUSE

HARVEY A. HOROWITZ, Special Editor

PRESIDENT'S PREFACE

Volume 18 of the Annals of the American Society for Adolescent Psychiatry continues the outstanding tradition of bringing together, in one volume each year, excellent papers dealing with the critical areas of adolescent development, psychopathology, and psychotherapy. Special sections dealing with specific interest areas augment these exceptional volumes.

The American Society for Adolescent Psychiatry is especially proud of this clinically rich series, which has consistently reflected a state-of-the-art quality of all that is unique to adolescents from normality to pathology. The American Society for Adolescent Psychiatry continues to be the only professional organization devoted exclusively to the adolescent age period and focuses on those issues particular to the adolescent population. *Adolescent Psychiatry* has become a ready and reliable source of reference for students and professionals dealing with the special issues of young people forging their way from childhood toward adulthood.

The American Society for Adolescent Psychiatry continues to grow in membership, in part, because it continues to focus on clinical issues and the psychopathology of adolescents. Clearly, biological psychiatry has greatly enhanced the clinician's diagnostic and therapeutic capabilities. Concomitantly, the spiraling costs of health care have imposed some serious restrictions on the utilization of mental health services for adolescents. These two forces have led some to the belief that intensive psychotherapy for adolescents will be relegated to the historical past and supplemented by new technologies, medications, and short-term goal-oriented therapeutic modalities. Many adolescents will be helped by these newer modalities, but many other adolescents will require time, patience, and careful treatment—the types of treatment exquisitely detailed in the contents of each volume of *Adolescent Psychiatry*.

RICHARD M. SARLES

IN MEMORIAM
JOHN BOWLBY (1907–1990)

John Bowlby, child and adolescent psychiatrist and psychoanalyst, pioneer in the emerging field of developmental psychopathology, and recipient of the American Society for Adolescent Psychiatry's 1986 Schonfeld Award, died September 2, 1990, at his vacation home on the Isle of Skye.

Born in 1907, the son of a London surgeon, John Bowlby was educated at Cambridge, where he read psychology and obtained first-class honors in natural science in 1928. After Cambridge, and prior to beginning his medical training, he spent six months working in a school for disturbed children and adolescents, an experience that greatly influenced his choice of career and led him to begin his training in psychoanalysis and a personal analysis with Joan Riviere even as he began his medical education. He studied medicine at University College Medical School in London, graduating in 1933. From 1933 to 1937, he took his specialty training in psychiatry at the Maudsley Hospital, in child psychiatry at the London Child Guidance Clinic, and in psychoanalysis at the London Institute of Psychoanalysis. During the years 1937–1940, he worked in London as a child psychiatrist and psychoanalyst.

Though believing prior to his psychoanalytic training that psychoanalysis was based on Freud's idea of a relationship between the child's real experience within the family and the adult's emotional problems, he quickly learned, most forcefully from Melanie Klein, his supervisor, that this premise had been abandoned in favor of the belief that the most significant psychic events of childhood took place in fantasy. Bowlby then as now disagreed. Impressed by his early experiences at the school for disturbed children and later at the London Child Guidance Clinic, he became convinced that many of the problems that he confronted in his child and adolescent patients had their origin in the actual experience of faulty and disrupted relationships between parent and child. This hypothesis, then controversial, created problems. One was how to account for the negative effects of disturbed parent-child relationships on personality development; another was how to demonstrate this proposed relationship to skeptical colleagues. Mindful of these difficulties, Bowlby undertook to study in depth the emotional and behavioral problems in children and adolescents resulting from prolonged maternal separation and deprivation in the first five years. By collecting a series of carefully researched cases, he demonstrated a profound relationship between this deprivation and the development of a personality incapable of making and sustaining affectional bonds, immune to praise and blame, and prone to repeated delinquencies. Thus, in these earliest studies, conducted in the late 1930s and published as "Forty-four Juvenile Thieves: Their Character and Home-Life" (*International Journal of Psycho-Analysis* 25 [1944]: 19–53, 107–128), was the attachment and loss paradigm gestating.

Then came 1940 and the war, and, as Bowlby recalled years later, "within six months I had said good-bye to child psychiatry. As an army psychiatrist for five years I fought my battles from Salisbury Plain and the Heights of Hampstead." The war ended, and, after leaving the army early in 1946, Bowlby was asked to direct the Children's Department at the Tavistock Clinic. He accepted the position and renamed the department the "Department for Children and Parents," remaining its director until 1972. At Tavistock, Bowlby was able to attract gifted people to join him in his research on the effects of the separation of the young child from his mothering figure. His first research assistant was the psychiatric social worker James Robertson. Already familiar with the separation problem from his work with Anna Freud at her wartime Hampstead nurseries, Robertson, using the techniques of the naturalist, made a series of studies of the unmistakable effects of brief mother-child separations occasioned by the hospitalization of the child. This work led to a film, *A Two Year Old Goes to the Hospital* (1952), which records an eight-day stay in the hospital of one child and vividly illustrates the distressful sequence of separation: first, protest and the attempt to recover mother; second, despair of doing so and depression; finally, emotional detachment from her.

While Robertson was engaged in this work, Bowlby accepted an invitation from the World Health Organization to write a report on the mental health of homeless children. This report, published in 1951 as "Maternal Care and Mental Health," was translated into twelve languages and led to far-reaching changes in the care of children in hospitals and institutions. Thereafter, Bowlby devoted himself to the theoretical implications of the observations made by his research team, which now included the developmental psychologist Mary Salter Ainsworth. Focusing on an understanding of the nature of the child's tie to the mother as the primary task of a developmental psychology and a developmental psychopathology, particularly one based on direct observations of the human mother and child, Bowlby reached beyond existing psychological and psychoanalytical theories to develop a new integration of concepts derived from ethology, cybernetics, systems theory, and cognitive psychology as well as psychoanalysis. Thus was the attachment paradigm born.

This work was courageously presented to the brilliant, yet divided and combative British Psychoanalytical Society of the 1950s and published in a series of papers between 1958 and 1963. The first of these was "The Nature of a Child's Tie to His Mother" (*International Journal of Psycho-Analysis* 39 [1958]: 350–373). The others were on problems of separation anxiety and mourning. These early papers, expanded and deepened, evolved into the seminal trilogy *Attachment and Loss* (vol. 1, *Attachment,* vol. 2, *Separation,* and vol. 3, *Loss* [New York: Basic, 1969–1980]), a work that may well be judged to be the most significant psychological writing of the period. As Sroufe has written, "The advancement of psychoanalytic theory, developmental psychology and developmental psychopathology by this effort is in each case fundamental. Bowlby's work has inspired new concepts, new methods, a new way of looking at basic phenomena in human development. As is always characteristic of development, whether in an individual or in a scientific field, Bowlby's work both integrates and transforms what went before, creating an alternative way of viewing the world without leaving behind critical insights contained in previous viewpoints" (L. A. Sroufe, "Appraisal: Bowlby's Contribution to Psychoanalytic Theory and Developmental Psychology," *Journal of Child Psychology and Psychiatry* 27 [1986]: 841–849).

Bowlby, child and adolescent psychiatrist and psychoanalyst, recast, with the *Attachment and Loss* trilogy, the central premises of psychoanalytic theory into the language and method of a modern science while at the same time bringing the complex and subtle vitality of human relationships into the sterile domain of behavioral psychology. By focusing again, as did Freud, on the centrality of vital relationships as the core of the human experience, and by reformulating these relationships within an evolutionary context, Bowlby has brought us to a more satisfactory theory of human behavior. His theory will surely be a major part of the science of human behavior for years to come.

In the decade following the publication of the final volume of the trilogy, John Bowlby traveled and taught around the world. Frequently coming to North America, he was tireless in his efforts to encourage and maintain the creative ferment that his ideas on attachment and vital relationships had inspired in this country. He was an enormously energetic and supportive mentor to many in the community of theorists, researchers, and clinicians who helped create the domain of developmental psychopathology.

It was on one of these lecturing visits to the United States that I first met John in 1983. He had accepted my invitation to come to Philadelphia to speak to the Philadelphia Society for Adolescent Psychiatry and to the clinical staff of the Institute of Pennsylvania Hospital. I learned when he arrived that during his two days in Philadelphia he was also going to meet with Aaron Beck and his cognitive therapy research group at Penn as well as see Martin Orne at the Unit for Experimental Psychiatry. All this in two days and at seventy-six years! John had time for all who wanted to talk with him and to learn from him.

John was also a wonderful guest to have in our home, so grandfatherly, white haired, and playful that our daughter, Rebekah, then age two, quickly became attached to "Doctor Bow-bee!"

In 1986, John was honored by the American Society for Adolescent Psychiatry with the Schonfeld Award. The subject of his lecture was Charles Darwin and the proposition that Darwin's repeated illnesses were the somatization of significant losses in childhood, particularly the death of his mother when Darwin was only seven.

While in Washington, my wife, Claudia, and I planned to visit John and Ursula in England that summer of 1986 and to meet for a day at Down House, Darwin's home from 1848 until his death in 1872. Surprisingly, although John had been a student of Darwin's life and work for many years, he had never made the one-hour drive from London to Downe, in Kent, to see the great biologist's country estate. Yet, as he walked the house and grounds, John informed and entertained us with stories of Darwin family members and events as well as anecdotes about the evolution of Charles's ideas as we retraced Darwin's "thinking path," where, on daily walks around his gardens, fields, and woods, he constructed some of the ideas so important to modern thought.

The last few years of John's life, following a stroke in 1987, were devoted to completing his book *Charles Darwin: A New Biography* (1990), which was published in June 1990 in Britain. Characteristically, he did not rest until his work was done. Also characteristically, he arranged with his publisher's Toronto office for gift copies of the work to be mailed to his friends in North America. My copy arrived in September, shortly before the news of his death. We will miss our friend, colleague, and teacher John Bowlby.

HARVEY A. HOROWITZ

PART I

ADOLESCENCE: GENERAL CONSIDERATIONS

1 PSYCHOTHERAPY OF BORDERLINE AND NARCISSISTIC DISORDERS IN THE ADOLESCENT: ESTABLISHING A THERAPEUTIC ALLIANCE

JAMES F. MASTERSON, JOHN BAIARDI, RICHARD FISCHER, AND CANDACE ORCUTT

The therapeutic alliance, essential to the successful psychotherapy of borderline and narcissistic disorders, is achieved by two different therapeutic interventions. The advantages of viewing this issue from this theoretical approach are that it provides an architecture of the patient's inner emotional life—in self- and object representations with their linking affects and ego defense mechanism and functions—that allows the therapist to identify and understand the ebb and flow of the patient's emotions; informs the therapist as to what emotional state must be dealt with and how to deal with it; and provides a tool for evaluating the effects of the interventions.

The therapeutic alliance can be defined as a real object relationship that is conscious and within which both patient and therapist agree to work together to help the patient develop better understanding and control. As a real object relationship, it is based on the capacities of both the patient and the therapist to see each other as completely separate figures, whole objects with both positive and negative attributes. In other words, the patient must be able to see the therapist as he is as well as to see his projections on the therapist.

The therapeutic alliance is a precondition for classic psychoanalysis, but it represents a substantial achievement in these patients. To understand why it is an achievement, we must distinguish the way a neurotic patient relates (i.e., transference) from the way borderline and narcissistic patients relate (i.e., transference acting out). The transference relationship is not conscious, and the therapist is utilized not as a real object but as a displaced object on whom unresolved infantile fantasies are projected. The transference relationship also requires the capacity for whole object relations, for how can a patient know he is displacing feelings onto an object unless he is able, at the same time, to recognize the independent existence of that object? In classic psychoanalysis, it is the therapeutic alliance that is operative at the beginning of treatment in the neurotic patient that forms the framework against which the fantasies, memories, and emotions evoked by the transference are measured, contrasted, interpreted, and worked through. The patient's awareness of the real object relationship—the therapeutic alliance—forms the essential background against which he can evaluate his displaced, unresolved, infantile fantasies.

The borderline and narcissistic patient, however, relates not by transference but by transference acting out, which is at the same time his style of relating to the therapist and his style of defense against underlying anxiety and depression. To understand the dynamics of transference acting out and its relation to working through we can refer to an article written in 1914 by Freud. To adapt this discussion to borderline and narcissistic patients we have only to substitute the words "transference acting out" for Freud's descriptive phrase "expressing what is forgotten in behavior" and splitting for repression.

Freud highlighted the following: "The patient remembers nothing but expresses it in his actions, in his behavior." He reproduces it not in his feelings and memory but in his behavior; that is, he repeats it in his transference acting out. The compulsion to repeat an action that defends against the impulse to feel and remember is activated in treatment. When it is curbed by therapeutic intervention, it is turned into a motive for remembering. The patient's repetitive reactions in the transference of affects, when not discharged by transference acting out, lead to the emergence of feelings and memories that set the stage for working through of the underlying anxiety and depression.

The developmental arrests of the borderline and narcissistic disorders, which produce the defensive style of transference acting out, also result in a weak and fragile capacity for a therapeutic alliance. There is little basic trust and capacity to use an observing ego to

4

understand the differences between past and present, reality and fantasy, and mature and infantile aspects of mental life.

The initial as well as continuing goal of psychotherapy is to establish, strengthen, and maintain a therapeutic alliance that will nonetheless routinely, inevitably, and repeatedly suffer transient breakdowns whenever the treatment impels the patient to give up defense and self-activate. These same breakdowns, however, properly managed, can lead many patients to understanding and mastery of their emotional problem.

The essential theme of this chapter is that different therapeutic interventions are required to establish the therapeutic alliance with these two disorders: confrontation with the borderline and interpretation of narcissistic vulnerability with the narcissistic personality disorder. It is the difference in the form and content of the intrapsychic structure in these two disorders that tells us why different interventions are necessary to establish a therapeutic alliance.

Borderline Personality Disorder

THE INTRAPSYCHIC STRUCTURE

The specific intrapsychic structure consists of the split ego and split object-relations unit. The ego structure itself is split into two parts, one functioning according to the reality principle and the other according to the pleasure principle. The latter can be called the "pathological ego." This contains defects in ego functioning, poor reality perception, impulse control, frustration tolerance, and ego boundaries. In addition, primitive mechanisms of defense such as splitting, avoidance, denial, clinging, acting out, projection, and projective identification are operative.

SPLIT OBJECT-RELATIONS UNIT

The split object-relations unit consists of two split self- and object representation part units that I have called the "rewarding object-relations part unit" (RORU) and the "withdrawing object-relations part unit" (WORU), each having its own self- and object representation and linking affect.

The rewarding object-relations part unit part object provides reward

5

or approval for regressive behavior, the self-representation is that of being a good passive child, and the linking affect is that of feeling good. The withdrawn object-relations part unit object representation is attacking or withdrawing at efforts to activate the self. The self-representation is of being bad, ugly, or inadequate, and the linking affect is the abandonment depression.

THE BORDERLINE TRIAD

I have called the relations between the split ego and the split object-relations unit—a key to understanding the psychopathology—the "borderline triad": self-activation leads to anxiety and depression, which leads to defense. The clinical vicissitudes of this triad reflect the essence of this disorder.

An alliance is formed between either the rewarding or the withdrawing object-relations part unit and the pathological ego that functions clinically as follows: any later-life separation stresses, efforts at self-activation, or improvement in treatment interrupts defenses and precipitates the withdrawing object-relations unit with its affect of abandonment depression. The patient then defends against these painful affects by activating his alliance with the pathological ego (with either the rewarding part unit, the withdrawing part unit, or each unit alternatively). If the alliance with the rewarding part unit is activated, the patient begins to behave in a regressive maladaptive fashion, but under the sway of the rewarding part unit his affective state is one of feeling good, and he is able to deny his maladaptive behavior. If the alliance with the withdrawing part unit is activated, he projects the withdrawing unit, does not feel the abandonment depression, but acts it out in a maladaptive manner that is also denied.

The defects in ego functioning and the primitive mechanisms of defense can be determined by history as well as by observation in the session; the rewarding and withdrawing object-relations part units can be observed in the history of relationships with the important people in the patient's life as well as in the transference acting out with the therapist.

Treatment

The therapist's task can now be more specifically defined: to help the patient convert transference acting out into therapeutic alliance and transference through the therapeutic technique of confrontation. Confrontation has several definitions. The first implies a lot of aggression, such as eyeball-to-eyeball confrontations. This definition is not what is meant. Rather, it is the second definition, that is, empathically, intuitively, but firmly bringing to the patient's attention the denied, self-destructive, maladaptive aspect of this defensive behavior. As the therapist confronts, lending his reality perception to the patient, the latter integrates the confrontation controlling his maladaptive defensive behavior and, thereby, interrupting his defense against his abandonment depression. The depression surfaces, and, following the borderline triad, the patient then defends again. The therapist then confronts again. This circular sequence eventually results in the patient overcoming defense and containing the depression.

The psychotherapy consists of three stages. First is the testing stage just described. In this stage, the adolescent tests the therapist's competence and trustworthiness preparatory to allowing a therapeutic alliance to be formed. Eventually, the patient controls his defense continuously, establishes a therapeutic alliance, and experiences fully his abandonment depression entering the second or working-through stage of the treatment.

In this stage, much less attention has to be paid to confrontation. The therapist can now use interpretation. It is vital to keep in mind that interpretation does not work unless there is a therapeutic alliance, unless the patient has that reality screen against which to contrast the interpretation. The last stage is the separation stage when the patient must work through the transference fantasies about the therapist as the object that provided support for self-activation.

Narcissistic Personality Disorder

INTRAPSYCHIC STRUCTURE

The intrapsychic structure of the narcissistic disorder contrasts with that of the borderline in both form and content. Rather than having split self- and object representations, the patient has fused selfobject representations. The content of these representations consists of a grandiose, self-omnipotent, object-defensive representation with the linking affect of being perfect, adored, and admired. Underneath is a fused aggressive unit consisting of an extremely harsh, attacking, aggressive, omnipotent object representation fused with a self-representation of being fragmented, inadequate, empty, and destroyed. These representations are linked by the affect of the abandonment depression. The ego structure of the narcissistic disorder is similar to the borderline in that it consists of split ego with primitive mechanism of defense. Clinically, the intrapsychic structure operates as follows.

The Exhibitionistic Narcissistic Personality Disorder

The patient's major emotional investment is in the grandiose self. He exhibits the grandiose self and seeks in his transference acting out perfect empathy and responsiveness from the therapist, that is, to be adored and admired, with the mirroring transference acted out. Failure to resonate and mirror his need for perfect responsiveness frustrates this grandiose self-defense, this failure triggers the underlying aggressive fused unit, the object representation is projected on the therapist, who is seen as disappointing and attacking, and the patient experiences his depression and fragmented self and then defends against this, either by devaluing the therapist or by avoiding the therapist altogether.

The Closet Narcissistic Disorder

If the major emotional investment is in the fused, omnipotent object representation rather than the grandiose self, the patient does not present as grandiose and looking for mirroring responses but rather idealizes the object, the therapist, and seeks his perfect responsiveness basking in the glow of the perfect therapist—that is, the idealizing transference acting out.

A very important and unusual characteristic of the defensive grandiose self of the narcissistic disorder, which is in dramatic contrast to the borderline, is its capacity to maintain continuous activation of the grandiose self and to coerce the environment into resonating with the grandiose self-projections or, where that is not possible, to avoid, deny, or devalue any stimulus that interrupts the grandiose self-projections. As a consequence, the narcissistic disorder, unlike the borderline, is extremely intolerant to experiences of depression.

Interpretations of Narcissistic Vulnerability to Establish a Therapeutic Alliance with a Narcissistic Personality Disorder

The patient begins therapy with either mirroring or idealizing transference acting out. The therapist cannot confront these projections since such a confrontation would trigger the underlying aggressive unit and the patient would see it as an attack and respond as he would to any other kind of attack, that is, projection, devaluation, or avoidance.

The only way to gain entrance to this seemingly solipsistic system is through the therapist's use of mirroring interpretations of the patient's narcissistic vulnerability to the therapist's failures in perfect empathy.

One does not confront a defense as in the borderline, but one interprets it as a defense against narcissistic pain. For example, one might confront a borderline patient who is late for a session by telling him that this is destructive to his objective—that is, he is depriving himself of time to do the work. In contrast, with a narcissistic personality disorder, one would interpret as follows: "It must be very painful for you to talk about yourself here, and you must have felt the need to withdraw to deal with that pain." In other words, the focus is always on the narcissistic vulnerability or pain. The goal of the psychotherapy is the same as with the borderline personality disorder—that is, using a therapeutic intervention to help the patient convert transference acting out into therapeutic alliance and transference. It is the type of therapeutic intervention that differs.

Treatment of the Parents

In both disorders, the designated adolescent patient's pathological behavior usually forms a linchpin for the whole family's system of communication so that it is difficult to treat the adolescent without also treating the parents. It is also preferable that the parents be seen by another therapist. The goal of the psychotherapy with the parents, however, is different: to encourage the substitution of verbalization as a means of communication for acting out; to teach the parents how to parent (many have personality disorders themselves and never learned how to parent); to help the parents contain their negative, regressive projections on the adolescent patient and instead provide support for

9

self-activation; and to find new and more self-activated, adaptive means of dealing with their emotions in their own lives.

Countertransference

One cannot consider psychotherapy of the narcissistic and borderline personality disorders without also saying a few words about countertransference. The reason countertransference is so prominent with these disorders, in our view, is a combination of the intensity of the patient's transference acted-out projections and the human vulnerability of a therapist. At the beginning of treatment, these patients are not there to get better since that would evoke depression. They are there to get the therapist to resonate with their projections. If it is the defensive projection, they feel better, and treatment stops; if it is the underlying pathological depressive projection, they get rid of all the rage they were unable to express as a child on the therapist, and treatment stops. For this reason, it is vital that the therapist maintain his therapeutic neutrality as a life preserver against the treatment being inundated by the tidal wave of these projections. The therapeutic neutrality provides the framework for the development of a therapeutic alliance.

Case Illustrations

FORMING A THERAPEUTIC ALLIANCE WITH A BORDERLINE ADOLESCENT IN CRISIS[1]

The patient I am about to describe is now twenty-four and is engaged in long-term, dynamic psychotherapy. Because of the current relationship, I have had the benefit of her comments on our initial, crisis-oriented work. She reaffirms that three components of the early treatment were especially important for her: I supported her validity as an individual; I called her to account when she avoided supporting herself as a valid individual; and she learned to identify and modify the defensive character pattern that was creating problems of adaptation beyond the presenting crisis.

INITIAL TREATMENT

Gerda, fifteen years old, came to her first regularly scheduled appointment with her hand in a cast. She had punched a wall during a frustrating discharge process from a psychiatric inpatient unit. It also occurred to her that she might have needed to create a crisis to relieve the anxiety she felt on leaving the unit. A month before, while leaving a party alone at night, she had been forced off the street and raped. Subsequently, she overdosed twice and was admitted to the hospital.

Gerda, a sophomore in high school, was a well-groomed, overweight girl with long, Alice-in-Wonderland hair. Her manner was engaging, although she described herself as "untrusting." She was intelligent and perceptive, and her speech was articulate and fluid, except for periodic silences. The silences occurred when she felt sad. She said she did not like to talk about sadness but, rather, would wait until it was "over." She believed that her problem had to do with "character," which she thought was not such a bad thing since character could be changed.

I had already spoken separately with Gerda's mother, an author of children's books who constantly traveled in search of ethnic source materials. The mother was attractive, thin, and dressed like a fashionable bohemian. She was quick, intelligent, and intellectualized. She told me that she felt as if her life had been "knocked out from under her" by her daughter's hospitalization. It occurred to me that Gerda seemed like one of her mother's fictional creations—even her name had a storybook quality. "I hate my name," said Gerda. "It isn't a real name, and nobody ever pronounces it right." Gerda's childhood was described to me by her mother. Gerda was the more reliable historian about her own adolescence.

Gerda had been a healthy baby who was weaned at nine months and had loved to eat. Her developmental milestones were achieved early, and, apparently, she toilet trained herself. She developed asthma at about three years of age, a year before her parents were divorced. When Gerda was four, her mother decided to move to Québec to allow herself "time to think." Gerda, uprooted from her home and friends, began to withdraw. Her mother sent her out to buy bread and milk so that she would have to deal with people and learn French Canadian; somehow Gerda managed. A year later, they moved again to New York City, and the mother's career took priority. At seven, Gerda was a latchkey child, with the door key on a string around her neck so that she could come and go by herself. When her mother arrived home from work exhausted, Gerda tucked her into bed. Gerda used to have "intricate, beautiful dreams" for her mother's benefit and would recount them in the morning to cheer her mother up. Gerda's latency period was fragmented by multiple moves, the mother's changing romantic attachments, and extensive trips abroad.

She was the clearest about her early adolescence. At eleven, she had begun what she called her "symbolic year," a period of expressing her anger at her mother in all possible indirect ways. For instance, she wrote "I hate you" in tiny letters on the walls in back of the furniture. By age twelve, she had declared open war, and she and her mother fought constantly.

By the time therapy started, Gerda had had one surrogate father as well as a series of surrogate mothers who took over her care when her own mother traveled. In school, she was maintaining an A average despite her troubles. Her compliance, social skills, energy, and humor helped her keep up the appearance of a model, outgoing, all-around student. Actually, she was constantly surprised to find that others perceived her this way. Her sense of herself was tenuous, and she told me that she had hid under her desk during her earlier school experience. Her relationships with both girls and boys had an intense, dyadic quality. She was offended at the idea of discussing her sexual activities with anyone of my generation, but she said that she believed intercourse should be saved for a deeply committed relationship.

On the night of the rape, she had left the party early when a girlfriend had unreasonably grown angry at her and had ordered her to leave. Gerda, upset, was searching for a cab when she was caught from behind by a man with a knife, who forced her into an empty lot and raped her. She walked home in shock and found that her mother was out. The phone rang, and it was an obscene phone call. Overwhelmed, she swallowed No-Doz washed down with rum and eventually began to vomit. Her mother arrived home and called the police, but Gerda locked herself in her room and refused to come out. Later, her mother took Gerda to the gynecologist for persistent vaginal bleeding. Gerda then overdosed again on flurazepam (Dalmane) and left a suicide note. This time her mother got her to the hospital, where her stomach was pumped, and she was admitted to the psychiatric unit.

COURSE OF TREATMENT

The treatment—shorter term and crisis oriented—lasted for over two years. For the first nine months, Gerda was seen individually twice a week and with her mother once a week. After that, she was seen individually three times a week for a year, then twice a week for the last nine months. Treatment ended when, at age eighteen, she graduated from high school and went away to college. From the outset, it was understood that her treatment would probably be time limited by her college plans.

The first phase of treatment focused on the crisis in Gerda's individual and family life. Although the work was heavily confrontational, it became increasingly insight oriented—especially when the family sessions ended and Gerda took increasing responsibility for her therapy.

In the family sessions, the mother and daughter argued, and they could be verbally devastating. At home, these arguments escalated into dramatic scenes with screaming and slamming of doors. Enmeshed in each other's anger, they could go on endlessly over such matters as the care of the cat's litter box.

I pointed out that, although they were both concerned with the issue of responsibility, neither was taking it. I labeled the arguments phony and nonproductive and wondered what it was they would have to face if they stopped arguing. Gerda agreed that the fights were useless and would surely put her "in her grave." Her mother said she feared there would no longer be any communication between them if the fights stopped. The theme of separation emerged (and, of course, the fighting had started when Gerda had begun to move toward adolescent independence). My job, then, was to promote constructive communication and confront phony litter-box talk until, one day, Gerda exclaimed, "We're running the session without you!" With a workable-enough truce declared on the home scene, it was possible to end the family sessions and give Gerda full attention and responsibility for her therapy.

Gerda had told me that these sessions with her mother were critical in forming the alliance between us. She felt that her mother was an expert in gaining emotional support, while Gerda somehow presented herself as incorrigible, and others were unable to get past this false self-presentation.

In her individual sessions, Gerda avoided her feelings by chattering entertainingly, more or less nonstop. I confronted this by asking how keeping me entertained was going to be helpful to her. In response, she told me about her "Pollyanna routine," which she had invented to minimize painful feelings in her social interactions. I said I was receptive to all her thoughts and feelings and that she would be maintaining herself at an impasse by leaving part of herself out of therapy. She then told me that she had always felt safer keeping her feelings "in little boxes" and was afraid of losing control if she did not.

My confrontations then focused on the silences that increasingly interrupted the "Pollyanna routine"—and each of these silences turned out to be "a little box" containing an unexpressed feeling. Gerda began to see how she inhibited her spontaneity by these silences. I began to realize how sensitive she had learned to become to meet her mother's need for constant cheering up.

Once Gerda began to observe her patterns of avoidance, she cautiously began to test how I would receive her expression of feeling. Anger came first, but obliquely. She began to criticize my office in fine detail. I responded to this in a light way, saying, "How can I help you get it together when I can't even put together my own office?" She became a little more direct, noting that I was from the suburbs with "all those little polyester people living in little polyester houses." I asked if she was worried about my being synthetic—a fake therapist. She then expressed her annoyance more directly, saying ruefully that I left her to take the initiative and have painful thoughts and feelings when she talked about herself. She also resented not having a choice about being in therapy. I pointed out that she had made a kind of choice through her suicide attempts and that she could make it easier for herself in the long run if she would learn to say what she wanted instead of doing it.

Gerda has confirmed that my confrontation of her avoidance not only increased her awareness of herself but also increased her appreciation of the therapeutic alliance. I could perceive her situation from a point of view that eluded her, and the sharing of this perception taught her how to observe and manage her actions in a more adaptive way. A sense of trust began to build, just a little, and the first concrete indication that the alliance was strengthening came when she brought in her poems and short stories to read to me.

One story had been written between the time of the rape and her second suicide attempt. It told about a grotesque circus—which was really the world—in which a woman behind a curtain of white silk was "the main attraction." In the story, the curtain is drawn aside, she "makes her one plea to the crowd," and then "a razor-sharp knife descends upon her." Gerda said she was frightened by the feelings in the story and of the feelings aroused in therapy. She was afraid she might be crazy and that, if she told me too much about herself, I would hospitalize her. This was more of a conviction than a fantasy, and it let me know how persuasively she had been taught the unacceptability of her feelings.

At this time, she grudgingly admitted that the family sessions were going well and sadly remarked, "My mother is not a grown-up." She spoke of finding it difficult to have her mother lean on her emotionally and began to feel guilty. She then wandered off the subject. I confronted her avoidance, wondering why she chose to create a diversion rather than accept her own feelings (a repetition of pleasing her mother rather than expressing herself). She got mad at me, saying that she did not want to get depressed again, as she had after the rape—that she would not be able to put the feelings away and would be stuck with them. I said, "You're stuck with them anyway; why not learn to manage them?" She got mad at me again, and I asked her why she was angry at me for believing she could handle her own feelings.

That she perceived this confrontation as evidence that I supported her capacity—and her rights—to deal with her own feelings was confirmed as she began to talk more about the rape. First, she tested briefly by bringing in an article about child molestation. The article stressed the importance of the child's being able to talk about what happened. She then directly began to reconstruct the memory of the rape.

At first she did this by drawing fragmentary, half-symbolic pictures that she brought to her sessions. The drawings contained certain repeated elements: malevolent eyes, a religious medal on a chain, a knife, a stuffed bear being torn apart, dissociated gears, and mechanical parts. The paper the drawings were done on was cut in an elongated, hexagonal shape.

She said that the drawing had to do with evil and the destruction of innocence. The rape was "the ultimate deceit that confirmed all other deceits." She said, "These are pictures of my head, filled with broken gears." She felt "fragmented, in pieces that don't fit together." It occurred to her that the paper was cut in the shape of a coffin.

She had more nightmares and a fear of being overwhelmed by a sense of guilt; she said that that was why she had attempted suicide. She said that she wished she had been beaten because people did not believe that she had wanted to resist. I said, "Your life was in danger.

If you had resisted, you might have been killed." She said that she recalled being grabbed from the back. When she started to run away, her sweater was torn off, and she experienced a brief amnesia—perhaps when she saw the knife. She next remembered being in the empty lot and gagged with her own sweater. She thought she was going to be killed and just wanted it to be over.

Gradually, she also became angry about the rape and at her assailant. She said that her pictures did not have enough anger in them. At home, she concentrated on drawing the rapist's face over and over. In time, she abreacted the trauma and followed that experience with an equally cathartic expression of rage. At the close of that particular session, she showed an expression of resolution and calm that was unique in my experience as a therapist.

Much working through was still ahead, but Gerda had learned, through the therapeutic alliance, to observe her old defenses and find that they did not meet her needs. She also discovered, by accepting a partner in the therapeutic process, that she could find the courage to break down the barriers of denial and silence that had kept her real self imprisoned.

ESTABLISHING A THERAPEUTIC ALLIANCE WITH AN ADOLESCENT WITH A CLOSET NARCISSISTIC PERSONALITY DISORDER[2]

Sean is now a nineteen-year-old white male who began treatment because of his feelings of worthlessness. At that time, Sean was a freshman at a New Jersey community college, where his lifelong history of dependency, passive-aggressive behavior, and underachievement was being replicated. He was without friends and failing in school because of his nonattendance. Sean resided with his aunt but remained in the middle of his divorced parents' ongoing hostility. His attempts to improve his situation were sabotaged by alternating feelings of inadequacy and entitlement.

Sean is an only child. His sixty-five-year-old father is a highly successful management consultant who emigrated from Eastern Europe. He views his father as an unyielding perfectionist who belittles everyone, especially him, for not meeting his standards. Sean acknowledged his homicidal rage toward his father.

The mother is a fifty-five-year-old native-born American who is employed as a school counselor. She is a gratifying and seductive parent who is constantly prepared to protect her son's fragile self-image by helping him avoid potentially dangerous situations like work, school, relationships, and getting out of bed. Sean is somewhat irritated by his mother's overprotectiveness but relates to her in a nonviolent manner.

The developmental history of early childhood is remarkable. His chronic asocial passive aggressivity began in preadolescence. Sean is of bright normal intelligence and did well in elementary school. At age seven, when his parents separated, Sean began what was to be his pattern of truancy, underachievement, and negativity in school. There were several expulsions that led to a three-year placement at the Oakmont Residential School, where he continued to do poorly. There was a period of marijuana and alcohol abuse and a period of violent acting out, but these issues have been resolved.

Treatment had been multifocal, individual, group, milieu, family, and pharmacological, but largely unsuccessful. He had been variously diagnosed as a dysthymic disorder and borderline psychotic, and there was a question of schizophrenia.

Sean appeared in our sessions to be a frightened, anxious adolescent whose fears of being devalued interfered with expressing himself coherently. It seemed as if he were projecting a sense of borderline helplessness. Sean felt like an inept unreal person whose fragmented self-image was of a "loser" or a "nerd" who was being scrutinized by other adolescent males who were awaiting, even expecting, his inevitable failure in order to humiliate or beat him as did his father. Feeling so incapable himself, he fantasized about women like his mother who could provide him with self-confidence.

Although the bulk of the sessions was spent in almost nonstop self-depreciation, Sean could usually and briefly allow me to view his other self-image. This grandiose side fantasized about someday achieving the highest levels of success in education, career, and material possessions. Women were expected to have a spontaneous need to gratify him. To be is to receive.

These grandiose fantasies suggest to me that his character structure was narcissistic, not borderline. Although he lacked the security of exhibiting his grandiosity for any period of time, there was clearly a sense that it was a well-defined part of his character structure. It was as if he were saving it like a bottle of fine cognac in a secret cabinet to share only with special friends.

In order to foster the development of a therapeutic alliance, I felt that it was necessary not only to interpret his disappointments empathically but also to tie them to his avoidant defenses. There was a sense that the pain of disappointment contributed to the secrecy of his grandiose fantasies. When early in the treatment Sean would lament as to his own ineptness—he felt like a mental case who would always be rejected by the kids in school—I would interpret to him that he felt so lacking in self-confidence and so unable to help himself that he sought to find it through the approval of others.

These mirroring interpretations of his personal vulnerabilities in self-activation led to the beginnings of a mirroring transference. Sean now felt secure enough to reveal his grandiose fantasies more fully. He was confident that someday, somehow, he would get that confidence (probably through some magic) that would enable him to get a job, go to Stanford, and have the power to destroy people who rejected him as he was driving by in a Mercedes. As Sean felt unsure that he could find a perfect pathway to success on his own, he protected himself from insecurity by seeking a guarantee. When guarantees, "breaks," and guidelines were not provided, it was so painful for him to act on his own that he felt unable to find his way. Thus, he "protected" his grandiosity by withdrawing from this unfair world that would confront it.

Ultimately, Sean decided that, as I understood him so well, and as my office had a view of the East River, I could provide him with this blueprint for success. The theme of personal vulnerability and the need for some idealized mentor recurred, only, on this occasion, Sean saw me as being a rejecting, withdrawing figure who lacked a perfect understanding of him.

I interpreted his disappointment in me as deriving from his feeling that, because it was so painful for him to find his own blueprint, he avoided the pain by turning it over to me. This led to a therapeutic stalemate. He pleaded, explained, felt disappointed, and resisted. I continued with the mirroring interpretations of his narcissistic vulnerability. Treatment was stalemated. Ultimately, Sean broke the pattern as he began to miss sessions. Further interpretations of the avoidance defense were unproductive.

As something of a mirroring and idealizing transference was already in place, I felt that the use of a more confrontational technique was necessary to deal with his passive-aggressive acting out. I noted to Sean that, although he showed a willingness to work in treatment, even he could not accomplish very much by not coming. In a more empathic confrontation, I reflected that the treatment had become a copy of his life, that when he felt angry and disappointed with someone like me, who did not meet his demands, he demonstrated that anger by withdrawing altogether.

Sean integrated these confrontations to acknowledge his own anger at a world that treated him like his father did and not like his mother did. He reported his grandiose fantasy that he should not have to manage his own life without perfect reassurance.

At this point, treatment began to focus more on his feelings about his parents and himself. His behavior improved, and there were far fewer demands on me. Although Sean's treatment remains somewhat "midstream today," the mirroring interpretations of his vulnerability to self-activation provided the framework for a mirroring transference and a therapeutic alliance.

ESTABLISHING A THERAPEUTIC ALLIANCE WITH AN ADOLESCENT WITH AN EXHIBITIONISTIC, NARCISSISTIC PERSONALITY DISORDER[3]

Danny was a fifteen-year-old from an upper-class family in New York when his parents sought treatment. His father, an extremely successful businessman, and his mother came from an aristocratic European family.

HISTORY OF PRESENT ILLNESS

His parents sought treatment because of his poor motivation in school and his dismissal from several boarding schools. Danny had a history of learning disabilities and poor grades and had been disciplined in several schools ïor drinking, smoking pot, and theft. Danny was described as a good-looking social charmer who got by on style. Danny's parents were concerned about his "Napoléonic complex," as he often spoke about getting even with authority and of being the dictator and leader of a chosen group of children. He often referred to his special destiny and voiced his contempt for ordinary people.

During the initial consultation, Danny's parents gave a frank account of their idealization of Danny and their consistent difficulty with providing appropriate limits for his behavior. The parents had been married in their forties and had adopted Danny and his younger brother. Danny's father was often absent from the family for long periods because of the demands of his business. Both parents described him as a "beautiful toy" and were unable to provide limits or interfere with any of his demands. They described him as a precocious infant who was perfect in every way.

His father said that there was "nothing that I wanted to change about him. He was gregarious, outgoing, and confident—everything that I wasn't." His mother gave a similar description but added that he was distractible, had a short attention span, and had temper tantrums when he was not gratified immediately. Danny's mother reported being depressed by her husband's long absences and of clinging to Danny to relieve some of her depression. Danny's father, on the other hand, was oblivious to the family's problems, claiming that he thought he had a perfect family. He was shocked and concerned to discover that Danny was having school-related problems. Both parents said that, "whatever Danny wanted, we did."

Danny was manipulative with his parents. When his father would try to spank him for transgressions, he would say, "If you were my real father, you wouldn't be this mean to me." These tactics would always disarm his parents. Both parents came from wealthy families that were cold, rejecting, and disinterested. They both admitted to using Danny to feel better about themselves and were proud of his casual, easygoing confidence. Despite this idealization of Danny, both sets of grandparents were rejecting toward Danny because he was not from an aristocratic bloodline.

COURSE OF PSYCHOTHERAPY

Danny came into this initial visit by knocking on all the doors in the waiting room and shouting, "Where the hell is this Dr. Fischer?" Dr. Masterson came out of his office and told him to sit in the waiting area until I was ready for him. When Danny came into my office, he immediately took off his shoes, sank into the couch, closed his eyes, and said, "One more boring shrink to put up with."

He told me that his problem was that teachers and other adults were not as smart as he was and that he was able to con the best of them. He went on to tell me that shrinks must love spoiled rich kids like himself to help pay the bills. He advised that I had better do as he said because he gave the orders and could cut off his parents' purse strings if I was not obedient to his wishes.

After fifteen minutes of his contempt and devaluation, I began to recover. I asked him what his present allowance was. He told me that the amount was not important because he could charm his parents into giving him any amount of money he wanted. He went on to tell me that obviously someday he was going to be president of the country and that the masses needed him. I laughed and told him that, from what his parents told me, it sounded like he was unable to cross the street by himself. I then told him to put on his shoes and get his feet off my couch. Danny sneered at me and said, "I call the shots with shrinks." I said, "You don't understand your parents. Since I told them that you are a wise-ass punk, they have now decided to listen to someone far brighter than you."

He said, "Who the hell do you think you are?" I told him that he was looking at his new boss. He said, "We'll see about that." I told him, "Don't press your luck, or I'll make sure that you become the poorest kid on the block." He began to protest, and I told him to leave my office and to be on time for our next session. As he walked out he said, "Holy shit! I really got myself into a fix this time."

Although confrontation is usually not the intervention of choice with the narcissistic personality disorder, it was deliberately employed with Danny. I felt that the lack of parental authority was responsible for his grandiose acting out and arrogant contempt. In order to become effective as a therapist with Danny, I had first to release myself from a position of contempt and possibly unleash some underlying idealizing needs for an object who could help him contain his behavior and affect. If such an idealizing relationship developed, then a therapist could become a valuable source of mirroring supplies.

During the next session, Danny was on time and was very careful with my couch. He told me that he told his friends that this shrink was a crazy drill sergeant. He then began to tell me that at times he was worried about his behavior and felt that his parents were scared of him. I told him that he felt reassured knowing that someone was now able to see through his front.

Danny spoke about acting like Superman but was really concerned about not doing well in school and not being able to live up to his parents' expectations. He said that "most people are unable to see through my front and need me to be a big shot." He went on to say, "You are a cool dude. My other shrinks were old fogeys. I think you can understand me."

This marked the beginning of an idealizing transference through which Danny was able to uncover his impaired real self. These transactions were addressed with interpretive interventions that would relate the grandiose self and its need to conceal an impaired real self.

The next session Danny came late with his pants unzipped. He said, "Sorry, dude, but I was getting laid." He then asked me to give him "skin" (a reference to being soul mates or a request for mirroring). He told me that, if women didn't give him sexual gratification, then he would physically abuse them. I told him that, although he acted like a man, it was nothing more than a facade because only weak boys had to be abusive to girls.

He then spoke in great detail about feelings of worthlessness, linking these to his adoption. He wondered if he came from an inferior genetic line. I interpreted his need to show off as being related to these other feelings and told him that his sensitivity to rejection had to be dealt with in a more appropriate way. Danny needed confrontation of his grandiose acting out as well as interpretation of the defensive grandiose self and its relationship to the impaired real self. These interventions paved the way for idealization and the use of "conditional mirroring," which is most useful in the short-term treatment of narcissistic personality disorder.

Several months into the treatment, Danny called me in a state of panic. He had had a dream in which everyone was admiring his beautiful bronzed body. He looked like a Greek statue on display. All of a sudden his body began to decay and fall apart. His limbs were weak and broken, and all his admirers left him. I interpreted the fear that without his front (grandiose self) he would be worthless and unacknowledged. He told me that I was a very wise man and he felt better. Usually, I do not conduct treatment on the telephone. This deviation of the frame is permissible in short-term treatment, however, because the therapist does not attempt to work through the grandiose self or promote separation or autonomy. The therapist must become an appropriate selfobject or extension of the patient's self by providing appropriate gratifications and mirroring responses in order to create a narcissistic equilibrium and to help the patient defend against painful self-esteem fluctuations, affective instability, and fragmentation of the self. With Danny, the idealization of the therapist was not interpreted or disrupted because it became a necessary vehicle and catalyst for change. This treatment typically was conducted on a once-a-week basis, but there were long breaks in the treatment when the patient's family took extensive vacations, which enabled the patient to deal with separation experiences and promoted self-containment.

As treatment progressed, Danny's behavior began to improve. His school grades were better, he put in more hours working, he accepted the limits that his parents had required of him, and he stopped abusing drugs and alcohol. He would come in talking about his accomplishments. I would smile and give appropriate positive remarks. He said, "I like to make you proud of me. Your opinion is important to me." This need to be mirrored for constructive behavioral change was gratified in the treatment and not confronted or interpreted. Periodically, Danny's defensive grandiose behavior would return, and the necessary confrontations and interpretations were given during those episodes, resulting in improved containment of behavior and symptomatic improvement.

Danny was graduating from high school and going away to college. During his last sessions, his idealization of me intensified. He told me that I must be the best therapist in the world, as I was able to help him. He brought in a camera and took a picture of me to keep with him when "things got rough." Danny wanted to become an actor. During his initial consultation, he had spoken about success without having to work for it—a clear expression of narcissistic entitlement. He now told me that someday after years of hard work he was going to be in the movies. He said, "You'll enjoy seeing your patient in the movies." I said, "Yes, I will." Danny and I parted with the understanding that he could call during times of stress and might return for treatment if necessary in the future. When Danny left, he said that he felt much better about himself but that he still had trouble with girls. He felt that he sexualized relationships because he had a problem with genuine feeling. He ended by saying, "What the hell, one can't be perfect.

Besides, I'm a teenager and don't have to worry about marriage for a while. I'll call you then for a major valve job."

Throughout the course of treatment, Danny's parents were seen by another therapist to help them manage his grandiose acting-out behavior and supply appropriate limits. The parents met with the therapist twice a month.

The closing phase of treatment was characterized by a number of treatment strategies. The need to incorporate the therapist (idealized object) through picture taking was permitted and not interpreted. This intensification of defense was supported to help him tolerate separation stress. It was important that the patient leave feeling appreciated and important to me—that I was as invested in him as he was in me—thus the need for the final mirroring response. Danny left with a beautiful description of short-term treatment goals. Separation was denied, and our relationship would continue at some point. There was an improved capacity to work without working through. Finally, the false defensive grandiose self was left intact with modifications and improved containment of affect and limiting of self-destructive acting out, but the capacity for intimacy was not developed.

Conclusions

Different therapeutic techniques are required to establish the therapeutic alliance with narcissistic and borderline disorders. Developmental self- and object relations theory helps us understand why the therapeutic alliance is crucial and how to go about establishing it: confrontation with the borderline personality disorder and interpretation of narcissistic vulnerability with the narcissistic personality disorder.

The difference in working with these two disorders goes beyond technique because the therapist must also shift his focus of observation and his alertness to countertransference. With the borderline, the focus in general is on maladaptive behavior outside the session, with the emphasis on confrontation. Countertransference vulnerabilities stress taking over for the patient, withdrawing from, or attacking the patient. In contrast with the narcissistic personality disorder, the focus is not on the behavior outside the session but on narcissistic vulnerability inside the session in the relationship with the therapist. The therapeutic technique is interpretation, not confrontation, and the countertransference vulnerabilities consist of failures in empathy—real or imagined. This difference in therapeutic atmosphere places a high premium on the therapist's flexibility and capacity to adapt his approach to these different disorders.

NOTES

1. Case presentation by Candace Orcutt.
2. Case presentation by John Baiardi.
3. Case presentation by Richard Fischer.

REFERENCE

Freud, S. 1914. Further recommendations in the technique of psycho-analysis: repetition and working through. *Standard Edition* 12:145–156. London: Hogarth, 1958.

2   THE TREATMENT OF EMOTIONAL
      DISTURBANCES IN ADOLESCENTS:
      PRACTICAL AND THEORETICAL
      CONSIDERATIONS

DEREK MILLER, HAROLD M. VISOTSKY, AND BARRY S. CARLTON

Recent Institute of Medicine (1989) studies estimate that in the United States 14–18 million children under eighteen years of age, or approximately 20 percent of that population, will suffer from a mental disorder and need psychiatric intervention. In an earlier study, 3 million of these children were estimated to have a serious mental illness lasting at least one year (Knitzer 1982). While these statistics demonstrate the need for services, access to care is not only limited by a shortage of resources but also complicated by the vast numbers of uninsured and underinsured (Gray and McNerney 1986). Thus, like all other types of mental health care, adolescent psychiatric care in the United States is partially dominated by a preoccupation with costs. Nevertheless, the evidence seems to be that the number of psychologically disturbed adolescents needing psychiatric help in hospitals has dramatically increased. For example, referrals for such care in the South Carolina state hospital system grew 50 percent in 1988 and a further 30 percent in the first five months of 1989 (A. McDonald, director, Hall Institute, Columbia, S.C., personal communication, 1989).

As well as the increase in the numbers of seriously disturbed young people, it seems that the nature of their disturbance has changed. Apart from formal etiological diagnosis and syndrome labeling, the number of young people who are able to make significant object relationships has apparently decreased. Thus, in care delivery, group relationships and the etiology of group disturbance has become more significant. Children with a limited capacity to form one-to-one trusting relationships with adults become highly involved with their peers in the impulsive expression of their disturbance. Their groups became highly vulnerable to contagion, and very often aggressive behavior is sparked off by one or two children—and not always the same ones. The leaders of these episodes of disturbance have to be appropriately contained; otherwise, the children find themselves quite unable to relate to staff in other than a mutually coercive way, however skilled the personnel. Thus, with the reduction of benefits that saving medical costs implies, and with an immense preoccupation with length of hospital stay on the part of regulatory and fiscal agencies, the accessibility of children to adequate therapeutic intervention becomes more and more impaired. Fashionable hospital stays of twenty days or less are of highly questionable value to these young people.

There have been two broad types of fiscal control. One is to reduce the amount of care offered in the variety of traditional modes: psychoanalytic, behavioral, and environmental (Goldman, Taube, and Jeneks 1987). Another is the production of commercially run treatment centers that, in a boutique-like fashion, depending on the funds available, deal with such symptoms as chemical dependence, eating disorders, depression, and, now, even delinquency. Finally, the costs of residential treatment are reduced by cutting off the availability of such centers by state regulation. It has been suggested that recent changes in adult psychiatric care have made hospitals less responsive than they have been to "broad community needs" (Dewart, Schlesinger, Davidson, Epstein, and Hoover 1991), and, from clinical observation, such changes have created a crisis in both the hospital and the residential care of seriously disturbed adolescents, whose needs have increased as the adequate care available has decreased.

Another attempt to reduce costs has been the use of the concept of the "least restrictive alternative." This constitutional concept (Hoffman and Faust 1977; *Shelton v. Tucker* 1960) is still used in some parts of the American community mental health care system. It can, however, become a substitute for adequate etiological diagnosis and treatment planning. In it, the justification for more intensive intervention is made on the basis of a failure to produce adequate symptomatic relief initially with minimal care—a concept that is unacceptable in other branches of medicine. The relatively new idea of "managed care" often looks only as far as whether symptomatic behavior is still present. Sometimes a recommendation may be made for residential treatment with no specificity as to what that entails. The recommendation to terminate hospital care may ignore the ease with which symptoms will recur under stress. To avoid psychic pain, the adolescent may return to previous techniques of inadequate coping. Such recommendations also tend to ignore the need for biological as well as psychosocial interventions, as many residential treatment centers are not well served with psychiatric intervention.

In outpatient treatment, which may become the only type of care available, social agencies are commonly not equipped for adequate biopsychosocial diagnosis, nor are they able to offer appropriate symptom control. They tend to put young people through a cycle of broken relationships as psychotherapeutic maneuvers fail. These repeat the rejection that is usually associated with developmental trauma for the large number of adolescents who nowadays have difficulty in making object relationships. For example, brief interventions are likely to be helpful only to those who have no significant biological vulnerability, who live in a relatively stable social system, who can make emotional investments in others, and who have temporarily been thrown off a developmental track because of stress related to acute conflict. When these criteria are absent, such interventions are likely to provide only temporary resolution at best.

The concept of continuity of care, which is particularly crucial for those who have difficulty in making object relationships, is widely recommended. Yet the fragmentation of services at the treatment level and the accompanying lack of an adequate educational support system is likely to produce a developmental impasse in the personality growth of the child as well as treatment failure.

This chapter will discuss an approach to the treatment of severely disturbed adolescents who require different levels of care. The principles of treatment are not different whatever the level of therapeutic intervention. We will describe an approach in which high-, medium-, and low-intensity care is offered by the same therapeutic personnel: psychiatrists, psychologists, nurses, child-care workers, teachers, occupational and recreational therapists, and social workers. Movement of the patients to a less intense level of care depends on the ability to control destructive symptomatology. This control is enhanced by the presence of continuous, stable, positive, meaningful, emotional relationships with individuals and with groups. As the patient improves, it also presupposes, through the different levels of care, a social system with a continuing ethos that values socially acceptable behavior. Whatever is thought and felt respects the integrity of others and reinforces and teaches empathy. As the patient improves, the personnel involved with his or her care do not change. The amount of personal responsibility handled by the patient is, however, considerably increased. Continuity of interpersonal relationships reduces the length of stay in a high-intensity care system in a hospital or residential treatment center, and, thereby, the overall cost of an episode of care is reduced.

High-intensity care requires the provision of a twenty-four-hour model of treatment. Medium care offers treatment during the equivalent of a school day, and the patient lives either at home or in a group home placement modeled on that described previously (Miller 1965). Low-intensity care encompasses traditional outpatient services.

The primary focus of care is based not on a hospital ward with a given number of available psychiatric beds but rather on a treatment center in which the therapeutic day takes place. This is conceived as the centerpiece of treatment. This concept is based both on a British model of a school for "maladjusted children" (Shaw 1974), with additional specialized services in the biopsychosocial field, and on the psychiatric day hospital (Creed, Black, and Anthony 1982). In our situation, the same setting provides therapy for children who live in a hospital, in a group setting, or at home. At our unit, the patients who are in the high-intensity program leave the hospital unit at 8:00 A.M., returning at 3:15 P.M. They and the day nursing staff move to the adolescent treatment center, which is three city blocks away from the main hospital. Children who are living at home or in community placement arrive at 8:00 A.M. All the facilities of the treatment center are available to both groups of children.

The treatment program we will describe is called the "campus model." It assesses the intensity of care required in a thorough diagnostic workup. Symptom remission, which may be temporary, leads to a transfer to another portion of the continuum of care area; a day program run by the same staff with the same school and therapeutic activities occurs in the high-intensity area. Ultimately, outpatient intervention, again with the same therapist who has treated the adolescent in the center, may be recommended as the patient returns to his or her home school. The model assures the proper level of therapeutic intervention and treatment. As the staff moves with the patients from the high-intensity treatment area to the less intensive partial hospital program, it provides a labor intensive cadre at cost-effective levels.

Movement based on the child's response to treatment is flexible. It is designed to meet the expected return to home, school, and community, yet, in those who temporarily regress to a less competent level of adjustment, a return to twenty-four-hour high-intensity care is possible, again with no change in therapeutic personnel. This is possible because nursing staff working in the afternoon start their day in the treatment center at 2:00 P.M. They are thus relating to their patients who will go home at 3:30 P.M. This model of programming, given the proper physical resources, is cost effective within an economically driven health care system. It is also exquisitely adapted to meet both the developmental stresses experienced by emotionally disturbed children and their therapeutic needs.

Indications for Intensity of Care

Adolescent psychopathology shows itself in behavior, aggressive or regressive. The former involves physical and psychological attacks on the self or others. Attacks on objects in the environment as a displacement of violence directed toward people, suicidal attempts or threats, homicidal intent or behavior, school failure or refusal, and antisocial activity are typical ways in which emotional disturbances in adolescents and children present themselves. Regressive behavior implies interference with personality development because of the withdrawal of emotional investment from objects outside the self, the abuse of drugs and alcohol and dietary manipulations, and passive compliance with the demands of the immediate social system (school, family, or neighborhood) with no true sense of personal autonomy. Psychological disintegration may occur as the result of aberrant responses to stress as in autism, schizophrenia, and mood disorders. Thus, subjective psychological symptoms such as depression, isolation, depersonalization, delusions, hallucinations, or personality fragmentation are produced. Splitting is particularly common, and nowadays peer support rather than one-to-one relationships with adults is sought. In those with limited relationship capacity, group contagion and antisocial behavior is likely to occur as an attempt to relieve stress. Symptomatic behavior that poses an acute threat to life calls for immediate placement in a high-intensity care area. Whatever its etiology, pathological behavior that does not remit on the basis of biopsychosocial intervention in the community requires a greater intensity of care. The indications for the type of placement also depend on the frequency, intensity, and quality of destructive behavior. The same applies to problems in interpersonal relationships at home, work, or school with the inability to perform in an age-appropriate manner.

If symptomatic behavior is not dangerous to the self or others and allows the adolescent to function so that there is no gross interference with personality development or underachievement in school due to a learning disability, attention deficit, or a mood disorder without suicidal intent, the indications will be for medium- or low-intensity care. If the adolescent feels intermittently suicidal and this behavior is personally acceptable, or if psychic pain is being attenuated with drug or alcohol abuse or school refusal, which the adolescent cannot or will not abandon, the indication will be for high-intensity care. Further, antisocial behavior may produce both realistic and instinctual gratification. This poses particular therapeutic problems. If its consequences are felt by the adolescent as irrelevant, high-intensity psychiatric care is required. The alternative is entry into the correctional system, which rarely appears to help the psychologically disturbed (Bartholomew, Brian, and Douglas 1967; Jewelka, Trupin, and Chiles 1989).

Sexual disorders do not generally require high-intensity care. However, sexual behavior that shows no respect for the integrity of the self or others may require intervention. Organic brain syndromes, especially conduction disorders in the brain, some neuroendocrine disorders, diabetes, and any illness requiring medication to which the adolescent will not conform, may also require a high level of care.

Since, during treatment, symptomatic behavior may recur from time to time, the prescription for the desired intensity of care may vary. It depends on the dangerousness of the symptoms both in reality and in their interference with personality development, community tolerance, the family's ability to contain the behavior, the responses of the school system, and the likelihood that the recurrence of symptoms will lead to premature termination of therapy. The intensity of care also depends on the ability of the adolescent to use a therapeutic relationship to lower internal tension and reduce the need for symptomatic acting out.

If adolescents are poorly treated, if adequate therapeutic intervention fails, or if no treatment is offered, the symptomatic behavior that stems from disturbance leads to a cycle of either rejection, coercion, or collusion by the social system impinging on the adolescent. Furthermore, if symptoms are not contained, the resulting developmental impasse produces characteristically disturbed individuals. The capacity to develop a therapeutic involvement may also become grossly impaired by treatment failure. At least a self-fulfilling prophecy that no one is to be trusted is created. Frustration then tends to be dealt with by inappropriate techniques of avoidance and the projection of responsibility onto others.

Principles of Care

Therapeutic intervention should also be designed to resolve etiological issues, and treatment programs should ensure that the development needs of adolescents are met. If this does not occur, then any psychological stress experienced by young people is enhanced, and care delivery becomes more complicated.

It may well be that the failure of some therapeutic settings is due to a failure to consider the social, psychological, and biological needs that all children require for successful personality growth. For example, it is a paradox that emotionally disturbed children and adolescents in hospitals are often offered less in the way of educational help than those who are developmentally well integrated (Nichtern 1974). This occurs even though almost all seriously disturbed adolescents have severe educational difficulties, frequently with a markedly lowered attention span. Many are concrete thinkers who are often prisoners of the present, with little capacity to predict how present actions affect the future. Some 48 percent of the children in our adolescent program suffer from a variety of learning disabilities. Thus, therapeutic environments that identify learning needs, blocks to learning, and current educational capacities and offer appropriate remedial help should be available to all children who require care.

One problem in the construction of those high-intensity therapeutic environments is that disturbed adolescents tend to be excessively destructive, not just of interpersonal relationships, but also of objects in the environment. If any damage is not rapidly repaired, permission seems to be implicitly given for further physical destruction. Even when every effort is made to preserve a decent ambiance, those adolescents who experience the explosive violence that may be associated with an altered state of consciousness may create damage. Individuals who have apparently withdrawn from any emotional involvement with external objects, with a grossly impaired capacity to make relationships, experience their world as an empty desert. They appear to do their best to create this in the outside environment, which becomes a manifestation of their inner emptiness. Thus, they may be untidy and dirty and unable to care for their own possessions. An occasional frenetic explosive experience appears to give them the illusion of being alive. Adolescents may create an environment that is a measure of their internal emptiness. Thus, staff may have to look after them, and their surroundings, in a manner that is more appropriate for much younger children. Further, staff need to be sensitive to the development of group turbulence and learn to identify those adolescents who, sharing the common problems of others, charismatically become leaders of antisocial behavior. Staff, who are themselves often young adults, may also easily allow the creation of a chaotic or barren environment that may then be implicitly colluded in by the administration of a hospital. It is not acceptable for a therapeutic setting to justify the provision of an inadequate environment with the attitude that disturbed adolescents ought to accept full responsibility for their own behavior.

Nonspecific Social Needs

All therapeutic systems for disturbed young people should offer two types of service: nonindividualized general services that are given to all patients to reinforce the biopsychosocial needs necessary for personality development (Knesper and Miller 1976) and individualized services applied to specifically diagnosed needs.

In all psychiatric treatment centers for adolescents, the resources of the community should be accessible. Free-standing closed units breed their own psychopathology (Easson 1969), particularly as obedience to institutional norms does not necessarily prepare adolescents to deal with the complexity of the world. Settings should perhaps best be described as living laboratories of human experience. They should titrate the stress young people experience by appropriate emotional and biopsychosocial support; they should incorporate the best of social

33

norms and be as open as possible, consistent with the child's capacity to handle responsibility. This is the genuine concept of a least-restrictive alternative.

Children should not be isolated from their families. Visits should be regarded not as a reward but as an essential part of a basic treatment program (Miller 1986).

Consistency of verbal and nonverbal communication and the stability of interpersonal relationships with staff expedite the ability to make personal identifications. Deviant behavior should have consequences that are clear and comprehensible; these consequences should not have the intent of being punitive. The situation is complicated because adolescents may not have control over their behavior. For example, violence that appears as a response to stress may be a genetically determined characteristic associated with neuroendocrine disorders (Miller and Looney 1976). The same applies to the isolation associated with severe depression. The problem is that many behavior modification systems respond as if the adolescents had learned only to make such behavioral responses. Initially, these responses may be biologically driven or the results of ultra psychic conflict, although the type of response is a function of psychosocial development and social system permission (Miller 1986). Ultimately, however, the response becomes learned and may particularly appear as a function of group pressures. The withdrawal of privileges as a tariff response to antisocial behavior invites manipulations. If the institutional demand for conformity is excessive, particularly in long-stay settings, temporary compliance may be created. Violent behavior is hidden from staff, and personality growth is impeded.

Single-sex settings, which are socially aberrant, are inevitably personality destructive, particularly if social isolation from the community at large is the institutional norm.

The advent of television poses particular social and psychological problems (Rubenstein 1983). In psychiatric hospitals, its presence appears to reinforce both passivity and a weakening of staff-patient relationships. From observation of many hospital settings, it is apparent that television is a filler of time. The staff and patients may sit together on such occasions, but interaction is at a minimum. On the other hand, television may protect staff from the particularly painful experience of working intimately with severely disturbed young people. In our setting, it is not used.

In therapeutic settings, there is often little respect for the significance of stable interpersonal relationships. Discharge from a treatment center or a move from a more closed to a more open setting should not mean losing significant others who become important in the child's life. Sometimes such therapeutic maneuvering may be life threatening.

Case Example 1

Catherine was a thirteen-year-old who, in the midst of a not yet diagnosed major depression, decided that she was intolerably ugly. She spent hours over homework, did not relate to other children, and began to starve herself. This gave her health maintenance organization, which would not pay for the hospital care of eating disorders, the excuse to refuse to allow her high-intensity care. She was in four hospitals (for brief periods of two days to two weeks) and one outpatient eating disorders program before being admitted to our treatment program. She was sixty-four inches tall, weighed seventy pounds, and had lost twelve pounds in the previous three weeks. She had halved her pulse rate, her blood pressure was hypostatic, and her serum potassium was dangerously low. She told her new psychiatrist that she was going to starve herself to death. After eight weeks in high-intensity care, she had begun to eat and was beginning to interact with other children. At this point, her insurance benefits expired. It was suggested that she move to another hospital. Her response to the proposed move was to refuse to speak to her psychiatrist. She stopped eating and drinking and curled up on her bed with her teddy bear, sucking her thumb.

Case Example 2

The treatment of individual adolescents without a diagnosis of family and parental psychopathology is inadequate. Sometimes, family therapy is provided as a sole prescription without adequate assessment. This can also be a most inappropriate intervention. A fourteen-year-old girl with problems of depression, alcoholism, and poor schoolwork was treated with family therapy for two years. At no stage was a diagnostic assessment made of the etiology of the child's illness or was much weight given to the intergenerational history of alcoholism. When a diagnosis was finally made, it was found that she was suffering from a biologically based mood disorder and that her capacity for object relationships was seriously limited. Family intervention did highlight her need to pose in the home as the good child, but it never dealt with her secretive dishonesty, her continued drinking, or her promiscuous behavior.

Nonspecific Psychological Needs

The drive toward socially acceptable autonomy poses particular problems in the psychiatric care of adolescents. Inevitably, in this age group, a degree of regression in the service of mastery occurs. The experience of feeling devalued is pervasive in those who are emotionally disturbed, and every effort should be made to enhance the individual's sense of worth. Maturationally appropriate productivity should, thus, be reinforced. Individual adolescents need to develop an acceptable sense of personal ethnic and social class identity. All children require educational and vocational learning and the provision of socially acceptable outlets for aggression. Staff should understand and respect the developmental needs of their charges, especially the need for integrity, privacy, and appropriate controls. The developmental shifts through adolescence are so rapid and so great that a high degree of staff sophistication in understanding group process in its particular relevance to this age is necessary. Apart from adequate cognitive development, a therapeutic setting should also reinforce creativity and imagination. Depending on the sociocultural environment, this will include everything from art, music, and drama to understanding the forces of nature. Group and family therapy can meet nonspecific developmental needs as well as being part of a specific treatment recommendation. They can help teach empathy, the importance of considering the implications of behavior, and respect for the integrity of others. The projections of the age group need to be well understood.

Case Example 3

The way the staff relates to adolescents in both specially designed therapeutic interventions and in generalized day-to-day relationships provides a model of interpersonal relationships with which the youngsters identify. A highly depressed schizophrenic girl of seventeen was seen daily by one of the unit nurses. The goal was to help her behave in a more organized fashion. The mother had been struggling with this issue for years and had suggested to her daughter that she list daily tasks (bed making, organizing clothes) and mark off each item as it was finished. The mother was never successful in this endeavor. Quite independently, the nurse-therapist made the same suggestion, and the patient responded. Not only did this model a known interpersonal relationship, but it also helped the processes of identification (Miller 1986) that previously had been difficult if not impossible for this girl. The nurse became a developmentally significant nonparental adult with whom the girl could identify without feeling that her sense of autonomy was being attenuated.

Nonspecific Biological Needs

All adolescents require adequate food, light, air, exercise, and the opportunity for both physical growth and development as well as the use of their bodies to enhance the capacity to sublimate. Recreational facilities should be available both indoors and outdoors and should be remedial as well as challenging and appropriately competitive. It is usually better to have competitive sports activities directed to those outside the system rather than directed internally to the group (Miller 1957).

The provision of adequate food is basic but sometimes quite difficult to achieve. There are many institutional settings that provide adolescents with the last meal of the day at 5:00 P.M. This is inappropriately early, as youngsters often continue to need to snack until bedtime. In an acute general hospital, there may be a repetitious seven- to ten-day meal cycle with which longer-stay young people become inevitably bored. Efforts have to be made to modify routine hospital fare. In our setting, the program had its own kitchen, and cooking was shared between a specially hired cook, unit staff, and patients.

Individual Services and Treatment Planning

Specific individualized services offer a variety of biopsychosocial interventions tailored to meet individual needs. Apart from the individual assessment of the patient, adequate evaluation includes the diagnosis of the etiology of disturbance in the impinging family and social systems. The decision as to whether high-, medium-, or low-intensity

37

care services are required depends on the balance between the stress experienced by the adolescent living in the community, the support that can be internalized from social systems, and the success of therapeutic interventions. Finally, the nature of the symptomatic behavior that inevitably occurs with the acting out of conflict to relieve immediate tension may be so stressful to others that their persecutory responses may mean that being in the community at large is no longer possible.

Psychological testing is needed to assess the intensity of the dynamic conflict, the presence of learning difficulties, and the possibility of organic brain damage. Test reports may also be necessary to ensure adequate educational placement.

Emotional support against the perception of stress depends on the capacity of the individual to make positively felt, meaningful interpersonal relationships with others. The ability to be trusting and contain ambivalence can be understood existentially within the context of the therapeutic evaluation and the child's biological sensitivity. Historically, it is based on the child's nurturing experiences. Significant developmental history does not necessarily include details such as the milestones of personality development, about which mothers are almost invariably confused. More significant is the evidence that the child bonded to the mother and was able to be dependent on her and thus make a meaningful, positive attachment (Bowlby 1977). The presence or absence of fathering in the first two years of life is highly significant in personality development (Wallerstein 1985). Child rearing by single-parent mothers, when they themselves are isolated from a network of mutually caring adults, is probably of increasing significance in the massive increase of the incidence of adolescent depression and the inability to make trusting relationships with others.

The aim of specific biopsychosocial interventions is to put the maximum weight of treatment in those etiological areas that will maximally affect the child's maladjustment. If the child suffers from a genetically based mood disorder and this is not treated, then psychosocial intervention will be less efficacious. If, on the other hand, all that is given is a pill, then it is less likely that appropriate characterological shifts will take place.

An individual diagnostic service of value is one in which problems are clearly stated. The treatment recommendation should specify both the nonspecific and the specific individualized services that should be offered. A specific treatment plan, which clearly states what the goals of treatment might be, is necessary, but there is as yet no adequate technique of assessing what the length of treatment might be. In the United States, a third-party imposition on the type and frequency of psychotherapeutic care and demands for statements about length of stay are serious barriers to effective care. The issue should not be whether an adolescent becomes asymptomatic. If biopsychosocial environmental needs are adequately met, the critical issue is rather what the adolescent's capacity to handle stress in the community at large and the family on discharge will be.

Problems in the Delivery of Therapeutic Services

Diagnostic assessment, even in a well-run psychiatric setting, may take up to two or three weeks. The recommendations as to treatment needs should then be made to the child's parents or responsible community agencies. Acceptance or rejection may, regrettably, sometimes be made on the basis of the parents' and communities' financial resources. The modification of recommendations on the basis of what can be afforded at the expense of a child's well-being is ethically questionable.

Adolescents in therapy must experience themselves in action, or no therapeutic movement takes place. The issue is the frequency and quality of symptomatic behavior. To assess this, developmentally normative behavior needs to be recognized. The goals of therapy are to enhance the development of relative freedom from infantile attachments, develop the capacity to tolerate frustration, contain antisocial behavior, and be loving. Adolescents who suffer from characterological disturbance may behave in a nonacceptable way as a manifestation of poor impulse control and an inability to tolerate frustration. On the other hand, this behavior may also represent a struggle for autonomy.

In outpatient care delivery, when behavior becomes conformist, particularly in a society where immediate costs appear paramount, therapeutic services are often withdrawn. This may then be an important reinforcement of symptomatic behavior if the youngster is using such behavior to seek an adult relationship as part of a developmental need. The reward for acting out is then more therapeutic intervention and more adult relationships. The reward for growth may be premature rejection.

39

In adolescents, gratification is often associated with disturbed behavior. The projection of helplessness onto and into others reinforces omnipotence. "Successful" antisocial behavior corrupts personality development. Drug abuse and alcohol offer peer acceptable and sterile regression; they also impair brain functioning. Interventions in which this behavior is allowed to continue are highly unlikely to be successful.

In therapeutic settings, staff at all levels require adequate emotional support and need to feel valued, particularly by more technically trained professionals. This is necessary because a particular problem is created by the inclination of disturbed adolescents to split the world into good and bad. At the same time, as staff may be exposed to attacking behavior, the patient may attempt to make the therapist an idealized object. This may be gratifying to the therapist but demoralizing to the staff. If therapists do not deal with these psychological splitting mechanisms, staff become angry at both the patient and the therapist. Further, unless there is good communication among all staff, the therapist may be ready to offer the patients more responsibility than they can handle. Neither staff alone nor therapist alone should control the patient's level of responsibility. This is a particular problem of systems that are modeled exclusively on behavior modification principles.

The time span of psychotherapy, its frequency, and the length of sessions are parameters that are often neglected when determining the type of therapy that may be needed: supportive, expressive, administrative, or behavioral. Action-oriented, emotionally deprived adolescents may not be able to sit in an office for a therapeutic hour, nor may they easily tolerate weekend or vacation separations.

Staff Development

Successful high- and medium-intensity therapy of disturbed young people is unlikely without ongoing staff development. In our setting, the children have a rest period late in the afternoon. This provides an optimum time for staff training. Staff development should minimally clarify the explicit philosophy of the institution and its consistence with the implied institutional message given to the patients. The most potent social system reinforcements of disturbance appear as a result of staff conflicts, or the institution may give implicit permission for a whole series of negative behaviors (Stanton and Schwartz 1954). Staff should be helped learn group counseling techniques and recognize the importance of group process and network relationships among both staff and patients. One-to-one relationships are highly significant but are not exclusively valuable.

Staff need to understand the nonspecific techniques that can be used to help reinforce the development of the individual child. Commonly, institutional expectations may not meet the developmental needs of the individual child. For example, long periods of inactivity and isolation from others are developmentally inappropriate. It is difficult to see the developmental value of chemical and physical restraint or punitive behavioral techniques. One child-care setting may have adolescents stand facing a wall for a day at a time. Isolation from others in "quiet" or seclusion rooms (Soloff 1985) does not seem valuable.

There is a tolerable level of staff tension that can be borne without the adolescent population becoming disturbed. If the tension becomes too great, disturbance takes place. Many attempts at developmental training collapse because of the social system in which they take place. If attempts at staff development, which represents a change of approach, are to occur, they should be done primarily with those members of the social system who are the most potent (Miller 1966).

Conclusions

Psychiatry will not impinge significantly on the care of disturbed young people until there is a general insistence on optimal standards of care that recognize those changes in developmental pathology that have probably occurred as a result of changes in the family and social systems. The relative failure of mental health care delivery in the United States means that the judicial and legal system is being allowed to claim that psychiatry has nothing to offer in the treatment of the disturbed young ("Radical Changes Urged" 1975). The pressure not to use hospital care has led to state systems being overwhelmed with very disturbed children and the correctional system becoming society's repository for nontreated disturbed youths. The young adults who fill the prisons were perhaps the adolescents to whom adequate care was not offered. Punitive social responses that reinforce violence thus become the norm.

REFERENCES

Bartholomew, A. A.; Brian, L. A.; and Douglas, A. S. 1967. A medico-psychiatric diagnostic review of remanded male minor offenders. *Medical Journal of Australia* 11:267–269.

Bowlby, J. 1977. The making and breaking of affectional bonds. *British Journal of Psychiatry* 130:201–210.

Creed, F. H.; Black, D.; and Anthony, P. 1982. Day hospital treatment for acute psychiatric illness: a critical appraisal. *British Journal of Psychiatry* 154:300–310.

Dewart, R. A.; Schlesinger, M.; Davidson, H.; Epstein, B. A.; and Hoover, C. 1991. A national study of psychiatric hospital care. *American Journal of Psychiatry* 148(2): 204–210.

Easson, W. 1969. *The Severely Disturbed Adolescent.* New York: International Universities Press.

Goldman, H. H.; Taube, C. A.; and Jeneks, S. F. 1987. The organization of the psychiatric inpatient service system. *Medical Care* 25(56): 551.

Gray, B. H., and McNerney, W. F. 1986. For profit enterprise in health care. *New England Journal of Medicine* 314:1523–1548.

Hoffman, A., and Faust, D. 1977. Least restrictive treatment of the mentally ill: a doctrine in search of its senses. *San Diego Law Review* 14:1113–1115.

Institute of Medicine. 1989. *Research on Children and Adolescents with Mental, Behavior and Developmental Disorders.* Washington, D.C.: National Academy Press.

Jewelka, R.; Trupin, E.; and Chiles, J. A. 1989. The mentally ill in prisons: a review. *Hospital and Community Psychiatry* 40:481–491.

Knesper, D., and Miller, D. 1976. Treatment plans for mental health care. *American Journal of Psychiatry* 133(1): 65–80.

Knitzer, J. 1982. *Unclaimed Children.* Washington, D.C.: Childrens' Defense Fund.

Miller, D. 1957. Treatment of adolescents in an adult hospital. *Bulletin of the Menninger Clinic* 1:189–198.

Miller, D. 1965. *Growth to Freedom: The Psychosocial Treatment of Delinquent Youth.* Bloomington: Indiana University Press.

Miller, D. 1966. Staff training in the penal system: the use of small groups. *Human Relations* 19(20): 151–164.

Miller, D. 1986. *Attack on the Self.* Northfield, N.J.: Aronson.

Miller, D., and Looney, J. 1976. Determinants of homicide in adolescents. *Adolescent Psychiatry* 4:231–254.

Nichtern, S. 1974. The therapeutic educational environment. *Adolescent Psychiatry* 4:432–434.

Radical Changes Urged in Dealing with Youth Crimes. 1975. *New York Times,* November 30, sec. 1, p. 1.

Rubenstein, E. A. 1983. Television and behavior: research conclusions of the 1982 NIMH report and their policy implications. *American Psychologist* 38:820–825.

Shaw, O. L. 1974. *Youth in Crisis: A Radical Approach to Delinquency.* New York: Hart.

Shelton v. Tucker. 1960. 364 U.S. 479, 81 S.Ct. 247, 5 L.Ed., 2d 231.

Soloff, P. H. 1985. Seclusion and restraint in 1985: a review and update. *Hospital and Community Psychiatry* 36:652–657.

Stanton, A. H., and Schwartz, J. S. 1954. *The Mental Hospital: A Study of Institutional Participation in Psychiatric Illness and Treatment.* New York: Basic.

Wallerstein, J. 1985. Children of divorce: recent research. *Journal of the American Academy of Child Psychiatry* 24:515–517.

3   THE FATE OF DON JUAN:

THE MYTH AND THE MAN

DAVID DEAN BROCKMAN

This chapter is devoted to the task of delineating some of the issues of adolescent character development (Deutsch 1965) in certain individuals who remind one of the dramatic and mythic character of Don Juan Tenorio, whose motives for control and power over others, as manifest in his sexual exploits, are legendary. Three important motivations in adolescence—mastery of sexuality, acquisition of power over others, and interest in accumulating money—may have appeared in some form earlier in development, but these motives certainly flower in adolescence and young adulthood. Motives such as these are less obvious than the externally more visible pubertal and maturational (physiological) changes of adolescence or the cognitive and intellectual changes, but they are nevertheless very important. Of these three, power and control or dominance over others have been sorely neglected in current psychoanalytic literature.

Fenichel (1945, p. 244) discusses these motivations in terms of libido theory and infantile sexuality, specifically in the anal phase or sadism and omnipotence. Horner (1989) claims that power of self arises as a mastery over childhood helplessness and powerlessness and is commonly repeated in adolescence in relation to parental control. When the opportunity occurred for studying the sexual motive in adolescence, commonly called "playing the field," I was stimulated to expand my understanding of this motivation.

Before describing any of the clinical phenomena, it seems appropriate to review the story of the classical figure of Don Juan from original sources. The original play was written by Tirso de Molina (Gabriel Téllez, a Mercerdarian monk) in the early part of the seventeenth century, during the golden age of Spanish drama, and published in 1630 along with some other plays by his mentor Lope de Vega. It is interesting to note that Tirso was in his early twenties at the time.

The title of the original play is *El burlador de Sevilla y convividado de piedra* (The jester of Seville and the stone guest). *Burlador* has been translated as "jester," but other meanings are "rake," "joker," "trickster," "rogue," "prankster," "seducer," "playboy" (Mandel 1963), or "mocker," all of which convey some part of the meaning. "Trickster" seems the most appropriate.

Don Juan is a late adolescent visiting his uncle, the Spanish ambassador to the king of Naples. He makes love to a series of women, beginning with the Duchess Isabella, who is betrothed to Don Octavio, and then, back in Spain, Doña Ana, who is betrothed to the marquis de la Mota. Her father, Don Gonzalo de Ulloa, is the commendatore of the Order of Calatrava and is killed by Don Juan in the act of defending his daughter's honor. In addition, there are two peasant girls who are seduced in the play.

An essential feature of Don Juan's seductions are his tricking the women into having sex with him and stealing them away from their betrothed or, in one case (Tisbea), a determined state of virginity. Don Juan is quite creative in devising the particularly successful tactics that he individualizes for each seduction. The second part of the story, which Tirso brilliantly merges with the legendary sexual exploits of Don Juan, concerns his mocking of the stone statue of the commendatore to sup with him. The commendatore agrees only if his slayer returns the favor. In the end, *el burlador* is carried off to hell in retribution for his sins, capping what is distinctly a morality play most likely designed to frighten off would-be imitators of Don Juan's life-style with eternal punishment. The rebellious, willful late adolescent behavior of Don Juan in the play brings consternation and exasperation to his father and the king of Seville, a story familiar to modern parents. But what is most striking is the fact that his mother is never mentioned.

I am using the term "legendary" here only in a descriptive sense, for Don Juan was really a mythic character (Worthington 1962), not a real living person. The play was put together from earlier Spanish legends. In the eighteenth century, a real person named Don Miguel de Manara imitated Don Juan's life-style only to repent later, become an ascetic, and donate all his money to build a children's hospital in Seville.

Parenthetically, the uncompromising outcome that was Don Juan's fate in the play has been neglected in psychoanalytic interpretations of the myth, except in the seminal work of Rank (1924). There are many versions of the story that have interested many writers: Molière, Byron, Shaw, Shadwell, Manara, Kierkegaard, Dumas, Maranon, Walcott, Zorilla, Tolstoy, and Camus among others. But many of them have diluted the essential character and turned Don Juan into a withered old man, an absurd hero (as in Camus; see Weinstein 1967), or a bland character not at all interested in sex (Shaw's 1903 *Man and Superman;* see Mandel 1963). Richard Strauss and Mozart have composed masterpieces of music around the theme of a proud and brave nobleman whose sole aim in life is short-term selfish pleasure (Maetzu 1968). The original play depicts Don Juan as a very erotic character who lives to make love, and, interestingly enough, women are delighted with his prowess and are willing partners. The popular appeal of both the play and the music shows that the idealization of exuberant adolescence is obviously not modern.

In the case example to be presented, control, subjugation, or dominance were experienced as a central problem in the transference situation of a clinical psychoanalysis, with many conscious and unconscious manifestations and meanings. For example, there were recurrent struggles over the appointment schedule and resistance to the process of free association. Furthermore, it was equally true in the real relationships with women as it was in the transference situation. A more detailed description follows in the case presentation. Control by subjugation as the paradigmatic defense is not, in my opinion, deployed (as Winter 1973 suggests) against the "chaos and confusion of incorporation"—a rather antiquated term that is borrowed from physiology. Instead, control measures are deployed against the loss or threatened rupture in the relationship with the idealized mother. In the transference, my patient was threatened with feelings of abandonment over weekends and vacations. He usually went into a rage and demanded his way about the most mundane issues. Motives for dominating control, subjugation, and power over others in the real person are seen as originating in early childhood, and these issues later on merge with adolescent phallic aggressiveness, sexualization, and exhibitionism in the form of a display of cavalier seduction of any and all those women the Don Juan character perceives as a challenge.

The motive for dominating control and power over others in group processes (Fenichel 1945, pp. 502–504) may emerge from similar sources, but group processes are much more complicated and deserve a separate study. I would only say at this time that exhibitionism and the love of power for its own sake and aggressivization take the place of sexualization processes. Fenichel also suggested that the desire for power may be derived from anal sadism and mastery of sphincter control (p. 283) or a defense against deep-seated or archaic anxieties about oral conflicts (p. 479).

To return to dominating sexual motivations, I would like to say that it seems reasonable to assume that various forms of hypersexuality occur along a continuum, at one end of which are the Don Juan (or Casanova) complex (Trachtenberg 1988), nymphomania, and certain instances of homosexual behavior and multiple partners in both sexes and at the other end are the phase-appropriate experimental efforts in adolescence to master and integrate sexuality on the way to adulthood. By this I mean those tasks of adolescence, as originally stated by Erikson (1959), to relish and integrate and not just tolerate intimacy with one person with whom a permanent commitment is made. Also, during adolescence, fantasies of living out a Don Juan life-style are very common and probably serve very important and constructive purposes.

The legendary and imaginary Don Juan derives the use of power from his pursuit of pleasure of the moment, while punishment by death is far away (*Tan largo me lo fiais*). He is creatively resourceful in using every trick in his bag of seduction games (Maetzu 1968) to accomplish his arrogant excesses. Through his rebellious defiance of the Everlasting, his father, and the king and his extraordinary vitality, creativity, sensuality, courage, and humor, Don Juan in the play expresses in general "man's challenge to the world of his limitations" (McClelland 1967). However, it is important at this point to differentiate the literary character from the clinical since the literary Don Juan is an imaginary person in whom certain human-like qualities are highlighted and exaggerated in the play and these qualities are not necessarily present in the same combination in real human beings.

Anecdotally, Anaïs Nin described her father and an opera singer friend she called Siegfried as Don Juan characters. She understood the typical Don Juan to be a charmingly lovable man who is attracted and devoted to women "always at the beginning, at the first moment of faith and love" (Nin 1966–1971, 2:272), but who never stays around to watch the relationship deteriorate. He is there only to satisfy his own pleasure. Simone de Beauvoir (1985) described Jean-Paul Sartre's many sexual adventures as similar to Don Juan's. The female (Doña Juana) and some homosexual counterparts present some interesting differences, but the essential quality of unbridled sensuality remains the same, and a similar formulation to the one presented here seems adequate to explain the phenomena. This presentation is a modest clinical contribution to a psychoanalytic definition of a person who in part resembled the inimitable Don Juan.

Clinical Example

While the outcome of adolescent character development is hard to predict in adolescence, studying the process of development retrospectively presents much less of a problem and is typically part of good clinical work. The following is a condensation of an ongoing analysis and suffers from the distortions of the effort to distill the essence of the pathological character formations and the specific defenses encountered. Much work yet remains, and this chapter must be considered preliminary and tentative.

Mr. H, a forty-year-old divorced professional man, came for analysis with symptoms of a long-standing depression, inability to form a lasting relationship with a woman, intense anxieties, and ruminative concerns about his erratic business successes and failures. He had trouble going to sleep and staying asleep. He is a handsome man with a swarthy complexion, slight in build but very muscular. Superficially, he is assertive and forthcoming so that it is easy to see that he is attractive to women. He smoked too much, and life held too few pleasures. His past history uncovered and revealed a Don Juan–type character beginning in adolescence. He claimed he had had relationships with some forty or fifty women, with whom he had brief encounters. He had been married briefly in his twenties, but that marriage ended in divorce. He had achieved some progress in a previous therapy by finishing a graduate degree in business and achieving some partial stability in his private and business life. However, this therapy had reached a stalemate, and he reluctantly and ambivalently terminated that therapy.

As we began our work together, it was apparent early on that his chief concern was his inability to effect a close relationship with a suitable woman. Considering his many sexual successes, he was tired of the emptiness and loneliness of that life, which no longer brought much excitement of the challenge or delight in the conquests he previously enjoyed.

After an extended diagnostic period, we decided on psychoanalysis as the treatment of choice. Very soon thereafter, he initiated a relationship with a woman. The death knell for the Don Juan behavior, however, had sounded some time before, when the underlying depression had surfaced.

What follows is a more detailed account of the middle phase of an ongoing analysis, beginning about a year after we started. He was angry when he felt controlled and manipulated by his fiancée. "She tries to make me into something I'm not. I told her I thought she was very demanding. She fights me on every point. I can't see why because other women give me my way." He was frustrated and angry when his most minute demands were not met. Similarly, he fantasized about getting control over me in the transference regarding appointment times and questioned me extensively about the analytic process, but then he became fearful that I would not like him and regressed to wanting to be coddled and comforted. He recalled that his mother overdid coddling, and we constructed a very confining early childhood situation. What frequently followed was a grandiose fantasy that he could surely please me by performing extraordinary business-related tasks and making a lot of money, but he was overcome in the transference with fear that I would be like God, who would "punish me and take it all away." Typically, during this period, interpretations were made to clarify what I thought to be the central transference meanings of the clinical data. For example, I pointed out his fears of competition in his business ventures, in his relationships with women, and particularly with me in the father transference. These interpretations had little or no effect on the transference or his symptoms.

Then his mother died unexpectedly. The character of the analysis came under the sway of the mourning process, even though he was unable to mourn at first. He said, "I can't cry. There just aren't any tears, and besides I have to keep up appearances for my father's sake.'' He dreamed of having sex with a man, moving in with his father, and in fantasy getting his mother's ring. He has always wanted to be a star for his father and now me in the transference. Accepting defeat, though, invariably led to symptoms of depression and self-defeating behavior. In a dream precipitated by a separation from me, he was afraid I would be angry that he was abandoning me. He acted out by performing many of his mother's domestic tasks for his father. The negative oedipal interpretation of these dynamics seemed cogent at the time, but, as the analysis proceeded and deepened, an entirely different picture emerged.

As he momentarily regained control over these regressive unconscious wishes to replace his mother, he contacted a previous girlfriend, who readily responded to his every whim. ''What I enjoy is the power of that experience.'' What he meant was that this woman was passively submissive and was content to satisfy his every need. After having sex, he would send her home in a cab. He fantasized about marrying a totally subjugated Oriental woman who would follow him around and cater to him. It gave him a powerful sense of dominating control. Physical tension was released by similar brief sexual encounters during which he was in complete control. However, he was more strongly drawn to women who physically and characterologically resembled his mother, that is, women who were petite but intrusive and reluctant to permit separations.

Each separation, whether generated by him or by me, led to feelings of angry helplessness and anxious depression and loss of sufficient energies to do his work—in a word, he collapsed. When his girlfriend became free after her divorce, he felt pressure from her to make a commitment. When he was married before and again now, he felt taken over and controlled by a close relationship that demanded a greater intimacy. These demands encroached on a hard-won equilibrium, consisting of his private free time to watch his favorite television shows and go to bed early. He claimed he needed much rest from the frenzy of his daily strivings, through which he hoped to impress his father and me in the grandiose transference. He was envious and angry with other patients, whom he felt got preferential treatment from me. This was interpreted to mean that he felt I was indifferent to his particular needs like his father had been.

Paradoxically, after major losses of income, it seemed that his head was clearer and he was able to pull himself together enough to recover some of his losses. Analysis of this paradox brought out a restitutional fantasy that he needed sympathy from me similar to what he had invariably got from his father to alleviate the shame and guilt of his failures. He dreamed of feeling strong enough to confront me as a belligerent adversary, but at the last minute stepped aside and excused himself. This abortive attempt at self-assertion, however, was infrequent. He was desperate to be a star for me. He discussed in detail his business problems, hoping to get some clue about his failures, but this invariably led to feelings of despair and defeat. This depressive cycle was deepened and further complicated by a sleep disorder.

Feeling as if he were second best made him very angry. As he ruminated about these feelings, he got more and more angry and more and more depressed. He hated himself and his failures to meet his grandiose goals. In his own words, "I'm always trying to hit a home run instead of just making dimes. I should be more aggressive without being wild and taking too big a risk. It's so sad that my father will die some day and I've never succeeded for him. It's more sad for him now that mother is gone."

He described the symptomatic onset of his neurosis seven or eight years ago. He saw women less frequently, and with only one or two would he have brief sexual encounters. There was no sense of permanence or stability. He no longer went prowling with his sidekick (his version of Catalinon or Leporello). As noted, it was as if the adolescent behavior pattern began to deteriorate and be replaced by a serious depression. He used to be more energetic in a regular sport activity. He said he had to have the ball all the time. A little later, he felt more confident to reveal other details of his neurosis: namely, that he was nervous in large crowds. "It has always been that way. I don't like to go out to parties and dress up—put on a suit and a tie. That's why I wear casual clothes all the time because I feel very shy and insecure. I think it all started when my father [repeatedly] told me I was second best. I've spent my whole life feeling inferior. In college people called me humiliating nicknames. That's when I started to smoke. This is another reason why I need a lot of rest. I started to take a lot of drugs and went to Europe for four months. Now, when I'm attracted to women, I can't get close. I chase them away, and I can't keep involved. What I want the most is to be number one with my father"—and me in the transference.

As the analysis proceeded into the third year, he continued to be preoccupied with his feeling manipulated and dominated by women who demanded that he do their bidding—for example, as to when they made love or to dress up to go out to dinner. He doubted his future would be any better, and he was obsessively angry about every instance of perceived manipulation. He withheld his love unless he felt he had complete control. At this point, he announced that he was leaving for a three-week winter vacation with his father.

When he recalled a childhood image of himself as a passive, wimpy, unaggressive little boy, he thought that image was an attempt to comply with his parents' unempathic admonition that he behave more like a neighbor girl, as if to say "put on a dress." This and similar humiliations were frequent. In contrast to his internal image of himself, he was told he was hyperactive as a small child—a "wild Indian"—because all the precious objects in the house had to be put up out of his reach.

As the analytic work proceeded, he reported that he had been feeling stronger, taller, and more aggressive. In fact, he reported that he had had a more financially successful year than previously. Telling me of his good fortune, however, was again followed by some costly business mistakes. He said, "Every time I reach for the stars, I come up with cobwebs." In a dream about his mother, the surface meaning was to replace his mother, but the deeper wish was to reestablish a close relationship with me in the idealized mother transference. This was acted out when he talked on the telephone with an aunt (his mother's sister) every day just as she had done with his mother before her death.

"In all the photos from my childhood, I'm on the outside next to my mother"—the unpreferred position. We reconstructed the early childhood experience of being overwhelmed with feelings of overstimulation and abandonment from his mother and humiliation from his father. Also, the father was not around to help him separate from the mother. He was a parent loss himself. My patient missed his mother and was for the first time deeply involved in the mourning process. A dream of looking for refuge from a storm revealed the transference meaning of expecting me like mother to magically relieve his distress, but he feared the worst. He was very sad and depressed, with no hope or prospect of recovery. He said, "Life has no meaning."

Another dream quickly followed with the similar meaning of being rescued but with an additional meaning of his fear of increasing involvement with women and me, as mother. In the idealized mother transference, he perceived me as forcing him into a helpless, submissive, and dependent but overstimulated relationship similar to what existed with his mother and from which he struggled to escape. He simultaneously feared and longed for this reunion with mother. As he prepared for another separation, he tried to minimize the disruption by shortening the time away. When he returned, he experienced another cycle of attempted closeness and withdrawal precipitated by his fears of being controlled and manipulated in the transference. He toyed with the idea of terminating therapy by talking about ending the relationship with his woman friend. He acted this out by reducing the frequency of the sessions as a way of restoring control over me in the analytic situation.

As though to calm himself about the increased tension in the analysis, he recalled how he was invariably successful in bar hopping with his buddy to pick up women. He believed he could never be the success that he thought his father or I demanded or, for that matter, acquire a healthy sense of self-worth. Fantasies of acquiring a family by marrying his woman friend (who had several lovely children) made him feel better because he expected that I (and his parents) would be pleased. In a romantic mood, he thought of giving her his mother's diamond ring. He dreamed of being very angry at me as his father for "busting my ass for him." He struggled to assert himself in the transference relationship by telling me off just before leaving for a vacation. These fantasies and efforts to assert himself were experimental efforts to move beyond the idealizing mother transference.

During the fourth year of the analysis, he began to feel more in control, and his image of himself improved significantly. He liked the image of being a family man and a father. There was no question that the woman friend was in love with him, though somewhat ambivalently and fearful of getting hurt.

When she withdrew out of anxiety and dated other men, it made him crazy with jealousy. He felt abandoned. Demanding exclusive rights over her made her balk. In desperation, he proposed, but she said it was too early and played for time. It seemed to him that she was acting like an adolescent girl rebelling against her mother, who had forbidden her to see other men, and unwittingly he had fallen into the same trap. As a matter of fact, she enjoyed the attention of several men.

In more ways than one, he had met his match. One could say that she was a kind of Doña Juana. With her behavior, she was declaring her independence from him and her mother. One way of looking at their relationship was that she and my patient were mirror images of each other.

When she went off for a weekend with other people, he got a dose of his own medicine, and, as he put it, he went "bonkers"—he really could not stand being abandoned by her. He was terrified by the thought that she was sleeping with other men. The sparks flew. They quarreled over who would control whom. He looked to me for direct advice on how to cope and solve such a dilemma of an impossible and uncontrollable woman. He was a very jealous lover who brooked no competition. He was frantic.

During this past summer's interruption in the analysis, both he and his woman friend became even more anxious about a permanent commitment to each other. This was followed by a brief interruption in the relationship. His response was that he felt that he could not trust her. He felt betrayed and disillusioned. On one or two occasions, he even followed her around to spy on her actions. He again sank into a depression and felt himself to be a magnificent failure. In this state, he felt helpless and out of control. He repeated his demand for an exclusive relationship with her. Controlling her actions and wanting her to submit to his needs were clearly major motivations in this man. When control failed, he withdrew. The woman friend responded with an infantile neediness that made him feel he was being converted into her mother, especially when she wanted to talk on the phone late at night. He spitefully refused. As both of them calmed down from this lover's quarrel, he feared he could never escape.

During this period of the analysis, he experienced a roller coaster kind of excitement and depression. In a word, he was floundering. Symptomatic of this state was the fact that he could not stop smoking. He had tried everything: hypnotism, nicotine gum, etc. He repeated that he considered himself a failure. He felt that he could not control anything or anyone, including me in the transference. The therapy was near another stalemate. Interpretations of the transference alone seemed to be insufficiently helpful.

At this point, we decided on adjunctive tricyclic antidepressant medication, which facilitated regaining inner control and allowed him to sleep better. The transference meaning of giving him something that he had not got from his father was clear. He stopped smoking for good. While control and power issues remained important concerns and potential sources of conflict, he was much less consumed with them. He was more in control of his rages and was more trusting. When he returned from a winter vacation, power struggles with me and his fiancée decreased significantly. Before, making love had been like possessing, dominating, and controlling her, but now there was more mutuality and trust. In the transference, he was more trusting and collaborating. Before, when he felt he was losing control, he got angry and contentious, but now he was more serene and confident. These changes were due mainly to the analysis and only in a minor fashion resulted from the medication. After four months, he is now in the process of gradually reducing the medication without any retrogressive symptomatology.

I prefer not to confine myself to a single case to illustrate my thesis. Therefore, I should like to mention some other data. For example, women who display Doña Juana behavior have been recently described by Kavesh and Lavin (1989). They referred to the type A woman, who, though married, toys with the idea of having an affair. She is always on the lookout for men and misses the chase. One woman said she liked "the tension and excitement of an early romance. I haven't felt that with my husband since our son was born three years ago." Similarly, the beautiful but vindictive noblewoman in the current movie "Dangerous Liaisons" (derived from Choderlos de La Clos's 1782 novel) is another analogous version of Doña Juana. She wreaks vengeance on her unfaithful lover, the viscount, who spends his life seducing new virginal challenges. But he loses out in the end since he too, like my patient, falls in love. With much guilt and sadness, he realizes that he loves the virginal novitiate. His fate is decided when he refuses to continue the duel.

In another clinical instance, having an attractive eye-catching, muscular physique became very important to a young man when he broke up with his lover. He enjoyed the admiring and envious glances of other men in the health club where he worked out daily. Getting this kind of attention became as important to him as success in his career. The only thing that exceeded this pleasure was the control and power achieved in taking over another person's lover. The essence of these dynamics, as discovered in the therapy, was a re-creation of his being his mother's darling throughout childhood and adolescence. By being

55

the model son, he disappointed neither of his parents. He achieved much scholastic success and became a very respected academic in a prestigious university. But he always felt weak, small, and inferior. Being admired for his startling physique and his social successes reinstated the ecstatic specialness he felt with his mother. Power and control in this case were also means by which he attempted to cope with threatened inner collapse due to the break up of a relationship with a lover whom he described as "the best person I have ever met." Mourning this loss occupied the first task of that therapy.

Another young man began a behavior pattern in adolescence that consisted of attempting to attract other men in a variety of settings. But, when he succeeded, he invariably escaped in a panic. His fantasies at this time consisted of getting even with his mother, whom he felt to be a very controlling person. Now he was in control and felt very powerful within himself.

Discussion

There are two sorts of data in a study such as this one about Don Juan and Don Juanism, namely, literary and clinical. From the standpoint of clinical observations, Fenichel (1945) said that the analysis of Don Juan personality types indicated "that their oedipus complex is of a particular kind. It is dominated by the pre-genital aim of incorporation, pervaded by narcissistic needs and tinged with sadistic impulses. In other words, the striving for sexual satisfaction is still condensed with the striving for narcissistic supplies in order to maintain self-esteem" (p. 243). Here, we see a predominately oedipal interpretation, but what is most important is the pointing the way to a deeper preoedipal configuration. Robbins (1956) essentially follows Fenichel's formulations, and his clinical material also emphasizes the narcissistic issues of a man who uses women to maintain inner cohesion and prevent collapse of a fragile self. Pratt (1960) refers to an essentially "infantile need for reunion with the mother" in Don Juanism and notes that the "philandering represents a flight from incest or perhaps from homosexuality" (p. 328). The data in my case as well as in the homosexual cases suggest a deeper narcissistic focus. The clinical data are rather sparse in Pratt's paper, and the main subject matter is anthropological in nature. Pratt does, however, take into account the punishment of the trickster as a function of the superego.

The clinical data that are described in this chapter are culled from

the transferences observed in psychoanalytic settings and are not literary or anthropological. Mr. H resembled the legendary Don Juan but
did not conform to the dramatic character in that he was potentially
capable of love and the capacity to grow, adapt, and develop a lasting
relationship. He was able to make use of his positive qualities of personal charm and convert his creative energies from pathological sexual
exploits to experiments in parenting, certain home improvement tasks,
and animal training. He started the analysis focused on himself and
his selfish needs, but he was able to make use of the analysis to re-
nounce to a significant degree this exclusive focus. He removed his
ultimatum for exclusive attention. Control and power issues were paramount in this man's every interaction with others, but especially with
those he had made a commitment to. The reason for this behavior was
to ensure continuing contact with the idealized mother and restoration
of inner cohesion through maintenance of narcissistic supplies. Frustration of his efforts to control me or some more serious interference
with the integrity of the transference or other significant relationships
led to loss of inner cohesion (feeling helpless and unable to prevent
his mother's death; his inability to prevent his father's angry disappointment in him; his father's advancing age; his father dating; his
woman friend dating or her childish neediness; and, most important,
separations or empathic failures in the analytic relationship). What
usually followed was a temper tantrum that his wishes be followed to
the letter. The next step was a grandiose fantasy of making large sums
of money, but, in the process of putting his fantasy into action, he
engaged in erratic, impulsive business practices. Withdrawal, feelings
of helplessness, depression, a sleep disorder, lack of energy, and a
pervasive sense of fatigue were coupled with a gloomy pessimistic
outlook of impending disaster and catastrophe. He felt abandoned and
unable to function. On weekends, he rarely set foot out of the house
except for brief excursions with his father for breakfast or to his aunt's
house for dinner. He felt disconnected from me and struggled to make
constructive plans for the future.

Years earlier, he had medicated himself with cocaine and marijuana,
but now he abused tobacco by smoking large quantities of cigarettes.
He was desperate to have a family life, but he was totally unprepared
for the compromises and adaptive tasks required of intimate adult relationships in a family. He was more given to trading one thing for
another—a kind of bartering: I'll give you this, if you'll give me that.

In the transference, he felt forced into a helpless, submissive, dependent relationship with me that was paralyzing. He was a jealous lover, and he thought that other patients were preferred over him. Control and power were, in fact, used to maintain the continuity of self-cohesion when the threat of regression, fragmentation, or loss of boundaries occurred owing to a real or imagined rupture in the primary relationship. My observations, furthermore, lead me to think that a massive resistance, clinically manifested as control, occurred in response to a break in the integrity of the wholeness of the self due to separation or, less frequently, failures in empathy in the transference.

What the Don Juan type of character, as clinically observed, strives to preserve at all costs is the internalized image of the idealized mother self-object, which process is acted out with a succession of conquests, none of whom can actually measure up to the idealized mother. The Don Juan behavior began as a sexualization of the repressed affective state that emerged later as an imperfectly obscured depression.

This formulation resembles very closely the one proposed for perversions (Goldberg 1975), but Don Juanism does not seem to be a perversion in the usual sense and more specifically in terms of traditional psychoanalytic theory (Socarides 1988), except that the unconscious conflicts in the clinical data presented could be characterized as predominately preoedipal in origin. What seems to be cogent is that the Don Juan character presents a kind of "pseudo-vitality"—a term that Kohut (1977) used to describe a defensive posture to counteract an "inner deadness and depression. As children, these patients had felt emotionally unresponded to and had tried to overcome their loneliness and depression through erotic and grandiose fantasies" (p. 5). Kohut referred to the frantic sexual activities of some depressed adolescents as arising under similar circumstances (p. 272). My patient was similar in many respects to this formulation.

On the other hand, the literary Don Juan, like Hamlet, Faust, and Don Quixote, is an imaginary and mythic character (Weinstein 1967) who continues to present a fertile source of continuing study. Deutsch (1937) characterized Don Quixote also as a narcissistic character, but it must be remembered that the man from La Mancha was asexual and was consumed with an idealized world. Mandel's (1963) collection of various versions of the play demonstrates that one can observe the changes in the literary Don Juan through the ages and in different cultures and in a way trace the history of Western mankind: "Always, he beats with the pulse of his epoch and the reason is that not one literary work concerning him is great enough to have forced a new note on its times or to have deviated into eccentric splendor. The fact must be faced: Don Juan as a type of man remains in the end more interesting than any of the plays, poems, or novels which gave him life" (p. 21). The essential feature of the classic character of Don Juan, according to Mandel, is "supreme sensuality," representing a kind of erotic triumph over other aspects of his character (p. 12). Mandel goes on to specify that this is not just one element in Don Juan's personality but the essence of his self—"rather it is his life's only business; whatever else he may be or do is incidental" (p. 12). Mandel probably was inspired by Kirkegaard's (1987, 31–113) emphasis on sensuality in Mozart's *Don Giovanni*. It has been said that there are as many versions of the legend as there were conquests (according to Lorenzo da Ponte—"one thousand and three" in Spain alone).

Similarly, psychoanalytic interpretations have changed over the years with each new theory. Rank (1924) was the first psychoanalyst to make a comprehensive applied psychoanalytic study of the Don Juan legend, using psychoanalytic concepts to bring informed understanding to this curious and fascinating story. He interpreted the story as primarily oedipal, wherein the seduced women represent the unattainable mother and the deceived men the father. The commendatore as father metes out retribution as a representation of the superego. Leporello (Catalinon) is seen as the ego ideal. Actually, Catalinon is a comic or jester whose name was known to the audience in sixteenth-century Spain as a feminine one. In the play, he is meekly submissive to Don Juan, even though he may warn Don Juan of the dangers of his behavior in ego-ideal fashion. Rank's study dealt with the version written by da Ponte, the librettist for Mozart's opera *Don Giovanni*. Parenthetically, it appears that both Mozart and da Ponte may have been given to Don Juan–like behavior (Davenport 1932). It is said, too (Nettl 1956), that Casanova added a few lines to the libretto (da Ponte 1961).

Ferenczi (1952) may have preceded Rank's contribution in his note on bridge symbolism and the Don Juan legend, which refers to a phallic interpretation. Winter (1973) is intuitively correct about many aspects of his psychological inferences of the Don Juan legend (pp. 168–200), and I agree with him that power and control are important, but there are some notable problems with his formulations. First, Winter claims that Don Juan's strivings for power over women are seen as defenses against "incorporation to control the chaotic and confused sources of pain and pleasure," by which he means that Don Juan defends himself against being swallowed up by the ambivalently loved mother. This Kleinian interpretation is but partially accurate. My patient was concerned about being swallowed up too, but, as I have stated, this is a rather superficial interpretation based on a physiological analogy. In the end, he was comforted by an increasing capacity for closeness and togetherness. Second, Winter's interpretations are derived and inferred from the literary Don Juan and sociopsychological research that is different from clinical observations. Finally, Don Juan, like other literary heroes such as Achilleus or Odysseus, was a figure of action (Don Juan was called the Hector of Seville), but action is not the main characteristic even in the literary character. He is a "spoiled brat" (a *senorito*) who always takes advantage of others and is not capable of taking the sacraments of marriage (Maetzu 1968). José Ortega y Gasset asserts that Don Juan is virility itself and is nothing until he performs sex with a woman.

As Mandel states, the original Don Juan, and the Don Juan of the entire classical period, was a powerful man. He shows this by being so often successful in his tricks, by an extraordinary adeptness with the sword, by (and this is usually overlooked) his wonderful luck, even by his excellent connections and his noble birth, and by his thrilling defiance of the forces of the supernatural, which the common man is always told to adore but which he does not mind having flouted by somebody else (Mandel 1963, p. 19).

Summary and Conclusions

The literary character of Don Juan has offered an opportunity to study certain characteristics in an adult man who began a behavior pattern in adolescence that resembled the legendary and mythical Don Juan. Power and dominating control issues were paramount defenses against a narcissistic depression in this man as seen in his relationships with women and in the transference relationship with me. The transference data have been put to use in providing a formulation for an explanation of the phenomena observed. Other clinical data concerning women and some homosexual men are presented in a more abbreviated fashion. This research effort is a retrospective construction of the dynamics that led to this man's neurosis.

In my opinion, a self psychological interpretation offers the more felicitous fit than the classic oedipal interpretation. In fact, at first I tried interpretations based on classic oedipal theory—concerning issues of competition with me as father and fear of retaliation and castration—but this strategy resulted in little or no response. More important than symptomatic response, however, the data minimally and weakly supported those interpretations. To be sure, there were and still are competitive and phallic oedipal issues. Moreover, when the patient's mother died, he was drawn into a closer relationship with his father, a relationship accompanied by wishes and fantasies of taking his mother's place. These wishes were quite real, but, as the analysis proceeded, this negative oedipal configuration occupied a much less prominent place in the dynamics. Power and control issues dominated the clinical picture, masking a depression emanating from a deeper narcissistic focus. Interpretation of these narcissistic issues provided my patient with the relief he was seeking, while the main effect of the antidepressant medication was to help him sleep. By giving him something, a deeply seated wish was gratified and was in keeping with an idealized mother transference.

REFERENCES

Beauvoir, S. 1985. *Adieux: A Farewell to Sartre*. Translated by Patrick O'Brady. New York: Pantheon.

da Ponte, L. 1961. *Don Giovanni*. Translated by W. H. Auden and C. Kallman. New York: Schirmer.

Davenport, M. 1932. *Mozart*. New York: Dorset.

Deutsch, H. 1937. Don Quixote and Don Quixotism. *Psychoanalytic Quarterly* 6:215–222.

Deutsch, H. 1965. *Neuroses and Character Types*. New York: International Universities Press.

Erikson, E. 1959. *Identity and the Life Cycle*. Psychological Issues, Monograph no. 1. New York: International Universities Press.

Fenichel, O. 1945. *The Psychoanalytic Theory of Neuroses*. New York: Norton.

Ferenczi, S. 1952. Bridge symbolism and the Don Juan legend. In *Theory and Technique of Psychoanalysis*. New York: Basic.

Goldberg, A. 1975. A fresh look at perverse behavior. *International Journal of Psycho-Analysis* 56:335–342.

Horner, A. J. 1989. *The Wish for Power and the Fear of Having It.* Northvale, N.J.: Aronson.

Kavesh, L., and Lavin, C. 1989. Married, but still wedded to the chase. *Chicago Tribune* (February 1).

Kierkegaard, S. 1987. *Either/Or*, pt. 1. Edited and translated by H. V. Hong and E. H. Hong. Princeton, N.J.: Princeton University Press.

Kohut, H. 1977. *The Restoration of the Self.* New York: International Universities Press.

La Clos, C. 1782. *Les Liaisons dangereuses.* Paris: Biblioteque de la Pleiade, 1951.

McClelland, I. L. 1967. Don Juan. In *Encyclopedia Britannica,* vol. 7. Chicago: Encyclopedia Britannica.

Maetzu, R. 1968. *Don Quijote, Don Juan y la Celestina.* Madrid: Espasa-Calpe.

Mandel, O. 1963. *The Theatre of Don Juan.* Lincoln: University of Nebraska Press.

Nettl, P. 1956. Casanova and Don Giovanni. *Saturday Review* 39:44.

Nin, A. 1966–1971. *The Diary of Anaïs Nin.* 4 vols. Edited by Gunther Stuhlmann. New York: Swallow.

Pratt, D. 1960. The Don Juan myth. *American Imago* 17:321–335.

Rank, O. 1924. *The Don Juan Legend.* Translated and edited by David G. Winter. Princeton, N.J.: Princeton University Press, 1975.

Robbins, L. L. 1956. A contribution to the psychological understanding of the character of Don Juan. *Bulletin of the Menninger Clinic* 20:166–180.

Socarides, C. W. 1988. *The Preoedipal Origin and Psycho-Analytic Therapy of Sexual Perversions.* Madison, Conn.: International Universities Press.

Trachtenberg, P. 1988. *The Casanova Complex.* New York: Poseidon.

Weinstein, L. 1967. *The Metamorphoses of Don Juan.* New York: AMS.

Winter, D. G. 1973. *The Power Motive.* New York: Free Press.

Worthington, M. 1962. Don Juan as myth. *Journal of Literature and Psychology* 12:113–124.

4   CULTS REVISITED: CORPORATE AND QUASI-THERAPEUTIC CO-OPTATION

SAUL LEVINE

The last decade has seen a remarkable shift in the public's perception of and preoccupation with cultlike organizations. During the 1970s, groups regarded as "fringe religions" were feared and vilified. To a large extent, many of those still viable organizations are often looked on by the mainstream as weird, to say the least, and dangerous, at worst. Of course, wrongdoing and skulduggery, even in established religions, have made the public more cynical about any groups promising either facile answers to life's existential dilemmas or guaranteed salvation. The last years have seen numerous mental health and behavioral science studies and publications on cults or related groups attracting young people (e.g., Appel 1983; Halperin 1983; Hutchins Center for the Study of Democratic Institutions 1982; Levine 1979a, 1979b, 1980, 1981, 1984a, 1984b). These, together with newspaper accounts and exposés, legal actions, books, and government commissions, have familiarized the academic, clinical, legal, and lay public with the nature of many of these groups. On the surface, their differences seem enormous, but, on closer study, their overwhelming commonalities are striking.

There is no doubt that these groups have the capability of attracting and swaying large numbers of older adolescents and young adults, at least for a while. The similarities in the approaches of the most successful cults merely corroborate Darwin's doctrine of the survival of the fittest. The common inherent properties of the successful groups indicate that only the strongest ones survive and thrive. While numerous crucial characteristics can be distinguished, there is no doubt that their major intrinsic (and vital) ingredients involve belief and belonging (e.g., Frank 1978; Levine 1984b). "Belief" refers to a powerful overriding ideology, a system of values and of perceiving the world, a unique mythology, and an outwardly directed (beyond one's own navel) belief system. "Belonging" typifies the sense of being an intrinsic part of an important group that unequivocally accepts, shares, and elevates the individual to a personal sense of significance and of happiness—a major issue. When these two crucial properties are included and presented in such a way as to be highly persuasive, the power over the individual that the groups wield, at least temporarily, is impressive indeed.

In recent years, however, curious developments have gradually, subtly, but unmistakably occurred. For one thing, some of the more radical antisocial or even dangerous groups have disappeared. Most of the others have attempted to put on a face of legitimacy and civic responsibility—eschewing coercion and violence, rejecting obviously disturbed members, encouraging family contacts, and doing as little as possible to incite police or legal actions against them. Members who wish to leave are discouraged by means of discussion and group pressure (inherent even if not purposeful), but, once committed to this course of action, they are free to go, even helped at times.

But even more surprising to professionals who have been heavily engaged in the study of such groups is the change in the nature of frantic telephone calls from worried kin. Heretofore, they have come from all over the world from concerned or frightened family members regarding a relative who has become a zealous convert to a new religious cause. Recently, the calls have, as often as not, been made by relatives of members, but the groups, while bearing remarkable similarity to some avowedly religious ones (like Hare Krishna, the Unification Church, or Scientology), have been either "quasi-therapeutic" or "corporate" in nature, as it were. In the former, the declared goal has been very much akin to Maslow's self-realization—to overcome or reduce stress in life, to achieve one's potential so as to get the most out of one's relationships, work, love, and self-esteem (Levine 1980). The latter's raison d'être, to achieve one's maximum potential, sounds somewhat similar, but this is either thinly veiled or, more usually, explicitly stated, in the cause of efficiency, productivity, and (always) profits (Haaken and Adams 1983; Hoffer 1951; Tucker

1987). These two types of groups make no claims to be religious in nature; thus, issues like tax-exempt status, freedom of worship, and religious orthodoxy or fundamentalism do not come up as areas of conflict. Yet two things about these groups are remarkable. (1) They have extracted from religious cults those approaches that have attracted and ensured the unwavering passionate allegiance of thousands of followers. (2) Families and friends of true-believing members can and do see through the therapeutic or corporate verbiage. They are the ones who invoke the word "cult" in describing the experiences of their loved ones, even in these socially sanctioned groups.

Examples of therapeutic groups would be offshoots of the human potential movement, Arica, EST, Gestalt, Alcoholics Anonymous, Therafields, Scientology, Overeaters Anonymous, Gamblers Anonymous, the Healing Workshop, Narcanon, the Sullivan Institute, and an enormous variety of intentional social systems, halfway houses, hospitals, group homes, farms, and other therapeutic communities designed to ameliorate a variety of emotional and behavioral woes (drug addiction, repetitive sexual misadventures, antisocial behavior, etc.) using an intense ideology and a communal program often based on the ubiquitous twelve-step model. Examples of corporate consulting groups include Krone, Access, Silva, Contact, Context, Lifespring, Miracle Management Technologies, Transformational Technologies, New Age Consultants, and Innovations-Associates. These are less often residential in nature, but they still use the group program and intense belief system to captivate and inculcate their message. These all have characteristics of religious/spiritual movements or of the human potential movement of the late 1960s and 1970s. What are the similarities and differences between these two types of groups and those popularly defined as religious cults?

Similarities

THE GROUPS

In the process of promulgating an intense ideology or belief system (believing), it is clear that homogeneity of thought is accomplished. A shared and private system of values and logic, using arcane terms or common English words used in unique ways, adds to the sense of importance and substance of their private language and thought. Just about all the groups have a tome, a literature that includes all the buzz words, highlighting the commonly used vocabulary repetitively, adding uniqueness, authority, and seeming credibility to the members, enhancing their fortunate (anointed, chosen, elite, blessed) status. There is a message promulgated that the members will have achieved a clarity of thought, a crystallization of meaning in one's life. The literature may be controversial, fatuous, or confusing, but this has no bearing on the degree of total belief manifested by followers. There is a heightened feeling of well-being brought about in large part by belonging, the shared experiences, learning emotions, and perceptions within the group, a group that seems to be on the exact wavelength as the individual members. There is tremendous social reinforcement adding to the cultish mystique, enhancing the feelings of uniqueness, specialness, and elitism.

All the groups have a well-defined, even rigid hierarchy with a strong, often charismatic leader at the top and a pyramidal structure beneath. The leader is imbued with all kinds of real or imagined talents. While it helps to be charismatic, it is not crucial since the movements themselves have charismatic properties. The leader is the chief proponent of the pursuit, and most of the fame (and fortune) accrues to him or her. As with so many other groups, the lieutenants, those executives below the titular leader, are less creative and flexible, more rigid, more humorless, and, paradoxically, more zealous about the cause.

Many have a certain number of steps, rungs, or stages toward the achievement of some ultimate goal or state (knowledge, happiness, truth, productivity, awareness, profit, whole clear, etc.; see, e.g., Halperin 1983; Levine 1981). The literature outlines this exact route to the desired goal in such a way that it is always perceived as profound and a revelation. Money is a universal commodity in all these pursuits in that a financial commitment, sometimes even a major commitment, is a prerequisite. Congruent with cognitive dissonance theory, the more money that is spent, the greater the perceived worth that is attached to the belief system. If a great deal is spent in a driven pursuit (aside from money, time, energy, and concentration expended), it is difficult to admit to oneself that it has not been a highly successful experience. The leaders (gurus) can amass extraordinary wealth in a short period of time. Money's complicated psychodynamic relevance to issues of life (like mastery, potency, and narcissism) is, in fact, heightened when the goal is avowedly profit and productivity. (Contrary to popular belief, money was and is an overriding goal of many of the religious sects, whose communal facade covered over a remarkable entrepreneurial and capitalistic ethic.)

Rituals play an important role in all those outlets for belief and belonging. They focus attention, impose structure, and ensure common and shared activities. They also give added emphasis to the belief system. The rituals become part of the "repetition compulsion" of the active group. They can be linguistic (chants), meditative (shared silence), or strenuous (exercises), but they all enhance the sense of importance and give a paradoxical perception of tradition, even though most of these groups are newly arrived on the scene. While singing and chanting is less common than in religious cults, there are frequent ritualistic incantations used repetitively in most of the groups, giving validity to the suasive power of music.

THE MEMBERS

The majority of members of these groups become "true believers," at least for a period (Noyes 1966). The new belief system gives them an all-embracing set of attitudes and values that define their perception of and relation to their world. These ethnocentric "articles of faith" color almost all other thinking and feeling at the time of maximal commitment. They have a heightened sense of well-being; they feel "high," even ecstatic. They have seldom, they say, been so happy in their entire lives. All ambiguity and existential dilemmas disappear. They have a new-found personal sense of growth, of health, and of having taken a quantum leap in self-improvement. There is a sense of clarity, of revelation, of the enhancement of a new truth, the answer (to any complicated existential questions). They are dedicated, devoted, inspired.

They are excited, with a sense of mission. In the guise of love, understanding, and tolerance, they are, in fact, less tolerant of doubters, nay sayers, skeptics, or those who do not understand. There is a perception of being different and better than. They suspend disbelief; there are no alternative ways to experience or interpret their new knowledge and insights. They often proselytize at the slightest opportunity with a new-found sense of mission. It is not enough that they have found their ideal state; it is seemingly incumbent on them to get others to join them. At times they can be, at best, boring and, at worst, downright offensive. To the uninitiated, there is an air of rote programming, of parroting, that makes the members sound eerily alike.

The stages that the members go through are similar for all the groups. Certainly, there is a stage of being committed to the group during which zealotry predominates. This is almost invariably followed by a period of doubt during which the group's ideology loses its magic and the member loses his or her zeal. This almost always is a prelude to leaving the group, and the aftermath can be jarring and upsetting for a few months. The turnover in membership is large and, for the vast majority of members, very predictable, although, during true-believer status, a member will not believe that this phase can possibly be temporary. The characteristics of the stages "after the group" are also often replicated. In addition to shame, sadness, and embarrassment, anxiety, depression, and flashbacks occur, with an apparent psychological diathesis akin to culture shock. It takes a few months for the former member to exorcise the group's intense tenets from cognitive and emotional consciousness. Memories persist, however, and, as with religious cults, many are positive and self-enhancing in nature. The final stage is almost inevitable. As with religious groups, as zealous as true believers are, more than 98 percent are out of the group and estranged from the belief system in under two years.

Differences

There are considerable differences between the socially sanctioned therapeutic and corporate groups and those religious groups popularly depicted as cults. The leaders of the therapeutic and corporate groups, as strong and charismatic as they may be, are never considered to be representative of or close to God or any other deity. But there is no doubt that temporary adulation does occur and that the leader has superhuman characteristics attributed to him by the membership. Members want to believe that their leader has extraordinary powers. This enhances the intensity of their involvement. God, however, is not usually invoked as the progenitor of the ideology, and worship is not demanded. While there may be rituals and even occasional repetitive incantations, there is little repetitive liturgical chanting, and there are not prayers to God on a regular basis in order to expedite the accomplishment of goals.

No fund-raising, hard-sell recruiting, or dedicated dishonesty on the part of the members is demanded. But, as mentioned, they often do proselytize and try to win converts to the cause. There is no overt encouragement to change one's identity radically or to become estranged from one's family and friends. However, estrangement is seen from time to time as the individual chooses on his own to break away from the traditional fold (seen by them as incarceration). It is, in fact, this very occurrence that prompts anxious phone calls to clinicians' offices. It is the suddenness, the unexpectedness, the unpredictability, the possible danger, but especially the estrangement that strikes fear and loathing in the hearts of loved ones.

The goals of these groups are more pragmatic and explicit, as opposed to the avowedly spiritual expectations of the religious groups. These groups do not use coercion or threats and tend to avoid taking in disturbed or emotionally vulnerable individuals. The truth is, however, that even the most egregious religious cults have moved in the same direction. They too do not want problems with litigation or prosecution. This is particularly paradoxical for those groups set up as growth environments with quasi-therapeutic aims; even they do not want individuals with emotional problems.

Finally, the corporate and therapeutic groups are not looked on with as much mistrust and hatred by the mainstream population. Somehow, the explicit goals, which seemingly fit in with current middle-class values, make them more palatable and less threatening. The fact that they are quite similar in many ways to the religious groups is irrelevant to this point; it is the "strangeness" of some of the fringe religious groups (cults) that makes them more derided, decried, and detested. When one looks closely at the ethic of many of these latter groups, however, their seemingly ideological zealotry often covers over fiscal priorities and psychological goals. In interviews with members in an earlier study (Levine 1981), the revered belief system was irrevocably and quickly superseded by the personal growth and gains achieved by members. The investments and entrepreneurial flare of many of these groups are truly astounding. The Maharishi International University, the academic arm of transcendental meditation, turns out more MBAs yearly than most prominent business schools. As with any true believer, it is not the cause that rivets the attention as much as the overwhelming personal factors: high energy and motivation, a feeling of happiness and potency, a zeal and dedication. They are all alike in this regard. We should not be surprised, then, by the recent developments dealt with here. It turns out that the so-called religious cults were never far from the corporate and therapeutic scene to begin with. Nor are the new entities distantly removed from their forebears.

Discussion

Certainly, utopian movements and cults are not new to the American and Canadian scene (Cohn 1957). The term "cult" is indeed a four-letter word, inherently pejorative, and the label is often largely within the mind of the beholder. It conjures up images of Jim Jones and Charles Manson at their worst, and perhaps of other figures and movements less dramatic and violent but equally weird and offensive to outsiders. A common definition of the term "cult" is a group of people that follows a dominant leader, who is imbued with omniscience, infallibility, and even deity-like powers and to whom total obeisance and loyalty is demanded. Admittedly, the new groups referred to in this chapter do not fit this literal translation exactly. While there are some that conform to the universal consensus on the term "cult" (e.g., Hare Krishna, Moonies, the Divine Light Mission, Rajneesh Bagwan, etc.), many others are, in fact, quite controversial. That is, what is one person's cult is another person's highly supportive, meaningful, significant, loving, caring, secure, and entirely laudable group. What is anathema to one might be salvation to another, and vice versa. Surprising examples of seemingly innocuous groups, which have been labeled as cults by highly concerned relatives, are Gestalt, Pritikin, Alcoholics Anonymous, Mormons, born again Christians, Bahai, Lubavitchers, Catholics, and many others. Preferable perhaps is the term "radical departures" (Levine 1984a), which, in effect, captures and encompasses the seemingly rapid and unexpected adoption of an apparently dramatically new and different way of thinking and living, with jarring effects on those around. Whether they engage in intrusive, coercive, and even illegal practices is important, of course, but this bears little relation to how involved or committed true believers become. One can use the term "autohypnosis" to describe the phenomenon whereby an individual "preprogrammed" to believe intensely succumbs to the ministrations and messages of mesmerizing and messianic groups. It is when the true believer becomes so enmeshed that he or she cannot see anything but the tenets of the group that the term "cult" is applied. Relatives get particularly perturbed when the move is totally unexpected and seems incongruent with the believer's past life. The total

70

conversion of the individual, the devotion of his or her life to the new group, the expenditure of money and energy, and the turning of his or her back on family and friends strikes pain and terror into their hearts, no matter what the nature of the group. What is of further significance is that, for all the avowed and promulgated differences and uniqueness, the commonalities among all these groups that attract true believers far outweigh their differences.

There is no doubt that these groups wield considerable power over their true-believing members during the period of maximal commitment. Or rather, a true believer suspends judgment and surrenders autonomy to such an extent that almost any leader and group can be imbued with characteristics of mind-controlling agents. Again and again, one hears the term "brainwashing," alluding to North Korean and Chinese torture techniques (ca. the 1950s), a purposeful, dedicated, malevolent, controlling totalistic approach to breaking down the ego strengths of the individual. It is intrusive, intense, and, most important, inflicted. But, during times of uncertainty, people come on their own in their quest for inner peace (Cohn 1957). In truth, contrary to what many of our colleagues say, the vast majority of true believers come to their chosen group of salvation during their own periods of heightened need for affiliation, a veritable critical period (alienation, demoralization, low self-esteem) providing motivation to succumb, and, by means of a cooperative and participatory process (autohypnosis), they develop a sense of personal enhancement and commitment.

These groups, like their religious forebears, serve important developmental functions for young people in the transition period between older adolescence and adulthood. As with the spiritual groups, a relatively young age group is attracted to these movements, partly because of their psychological state, their personal needs at the time, and partly because of the psychodynamic work that they are doing. In earlier publications, I described the state of ennui in which the potential members find themselves as a critical period in their lives. It was typified by feelings of alienation, demoralization, and low self-esteem. In addition, for most of the members, the work on separation-individuation had somehow been stymied. The groups, irrespective of their lofty messages, provide an effective counterbalance to the critical period. By providing belief and belonging, the feelings of alienation, demoralization, and low self-esteem are supplanted. The process of coming to grips with one's identity is accelerated again, usually after a prolonged stagnant position. In addition, the individual often uses the group as a vehicle for separation from parents and achieving more autonomy and independence.

There are documented problems of certain intense demanding groups affecting members deleteriously. Certainly, those that are more intrusive, coercive, messianic, charismatic, and pressured do prove inimical to some members. Those who are most vulnerable are individuals who are in crisis, have rigid, obsessional personalities, magical expectations, or individual psychological needs, or have psychiatric histories. There is no doubt, however, that, for all the inherent and real dangers, benefits of radical departures can and do accrue to these groups' members. They do feel happier and better, at least for a while. They tend to be drug free, dedicated, committed, and enthusiastic during their believing phase. Feelings of alienation, demoralization, and low self-esteem are overcome. They feel good about their lives, their goals, and themselves. Their psychological symptoms, especially related to anxiety and depression, are dramatically diminished. One of the many reasons for corporate and therapeutic groups to adopt intense group techniques is that they are, at least temporarily, effective. During periods of rapid change and uncertainty, "cults of unreason" have always flourished. Their magic has resided in the powers of belief and belonging. If these groups were not established, many individuals would (and do) find their own cause célèbre to identify with and proselytize for (e.g., the right to life movement, antivivisectionists, fundamentalists, etc.). It is, therefore, no accident that groups have adopted techniques that have been proved to be more effective than traditional psychotherapeutic methods in overcoming the anxieties and stresses of life. While those on the outside find true believers to be offensive, from a psychological perspective they might take heart in knowing that the members are being protected or even helped psychologically, at least temporarily.

Conclusions

There is no doubt that therapeutic agencies and corporate consultant groups use these cultlike techniques because they work—so much so that for work with certain clinical populations they are seen to be the sine qua non of success (especially for addicts, alcoholics, antisocial youths, and repetitive deviant behavior). In the business realm, profits actually increase, at least for a period of time, after the introduction of group and ideological techniques (Japan is a good example on a larger scale).

If any of these groups are breaking any laws, they should be charged forthwith. But, unless this can be established, we have learned through bitter experience that, no matter how we might decry mercenary motives, ridiculous theory, invalid or messianic claims, or high-pressure techniques, groups like these will come, go, and flourish in any society where change and ambiguity are part of the context of living.

REFERENCES

Appel, W. 1983. *Cults in America*. New York: Holt, Rinehart & Winston.

Cohn, N. 1957. *The Pursuit of the Millennium*. New York: Essential.

Frank, J. D. 1978. Sources and functions of belief systems. In P. E. Dietz, ed. *Psychotherapy and the Human Predicament*. New York: Schocken.

Haaken, J., and Adams, R. 1983. Pathology as personal growth, a participant observation study of lifespring training. *Psychiatry* 46:270–280.

Halperin, D. 1983. *Religion, Sect and Cult*. Boston: Wright PSG.

Hoffer, E. 1951. *The True Believer*. New York: Harper & Row.

Hutchins Center for the Study of Democratic Institutions. 1982. Cults and the Constitution. *Center Magazine* 15(2): 17–28.

Levine, S. 1979a. Adolescence: believing and belonging. *Adolescent Psychiatry* 7:41–53.

Levine, S. 1979b. The role of psychiatry in the phenomenon of cults. *Canadian Journal of Psychiatry* 24(7): 593–603.

Levine, S. 1980. *Study of the Mind Development Groups: Sects and Cults in Ontario*. Report to the Attorney-General's Office. Toronto: Government of Ontario.

Levine, S. 1981. Cults and mental health: clinical conclusions. *Canadian Journal of Psychiatry* 26:534–539.

Levine, S. 1984a. Alienated Jewish youth and religious seminaries—an alternative to cults? *Adolescence* 19:185–198.

Levine, S. 1984b. Belief and belonging in adult behavior. *Perspectives in Psychiatry* 3(8): 1–6.

Noyes, J. H. 1966. *Strange Cults and Utopias of 19th Century America*. New York: Dover.

Tucker, R. 1987. *New Age and Mind Control Training Programs*. Toronto: Council on Mind Abuse.

5 MOVIES AND THE ADOLESCENT: AN OVERVIEW

SCOTT SNYDER

Motion pictures can serve as a powerful socializing influence on the developing adolescent. Movies can circumvent established socializing agencies in our society (school, church, and parents) and directly affect the individual (Jowett and Linton 1980). No segment of society is more prone to such influence than adolescents. The response of an adult to a particular movie will be tempered by the experience of that individual, including traditional social and cultural influences. The adolescent, however, does not have an equivalent amount of experience in these areas and can be even more sensitive to the effects of the movies.

There has been little change in the influence of films since 1917, when the National Council of Public Morals (1917) in Great Britain stated that "in the course of an inquiry we have been much impressed by the evidence brought before us that moving pictures are having a profound influence upon the mental and moral outlook of millions of our young people—an influence the more subtle in that it is subconsciously exercised—and we leave our labours with the deep conviction that no social problem of the day demands more earnest attention."

Movies can be a medium more for adolescents than either children or adults. The bulk of the American movie audience is in its teens or early twenties. In 1981, 40 percent of all people attending American movie theaters were between the ages of twelve and twenty, despite the fact that this age group accounted for only 19 percent of the population at that time (Squire 1983). These percentages were remarkably similar in surveys performed in 1957 and 1972 (Jowett 1976). Filmmakers often tailor their productions to adolescent audiences of these demographic factors.

This chapter will examine how movies influence adolescents. An impressive literature on the social and psychological effects of movies on adults has evolved since the advent of the film industry. However, research and commentary on the interplay between the adolescent and films is sparse. A review of the literature spanning the years 1966 to the present revealed only twenty-six references pertaining specifically to teenagers and the movies. The majority of these studies occurred in the laboratory as opposed to analyses of real life effects of motion pictures. Also, many of these studies had subjects in the age range of youths, eighteen to twenty-two, rather than younger adolescents. The role of identification, group influence, fantasy, dreams, and related factors that affect adolescents will be explored in movies that emphasize these themes and present adolescents in key roles. This will be followed by an overview of empirical research devoted to the actual effects of films on various aspects of adolescent behavior and thought.

How Movies Affect Adolescents

Much of the existing literature describes how motion pictures may adversely affect the socialization and personality formation of youths or cause deviant group behavior. But movies may also have an important contribution to make toward the development of healthy socialization and character structure. Haley (1952) suggested that, as the traditional family structure disintegrated, youths would rely more heavily on all the mass media to "provide an interpretation [of life] that was once the province of family and cultural traditions." Movies can act as sources of ideas and attitudes, especially when the viewers have gaps in their experience, as is often the case with the adolescent. The movie may move the adolescent audience outside of its parochial cultural experience and into one with a broader range of possibilities.

The adolescent moviegoer may be especially impressed by the vivid visual presentations characteristic of movies in which images are developed, identified, and followed easily. Even the intellectually, educationally, or socially impaired adolescent can readily comprehend these images on an elementary level. Such ease of comprehension helps the viewer identify with the roles of the characters. This identification is encouraged by groups ranging from the movie producer to the movie

75

audience itself. Most movies, especially those dealing with adolescent themes, depend on appeals to the primary emotions in order to increase the likelihood of such identification. Examples of this utilization of affect include *East of Eden* (1955), a film about intense sibling rivalry and father-son conflicts presented in a powerful manner. Intense emotions are seen in this portrayal of an adolescent who initially hates his father and rebels against him but who eventually learns to understand, forgive, and even accept him (Goldstein and Zornow 1980). Family relationships, generation conflicts, and love and sex are presented with great depth and insight in *The Last Picture Show* (1971). Boredom, alienation, and despair are vividly presented in this film. The more recent *Breakfast Club* (1985) is another example of a movie presenting teenagers in a realistic manner such that the adolescent viewer can readily identify with the emotions and sentiments of the characters. In films about adolescence, emotions, passions, and sentiments may at times be overdramatized compared to other forms of drama. Thus, films dealing with adolescents often utilize affect as the final common pathway in order to appeal to the largest possible teenage audience.

The Role of Identification

One of the main goals of the moviemaker is to persuade the viewer to experience vicariously the events that occur on the screen. Lynd and Merrell (1928) quoted a mother as saying, "I send my daughter [to the movies] because a girl has to learn the ways of the world somehow, and the movies are a good safe way" (p. 268). This vicarious involvement with film is brought about by many factors, one of which, identification, is especially relevant for adolescents. The two principal forms of identification in film are similarity and wishful identification. In the former, the viewer identifies with the characters in the film that are most like himself. Wishful identification occurs when the viewer desires to be like certain characters in the film (Feilitzen and Linne 1975). Tudor (1974) refers to identification as "the central factor in the psychology of the movie audience" (p. 76). Identification with the type of story is usually secondary.

The adolescent can learn from movies because they are modeled after life situations the adolescent will eventually face. Although the manner in which the screen actor handles these situations is sometimes less than ideal, the ability to anticipate such predicaments is valuable.

Mendelsohn (1966) proposed several ways in which such learning can take place. In reference group theory, it is believed that groups to which the audience would presumably aspire to belong (i.e., the rich, the powerful, the successful) serve as reference points for the movie-goer. If a film subject is even remotely plausible, it is theorized that this will make the characteristics of the reference group realistic for the audience. This concept is exemplified in *Red Dawn* (1984), in which a group of adolescents forms a guerilla unit fighting a hypothetical Soviet invasion of the United States. At one point in the film, a teen-age, intellectual liberal and an athletic, powerful conservative win and establish an authoritarian leadership based on the belief that those with the greatest force or power should prevail. Ryan and Kellner (1988) felt the film essentially endorses a right-wing ideology based on author-itarian, almost totalitarian, leadership principles. *Rambo* (1985) is another example of militarism. The figure of Rambo may also be in-dicative of how the options of American working-class youths are somewhat limited. Militarism and nationalism can provide some self-worth for youths who are undereducated and offered the military as the only way of validating themselves. The violence and aggression of these films can also serve to enhance the masculine, strong, indepen-dent image of its hero, Rambo, according to Ryan and Kellner (1988).

Powdermaker (1950) stated that "audiences tend to accept as true that part of a movie story that is beyond their experience" (p. 13). In status aspiration, the movie will portray a way of life associated with high status. A recent example is *Stand and Deliver* (1988), which pre-sents a heroic portrait of a high school teacher who takes a group of underachieving, lower-socioeconomic-status high school students and through extreme dedication and perseverance teaches them calculus, a feat considered impossible by his fellow teachers. He becomes an inspirational example to the entire community.

Mendelsohn (1966) also proposed the concept of anticipatory social-ization. Moviegoers of lower social status can learn from films how members of the groups to which they aspire behave and can begin to pattern their own behavior after such cinema examples. Ryan and Kellner (1988) believe that films such as *Saturday Night Fever* (1977) and *Flashdance* (1983) demonstrate that people can transcend their working-class background and cross over into a world of upward mo-bility. The means of cultural escape in these movies is dance, an exam-ple of the type of physical activity (sports being the prime example) that for some represents their only avenue for advancement. Each movie also presents characters who are already successful models of what can be achieved. A related phenomenon is that of reinforcement of values, in which working-class people approve working-class values and shun middle-class values. These issues would be especially relevant for adolescents who are already struggling with issues of power/authority, status, and values.

Interaction among the Movies, the Adolescent, and Group Phenomena

It is well known that phenomena such as identification, status, and peer influence are important in growth and development. The concept of the group itself and how the group can exert its influence on the individual is important in the development of identification, status, peer influence, and related phenomena. Peer pressure to be strong, masculine, and loyal to your friends is evident in such films as *Lords of Flatbush* (1974). *Foxes* (1980) presents a female perspective on friendship and honor. It shows how fiercely devoted to each other four teenage girls can become. The girls form a substitute family, mutually attempting to protect each other from the challenges of drugs, sex, and broken homes they are surrounded by in Los Angeles.

The relation between the film, the adolescent, and group phenomena is very significant. The audience for movies has been called "an unstructured group" (Jarvie 1970, p. 89) in that it has "no social organization, no body of customs or tradition, no established set of rules or rituals, no organized group of sentiments, no structure of status roles, and no established leadership" (Blumer 1951).

Jarvie (1978) proposes that one of the main socializing influences for the teenager is the peer group. While rock music concerts may have similar patterns of attendance and socialization influences, they are less frequently attended.

The adolescent peer group makes the movies its medium of choice because they are removed from the home, other adolescents are likely to be in attendance, cinema is a freer medium to examine varieties of human experience, and the movie itself is relatively short in length, leaving time for discussion and reflection. The adolescents may relate to each other in terms of which films they have seen, which films they enjoy, and which actors or actresses they admire or dislike.

The cinema may act as a "social lubricant" and provide an opportunity for "trying out," utilizing the film content in group interactions. Middle and late adolescents see films at a time when they are beginning to form intimate relationships. Films may assist in this socialization process. Mendelsohn (1966) wrote that teenagers share an interest in the same kind of experience, such as the movies, which helps establish feelings of mutual rapport. The teenagers in the movie audience can be quite heterogeneous and may have had a variety of reasons why they chose to attend a particular movie, but they end up forming an informal group that assists the adolescent in facilitating his relationship with those adolescents whose support he so actively seeks.

Subliminal and Escapist Effects of the Movies on the Adolescent

The movie may also exert a dreamlike influence on the adolescent (Munsterberg 1970). Tudor (1969) suggested that the darkened theater, combined with the heightened intensity of the message stimuli, the increased sense of social isolation that it creates, and the relaxed posture of the movie viewer, makes the message more potent emotionally and the viewer more easily influenced than does television. Movies may create a visual fantasy for adolescent viewers, who are already susceptible to such influences. Jowett and Linton (1980) state that movies are similar to dreams in that they can fulfill the dreams of the audience through fantasy, can act in a more profound psychological sense to symbolize hidden fears and desires and act as a type of "conscious dreaming," or can act as a source for dreams themselves, especially when there might be a strong identification with a movie star or a specific incident. Movies can become the "shared daydream" for millions of adolescent viewers for, "where a group of people share a common culture, they are likely to have certain daydreams in common" (Wolfenstein and Leites 1950). Jowett and Linton (1980) propose that, for the adolescent, such daydreams may focus on our "material culture" (the visual aspects of modern culture that have been profoundly influenced by the images created and fostered by the movies).

Horror films are one example of a film genre popular among adolescents that may consciously and unconsciously reflect their fears and anxieties. Ryan and Kellner (1988) believe that films dealing with the occult reappeared in the 1970s to represent threats to the existing

American social and institutional structure. They wrote that the *Omen* trilogy consisted of three movies released between 1976 and 1981 that traced the life of the devil from his infancy to adulthood, when he becomes an evil corporate chief and power broker who plans coups and disasters for profit. This series of films was released at a time of economic recession in America, affecting adults and adolescents alike. These films may have achieved popularity as a vehicle through which youths could vent their hostility against the financially and politically powerful.

Another major type of horror film of recent times has been the "slash and gash, slice and dice" genre. Adolescents are frequently the victims of murder and cannibalism (e.g., *The Texas Chainsaw Massacre*, 1974), the modern prototype of this film. Obsessive male fantasies of violence against women, especially adolescent girls, is evinced in films such as *Halloween* (1978) and the *Friday the 13th* series. Violence and satanic themes are often combined in these movies, with liberated, sexually independent teenage girls ending up brutally killed. Some feel these films represent a puritanical, repressive, male-dominated reaction to the sexual and women's revolution that gave women more power and influence in a wide array of behaviors, including teenage female sexuality (Ryan and Kellner 1988).

Finally, the movies may serve as a form of escape from the stress of adolescence itself. The world of movies is one in which, unlike dreams, there is a resolution no matter what we do. The developing adolescent can release emotional and intellectual reactions and be exposed to sublimation and repression through the movies. Movies can provide a few hours of shape and even meaning to adolescents who are often struggling with structure and the meaning of life itself.

Limited Review of the Effects of Movies on Mood and Behavior in Adolescents and Postadolescents

MOOD

Films have been shown, in various studies, to exert a significant effect on adolescent mood and behavior. The effects of film on the mood of normal adolescents and postadolescents have been studied since the early 1960s. An example is the pioneering work of Lazarus, Speisman, Mordkoff, and Davison (1962), who exposed undergraduate students, with a median age of nineteen, to a stressor film that vividly portrayed a sequence of crude operations performed on the genitalia of adolescent boys and to a neutral control film depicting corn farming in Iowa. The stressor film produced increases in the measures of skin resistance, heart rate, and tension and in a variety of objective scales measuring stress. Anxiety, unpleasantness, social unaffection, and depression were most affected by the stressor film. Narcissistic subjects demonstrated fewer physiological effects, whereas the stressor film produced more profound physiological effects on those subjects described as mature and responsive to the plight of others. Subsequent studies have shown that exposure to motion pictures can produce anxiety and depression (Marston, Hart, Hilleman, and Faunce 1984; Zuckerman, Lubin, Vogel, and Valerius 1964), elation (Govax 1971), or obsessive-compulsive thoughts (Wilner and Horowitz 1975) in late adolescents and young adults in laboratory environments.

A more recent study (Cantor and Reilly 1982) examined the effects of frightening films viewed by sixth- and tenth-grade students in movie theaters. Thirty-five percent of the tenth graders reported enduring fright reactions to films they had seen when they were younger than six years old. In the preceding two years, 18 percent of the tenth graders had enduring fright reactions to films. The sixth graders reacted even more strongly to frightening films. Boys like to see frightening films significantly more often than girls and are less reactive to such films than girls are. Cantor and Reilly found that parental restrictions on viewing such films decline with the age of the child.

SUICIDE

Suicide has not been examined in relation to theatrical film viewing, but a number of studies have explored the effects of televised movies. Gould and Shaffer (1986) studied the effects on adolescent attempted and completed suicides in the greater New York City area after four fictional films dealing with adolescent suicide were broadcast on television. The number of attempted suicides was significantly greater in the two-week period after the broadcast compared to the two-week period prior to the broadcast. The number of completed suicides increased significantly after three of the four movies were shown. Extensive educational and preventive materials were shown after the one film not associated with increased suicide rates. The authors concluded that television movies may have either a provoking or an inhibiting effect on adolescent suicide. Others reported similar findings (Phillips 1982; Wasserman 1984).

A replication study of Gould and Shaffer's research found no evidence of an increase in teenage suicides in Pennsylvania and California after presentation of the same films (Phillips and Paight 1987). Using a nationwide sample of completed suicides, Berman (1988) found no evidence for increased numbers of suicides. There was evidence, however, that a significant imitation effect of the method of suicide (carbon monoxide poisoning) employed in one of the films was occurring.

VIOLENCE

The relation between films and violence has also been studied extensively. Feshbach (1955) proposed the "symbolic catharsis" doctrine, which stated that the symbolic expression or vicarious enactment of aggression could reduce the likelihood of subsequent aggression when instigated. Numerous studies since the early 1960s have disproved this theory by showing that experimental situations, in which fantasy aggression was justified, generated greater hostility and violence in subjects by lowering inhibitions against aggression. Such findings have been found repeatedly not only in middle-class university students but also in juvenile delinquents (Parke, Berkowitz, Leyens, Weste, and Sebastian 1977).

Most previous studies had not explored social class differences. A recent study did examine whether social class, gender, or personality can affect physiological responses to filmed violence (Frost and Stauffer 1987). A group of affluent undergraduate students (mean age 19.7 years) was compared to a racially mixed group of residents of an inner-city housing project (mean age 20.1 years). Each group had half males and half females. Each group was shown two minutes of nonviolent material followed by ten excerpts from theatrical films, each depicting one of ten different forms of violence. Skin conductance response and blood pulse volume were measured. Inner-city residents were significantly more aroused by viewing filmed violence than the college sample. Depictions of rape caused the highest response by inner-city subjects but only the fifth highest by the college sample. The most arousing types of filmed violence depicted the killing of another human being. Accidental death and assault caused less arousal in both samples. Gender was not found to be a significant factor in arousal to violence portrayed on film. Personality variables were not related to physiological arousal. The authors suggested the concept of "resonance" to explain their findings of different social class responses to filmed violence: "When what people see on television is most concurrent with everyday reality (or perceived reality), the combination may result in a coherent and powerful 'double dose' of the television message" (Gerbner, Gross, Mogan, and Signorelli 1980, p. 15). This may produce enhanced physiological arousal. This study examined a post-adolescent or young adult population as opposed to actual adolescents. The authors cautioned against generalizing the findings to naturalistic settings in the real world.

Viemero (1984) showed two violent youth films and a cartoon to 288 students aged ten to seventeen to test the relation between aggression and moral judgments about the behavior of film characters and events. Subjects accepted the behavior of movie characters on a moral level, even if it was violent or antisocial, as long as they identified with the characters. The age of the actor was found to be one of the most important factors in the acceptance and possible imitation of the film character's behavior by the subjects. The more aggressive the viewers, the easier it was for them to accept the violence of the film actor.

Another way to examine this relation is by means of actual episodes of film-inspired violence. Wilson and Hunter (1983) examined a number of such episodes and concentrated on those with grave outcome. The term "victim chosen" was used for episodes of violence involving one offender and one victim and "victim inspired" for episodes in which violence was self-inflicted. The authors found that motion picture viewing was involved in thirteen out of twenty-three victim-chosen incidents and thirty-two out of thirty-five victim-inspired incidents. Victims were between the ages of thirteen and twenty-four and offenders in their teens and twenties. Four films, *The Deer Hunter, Magnum Force, The Warriors,* and *Taxi Driver,* accounted for the majority of the incidents.

Wilson and Hunter proposed a three-step model consisting of (1) identification, (2) perseveration of beliefs, and (3) execution of those beliefs to explain the connection between pretend violence in the film and real violence. In the first step, the person may identify with a character in the film or a graphic scene of violence from the film. Russian roulette was depicted in *The Deer Hunter,* a technique mimicked by many real life victims. John Hinckley presumably identified with the protagonist of *Taxi Driver,* Travis Bickle, in his attempted assassination of President Ronald Reagan. He seemed to develop an obsessive attachment to Jodie Foster, who portrayed a teenage prostitute in the film, after viewing the film at least fifteen times. Wilson and Hunter (1983) recalled, however, that the prosecution felt that the news media and suggestibility of media influences during psychiatric sessions may have greatly contributed to such identification.

Step 2 involves the perseverative effect of the movie. The person accepts certain strategies that allow his or her views to persist even if they are in error or encounter strong opposition. The film may focus already existing problems or allow the viewers a rationale, which they believe will solve their problems. Drugs, rejection, loss of a job, or other factors may combine with the film viewers' beliefs if they reach for confirmation, invent a weak explanation in order to maintain the validity of their beliefs, or have a strong emotional commitment to the issue (Nisbett and Ross 1980; Ross and Lepper 1980).

Step 3 involves the actual transition from violent thought to violent action. The troubled viewer may need to believe that a particular movie supports violent action (Malamuth and Donnerstein 1982). For example, in *Taxi Driver,* Travis Bickle first considers assassinating a political candidate at a rally. When his plan fails, he begins to attack the pimps and degenerates who control Jodie Foster and becomes a hero.

Malamuth and Check (1981) believed that these effects can occur either immediately or after a considerable lag time. The deaths reviewed by Wilson and Hunter (1983) occurred during the actual viewing of the film, in the case of *The Warriors,* when murders occurred in the movie theater itself, to five years later, in the case of a girl who shot and killed her sister under Satan's orders years after viewing *The Omen.*

A criticism of this study is that it examined a highly selected sample, ignored minor incidents of violence, and focused on those with a fatal outcome. The three-step theory of identification is highly speculative, yet it does provide a theoretical framework that can be tested more vigorously.

A similar relation may be found between sexual violence depicted in movies and subsequent behavior. Exposure to aggressive pornography and "slasher" films (in which a woman is tortured, often sexually, at the hands of a stalker) may cause viewers eventually to become desensitized and to stop believing that such activities are violent. Viewers become more sympathetic toward myths about rape and impose weaker sentences in fictional experimental trials held for the rapists (Comstock 1981). Postadolescents exposed to depictions of rape in films created more violent sexual fantasies as measured by both penile tumescence and self-reports of arousal compared to controls (Malamuth 1981). These results were consistent with earlier findings that certain portrayals of rape stimulate relatively high sexual arousal in nondeviants in an experimental situation (Malamuth, Haber, and Feshbach 1980; Malamuth, Heim, and Feshbach 1980).

A study of fifty-two college males exposed for two hours each day for five consecutive days to feature-length R-rated movies that depicted violence against women demonstrated compatible findings (Linz, Donnerstein, and Penrod 1980). This study differed from previous research in the amount of exposure subjects received to filmed violence. There were four phases to the experiment: an initial pre-screening, a film viewing session, a simulated rape trial, and an extended debriefing. Subjects were significantly less depressed and anxious on the final day of the film viewing and more likely to enjoy the films by day 5. Men who viewed the films felt that the victim of a violent assault and rape was less injured and less worthy compared to a central group who viewed no films. One criticism of the study is that subjects participated as mock jurors and evaluated the rape victim almost immediately after viewing the films. Some theorists believe a longer time interval is needed between the last film exposure and evaluations of the rape victim (Berkowitz 1984). Age, sex, and social class differences were also not considered in this study.

Goleman (1985) reviewed several interesting findings in this area. He observed that women also became more callous and were likely to believe that a woman who was raped sought it out. It was formerly believed that these attitudes and patterns of behavior were found only in actual rapists. Adolescent sex offenders and most young rapists actually have had little or no exposure to pornography. Straightforward film pornography without violence did not induce these same effects on peoples' attitudes toward women. But films showing violence against women sexually stimulated one-third of the normal men who watched them, even though the films contained relatively little that was explicitly sexual.

Goleman (1985) also commented that the amount of exposure to violent pornography is rapidly increasing, with one in eight commercially released films in 1983 showing violent acts committed against women, compared to one in twenty in 1982. He felt that there was a clear link between aggressive pornography and violence and that the reason that the U.S. Commission on Obscenity and Pornography (1970) reached a different conclusion is that, during that period, violence as a component of pornography was rare.

Conclusions

Adolescents constitute a major proportion of the motion picture audience. Contemporary movies are often geared to an adolescent audience owing to demographic and economic factors. Although a vast literature on the effects of television on youths has developed, there has been relatively little scientific inquiry on the effects of movies on youths. There is a need for controlled scientific studies of how and to what degree movies affect contemporary adolescents. The type of movies adolescents are drawn to and why could also be an important subject for investigation. An analysis of the recent popularity among youths of films dealing with horror, satanism, or the victimization of women would be of particular interest.

The adolescent of today, perhaps as much as any generation, is in search of identity. Motion pictures may provide either acceptable or inappropriate role models that youths utilize as examples for social learning. Subliminal and escapist effects of the movies may be especially relevant for modern adolescents, who are flooded with information about AIDS and other sexually transmitted diseases, drug and alcohol abuse, teenage suicide, divorce, and related affect-laden issues. The teenager can even escape in his own home via the ubiquitous VCR and cable television, which provide a wider array of films than ever before.

Youths that are already psychiatrically impaired may be even more vulnerable to the effects of movies. In such at-risk adolescent populations, movies may serve as the final common pathway for a variety of aberrant behaviors ranging from violence to suicide. More subtle effects on affect and personality formation may result from movie viewing. Narcissistic and borderline personality traits of film characters may too often be mimicked by adolescents and incorporated into their own personalities.

Positive social learning about adolescent phenomena such as peer group, family systems, sexuality, etc. may occur by viewing films. Prosocial behaviors such as sharing, sympathy, cooperation, delay of gratification, empathy, etc. may be fostered by the exposure of youths to motion pictures dealing with these themes. There is a vast potential for the use of movies to assist both normal and psychiatrically impaired youths in learning adaptive behaviors and social skills.

A much more detailed theoretical and scientific analysis of movies will be necessary before this potential can be realized. I hope that this chapter will assist in stimulating further inquiry into this important topic for adolescents.

REFERENCES

Berkowitz, L. 1984. Some effects of thoughts on anti- and prosocial influences of media events: a cognitive-neoassociationist analysis. *Psychological Bulletin* 95:410–427.

Berman, A. L. 1988. Fictional depiction of suicide in television films and imitation effect. *American Journal of Psychiatry* 145(8): 982–986.

Blumer, H. 1951. Collective behavior. In A. M. Lee, ed. *New Outline of the Principles of Sociology.* New York: Barnes & Noble.

Cantor, J., and Reilly, S. 1982. Adolescents' fright reactions to television and films. *Journal of Communication* 32:87–99.

Comstock, G. 1981. Sexual fantasies as a function of exposure to violent sexual stimuli. *Archives of Sexual Behavior* 10(1): 33–47.

Feilitzen, C., and Linne, O. 1975. Identifying with television characters. *Journal of Communication* 25(4): 51–55.

Feshbach, S. 1955. The drive-reducing function of fantasy behavior. *Journal of Abnormal Social Psychology* 50:3–11.

Frost, R., and Stauffer, J. 1987. The effects of social class, gender, and personality on physiological responses to filmed violence. *Journal of Communication* 37(2): 29–45.

Gerbner, G.; Gross, L.; Morgan, M.; and Signorelli, N. 1980. The "mainstreaming" of America: violence profile no. 11. *Journal of Communication* 30(3): 10–27.

Goldstein, R., and Zornow, E. 1980. *The Screen Image of Youth: Movies about Children and Adolescents.* Metuchen, N.J.: Scarecrow.

Goleman, D. 1985. Violence against women in films. *Response to the Victimization of Women and Children* 8(1): 21–22.

Gould, M. S., and Shaffer, D. 1986. The impact of suicide in television movies: evidence of imitation. *New England Journal of Medicine* 315(11): 690–694.

Govax, C. 1971. Induced affective states and interpersonal attraction. *Journal of Personality and Social Psychology* 20(1): 37–43.

Haley, J. 1952. The appeal of the moving picture. *Quarterly Journal of Film, Radio and Television* 6:361–374.

Jarvie, I. C. 1970. *Movies and Society.* New York: Basic.

Jarvie, I. C. 1978. *Movies as Social Criticism.* Methuchen, N.J.: Scarecrow.

Jowett, G. 1976. *Film: The Dramatic Art.* Boston: Little, Brown.

Jowett, G., and Linton, J. M. 1980. *Movies as Mass Communication.* Beverly Hills: Sage.

Lazarus, R. S.; Speisman, J. C.; Mordkoff, A. M.; and Davison, L. A. 1962. A laboratory study of psychological stress produced by a motion picture film. *Psychological Monographs* 76(no. 34, whole no. 533): 1–35.

Linz, D.; Donnerstein, E.; and Penrod, S. 1980. The effects of multiple exposures to filmed violence against women. *Journal of Communication* 34(3): 130–147.

Lynd, R. S., and Merrell, H. 1928. *Middletown.* New York: Harcourt Brace.

Malamuth, N. M. 1981. Rape fantasies as a function of exposure to violent sexual stimuli. *Archives of Sexual Behavior* 10(1): 33–47.

Malamuth, N. M., and Check, J. V. P. 1981. Sexual fantasies as a function of violence against women: a field experiment. *Journal of Research in Personality* 15:436–446.

Malamuth, N. M., and Donnerstein, E. 1982. The effects of aggressive-pornographic mass media stimuli. In L. Berkowitz, ed. *Advances in Experimental Social Psychology,* vol. 15. New York: Academic.

Malamuth, N. M.; Haber, S.; and Feshbach, S. 1980. Testing hypotheses regarding rape: exposure to sexual violence, sex differences, and the "normality" of rape. *Journal of Research in Personality* 14:121–137.

Malamuth, N. M.; Heim, M.; and Feshbach, S. 1980. Sexual responsiveness of college students to rape depictions: inhibitory and disinhibitory effect. *Journal of Personality and Social Psychology* 39:399–408.

Marston, A.; Hart, J.; Hilleman, C.; and Faunce, W. 1984. Toward the laboratory study of sadness and crying. *American Journal of Psychology* 97(1): 127–131.

Mendelsohn, H. 1966. *Mass Entertainment*. New Haven, Conn.: College and University Press.

Munsterberg, H. 1970. *The Photoplay: A Psychological Study*. New York: Dover.

National Council of Public Morals. 1917. *The Cinema: Its Present Position and Future Possibilities*. London: Williams & Norgate.

Nisbett, R., and Ross, L. 1980. *Human Inference: Strategies and Shortcomings of Social Judgment*. Englewood Cliffs, N.J.: Prentice-Hall.

Parke, R. D.; Berkowitz, L.; Leyens, J. P.; West, S. G.; and Sebastian, R. J. 1977. Some effects of violent and nonviolent movies on the behavior of juvenile delinquents. *Advances in Experimental Social Psychology* 10:135–172.

Phillips, D. P. 1982. The impact of the fictional television stories on U.S. adult fatalities: new evidence of the effect of the mass media on violence. *American Journal of Sociology* 87:1340–1359.

Phillips, D. P., and Paight, D. J. 1987. The impact of televised movies about suicide: a replicative study. *New England Journal of Medicine* 317:809–811.

Powdermaker, H. 1950. *Hollywood—the Dream Factory*. Boston: Little, Brown.

Ross, L., and Lepper, M. 1980. The perseverance of beliefs: empirical and normative considerations. In R. Sweden, ed. *Fallible Judgment in Behavioral Research*. San Francisco: Jossey-Bass.

Ryan, M., and Kellner, D. 1988. *Camera Politica: The Politics and Ideology of Contemporary Hollywood Film*. Bloomington: Indiana University Press.

Squire, J. E. 1983. *The Movie Business Book*. Englewood Cliffs, N.J.: Prentice-Hall.

Tudor, A. 1969. Film and the measurement of its effects. *Screen* 10 (4/5): 148–159.

Tudor, A. 1974. *Image and Influences*. London: Allen & Unwin.

U.S. Commission on Obscenity and Pornography. 1970. *The Report of the Commission on Obscenity and Pornography*. New York: Bantam.

Viemero, V. 1984. Aggressivilsuss ja filmlsankareiden kayttaytymisen moralen arviointi (Aggression and moral acceptance of the behavior of film characters). *Psykologia* 19(6): 420–426.

Wasserman, I. M. 1984. Imitation and suicide: a reexamination of the Werther effect. *American Sociological Review* 87:427–436.

Wilner, N., and Horowitz, M. J. 1975. Intrusive and repetitive thoughts after a depressing film: a pilot study. *Psychological Reports* 37:135–138.

Wilson, W., and Hunter, R. 1983. Movie-inspired violence. *Psychological Reports* 53:435–441.

Wolfenstein, M., and Leites, N. 1950. Film and the measurement of its affects. *Screen* 10(4/5): 148–159.

Zuckerman, M.; Lubin, B.; Vogel, L.; and Valerius, E. 1964. Measurement of experimentally induced affects. *Journal of Consulting Psychology* 28(5): 418–425.

6 RISK FACTORS FOR THE DEVELOPMENT OF EATING DISORDERS

REGINA C. CASPER

To fast—to study,—and to see no woman,
Flat treason gainst the kingly state of youth.
Say, can you fast? Your stomachs are too young,
And abstinence engenders maladies.

Shakespeare, *Love's Labors Lost*

I first encountered anorexia nervosa as a medical student, when I played second violin in the student orchestra in Freiburg, Germany. One Sunday afternoon, we played in a villa that was reserved by the Department of Medicine to treat chronically ill patients. Among these were three or four patients with anorexia nervosa. As they descended the staircase, ghostlike but obviously conscious and proud of their appearance, all of us had but one thought—"how bizarre." Most people's reaction to anorexia nervosa is still the same—how bizarre and, perhaps, how sad.

When I started working in the field of eating disorders about fifteen years ago, there was only anorexia nervosa. Over the years, we discovered that anorexia nervosa appeared in at least two forms (Casper, Eckert, Halmi, Goldberg, and Davis 1980; Garfinkel, Moldofsky, and Garner 1980). In the first, food-restrictive form, patients simply eat less and less. In the second, patients are periodically overcome by hunger and end up overeating. This frightens them, so they seek ways to get rid of the food. Studies have shown that each form corresponds

The Wirszup Lecture, presented at the University of Chicago, April 1990.

to a different personality type (Casper 1990; Casper et al. 1980; Strober, Salkin, Burroughs, and Morell 1982).

To these two types of anorexia nervosa, the restricting and the bulimic, we need to add another disorder that has increased dramatically during the past ten years, namely, bulimia nervosa (Russell 1979). In bulimia nervosa, body weight essentially remains within normal limits even though there may be large weight fluctuations.

Medicine classifies illnesses by symptoms, by observable signs, and, in the case of an emotional illness, by changes in behavior. For anorexia nervosa, DSM-III-R (American Psychiatric Association 1987) recognizes the following symptoms: (1) refusal to maintain a normal body weight; (2) intense fear of gaining weight despite being underweight; (3) disturbance in the way body size is experienced, that is, patients do not feel thin; and (4) loss of menstrual periods. The mentioned subtypes will be included in the upcoming DSM-IV manual. The following symptoms characterize bulimia nervosa: (1) recurrent episodes of binge eating with at least two binge-eating episodes per week for at least three months; (2) a feeling of lack of control over eating; (3) different maneuvers to prevent weight gain; and (4) persistent overconcern with body shape and weight.

Why 95 percent of patients with anorexia nervosa are female and less than 5 percent are male we still do not know. Certainly, cultural expectations play a role. In contemporary society, females want to be thin. In a recent study in schoolchildren and teenagers, we found that boys or male teenagers rarely want to lose weight (Casper and Offer 1990; Richards, Casper, and Larson 1990). Nevertheless, the psychopathology in males is little different from that in females (Andersen 1990; Falstein, Feinstein, and Judas 1956). Another important fact, despite all the publicity, anorexia nervosa in Western society is still a rare illness afflicting about one in 150 teenage girls or one in 10,000 in the population at large.

A first hazard is the conditions germane to our society and culture that tempt people to eat more than they need. Nearly everybody has access to an abundance of rich food. Eating disorders are unusual during famine and in societies where food is scarce or expensive; conversely, surplus food increases food consumption and food perversion. Rats maintain their weight on Purina chow but will become obese on a "cafeteria" diet consisting of gourmet food (Grossman 1984). The introduction of fast-food chains has changed eating habits in Japan, where bulimia nervosa is an increasing health problem. In comparison, not so long ago earnings would barely feed a family. The history of one of the food staples that is a major source of calories, sugar, chronicles some of these changes. Fourteenth-century French records of purchases made for the households of the nobility indicate that sugar was used as a spice, only in dishes for the sick, just like salt (Laurioux 1985). Even as a seasoning, sugar was not available in Europe at large until the fifteenth century. In eighteenth-century Europe, sugar remained a luxury, delivered in large rocklike cones. A century later, Tolstoy recounts, in *Anna Karenina,* how Princess Maria offered one morsel of sugar to the peasants with their tea as a special treat. Perhaps, we need to be reminded that, into this century, famine mostly due to crop failure was commonplace in northern Europe and Asia and still is present in Africa. As recently as 1919, Russia suffered severe famine and received $60,000,000 in food aid from the United States.

The abundance of food in contemporary society turns a genetic disposition toward excess body weight into a risk factor for bulimia nervosa; some people seem to have a harder time resisting the temptations of good food and gain weight in consequence. This is less of a problem for anorexia nervosa. In a collaborative study, only 10 percent of girls were found to be overweight before developing anorexia nervosa (Casper et al. 1980).

Another risk factor is the gradual dissolution of the family as the social unit where meals are shared at expected times. Without being offered a regular meal, young children are left to their own devices and a responsibility to feed themselves. Left alone with a full refrigerator, some children tend to eat beyond their physiological needs. For a patient of mine who developed bulimia nervosa, family meals disappeared when her parents divorced when she was thirteen years old; her mother never cooked a meal again. Not until she met her boyfriend, whose family treated her with invitations to dinner, did she eat again in company. The times when food was scarce and, of necessity, had to be shared with other family members seem to be long past in Western society.

Another rather obvious hazard is the extreme standards for feminine beauty conspicuously displayed by fashion models. Unlike the women of a century ago, for whom to be pink and plump was *en vogue,* contemporary young women espouse the pale, not only slim, but lean look, as if, with regard to body shape, women were meant to be created equal and all should fit into one size.

I will, for the most part, discuss anorexia nervosa because its psychopathology is so much further removed from ordinary life and it remains a puzzle. Anorexia nervosa is by no means a novel phenomenon; the disorder is well documented as far back as the twelfth century (Bell 1988). For bulimia nervosa, we are less certain because the terms for the syndrome vary. The current term "bulimia," which literally means "ox hunger," was synonymous with dog hunger, or *fames canina,* or kynorexia, and the existence of still other expressions that denote the symptoms makes it much more difficult to trace bulimia nervosa (Casper 1983).

The factors I have mentioned, slimness as a beauty ideal, easy access to rich food, and the loss of structured family meals, affect many people in our society, yet most are spared from eating disorders. Which other mechanisms then increase the risk for eating disorders?

For once, too much good food makes it harder to keep one's body weight stable. Twenty-five percent of the American population are overweight (they exceed their upper weight limit by at least 15 percent), and studies show that 80–90 percent of teenage girls have made one or more efforts to reduce. This means that, through deliberate dieting, a common pathway and foremost risk factor for the development of anorexia nervosa, namely weight loss, is triggered more frequently. Without substantial weight loss, anorexia nervosa would not develop. By the same token, omitting meals increases hunger and, subsequently, the chance for overeating. From data obtained in our follow-up study, we found that women with anorexia nervosa had thought about wanting to diet as early as age twelve as opposed to age fourteen to fifteen for sisters and other women who had no eating disorder (Casper and Jabine 1986). Thus, the wish to diet at an early age puts girls at risk. From reviewing patients' histories, we observed that the first manifestations appear when weight drops by about 15–20 percent of previous body weight (Casper and Davis 1977). This means that, if someone normally weighs 100 pounds, at about eighty to eighty-five pounds, given the disposition, signs of anorexia nervosa may appear. To be sure, many factors other than dieting can bring about the initial weight loss. A physical illness, sometimes a depression, can lead to loss of appetite and weight; nowadays, however, persistent dieting seems to be the most common precipitant. The term "anorexia," therefore, is a misnomer because most anorexia nervosa patients really do not lose their appetite.

No matter how the weight loss comes about, peculiar to anorexia nervosa is that the person considers weight loss a desirable goal. This gives the weight loss struggle a personal touch; ultimately, dieting becomes intertwined with each individual's personal conflicts, whatever these may be. This personal investment in the bodily changes is invariably present. The tenacity with which thinness is defended is a rough measure of the seriousness of the psychological problems.

Of course, the attitude that weight loss is a good thing is hardly surprising given our society's aspirations, but, if you grew up a hundred years ago, a solid weight conveyed status and beauty. Indeed, most cases of anorexia nervosa a hundred years ago began with indigestion or an upset stomach; few girls dieted. Several hundred years ago, the most common pathway seems to have been religious fasting.

Let me digress here for a moment because fasting as a periodic abstinence from food is a universal human practice, found in most ancient civilized and primitive societies. The various functions attributed to fasting recur at times in fantasy or as a motif in anorexia nervosa. Food abstention served as a religious rite of preparation based on the idea that fasting voids the body of impurities and thereby liberates the soul. The Egyptians fasted before entering the temple. Orthodox Jews fast during Yom Kippur. Lent, in commemoration of Christ's forty days of fasting, precedes Easter. In Muslim countries, Ramadan, a month of fasting from sunrise to sunset, is observed annually.

Fasting has been part of the process of ritualized mourning, independent of the loss of appetite often associated with grief and sadness. Food restriction practices following death have been reported by the Egyptians, the Greeks, the Chinese, and many other cultures. In Japan, the family may eat a vegetable diet only for fifty days after the death of a parent.

Fasting can serve as an act of penitence, as on Yom Kippur and during Lent. The person who refuses food suffers privation or pain for a wrong done and to ward off unknown and more dreaded punishments. The Egyptians, Babylonians, Hebrews, and Christians all fasted to expiate sin. Paradoxically, most girls with anorexia nervosa whom I have encountered undermined the purpose of repentance on

Yom Kippur; they enjoyed a sense of superiority over other family members because their habitual fasting made it so much easier for them to abstain from food as prescribed.

Finally, fasting is an expression of asceticism, the practice of self-discipline for a personal or spiritual ideal. Asceticism for a spiritual goal presupposed a dualism between the evil body and the pure soul. Thus, abstinence from either excessive or normal bodily desires made a person virtuous. Parenthetically, the term "virtue" derives from manliness, so perhaps we should say that fasting conveys moral excellence. In Egypt, in Greece, in Judaism, and in Christianity, we find ascetic groups whose members ate nothing before sunset or fasted for months and years in order to free themselves of bodily needs and to gain spiritual strength. The not so uncommon asceticism of puberty may be considered a benign counterpart of anorexia nervosa.

Fasting involves sacrifice. As Rudolph Bell (1988), a historian, has recently documented, eating the minimum, along with other ways of self-mortification, led to an epidemic of anorexia nervosa among Italian women saints. Bell reviewed documents for a total of 261 women saints in Italy from the thirteenth up to the twentieth century. Among those who fasted rigorously, 30–50 percent developed behavior that resembled anorexia nervosa. Yet how do we know that these women suffered from anorexia nervosa? Eating crumbs of bread and drinking water, they insist that they feel well and feel no need to eat more. Actually, they profess a horror of eating. They are constantly on the go and indifferent to the degree of their emaciation. Here, we recognize two more features, a continued sense of relative well-being and a higher than expected energy level; both symptoms still puzzle researchers. To be sure, the women saints' austerities included other forms of self-mortification, such as self-flagellation, scalding, or sleeping on a bed of thorns. By and large, Christian doctrine explicitly condemned excessive fasting. These women, therefore, were an embarrassment to the clergy and not infrequently were accused of collaboration with the devil. Moderation was the desired goal. According to John Cassian, a fifth-century writer (Bell 1988, p. 20), gluttony was only a hairbreadth from moderation. Gluttony manifested itself in three distinct ways: eating before the prescribed time for communal meals; satiating fully one's hunger; and seeking especially delicate and succulent food.

Another risk factor becomes apparent when one examines the lives of these saints, a risk factor that we have only recently begun to recognize, the contribution of the personality. From an early age on, these young women, seemingly obedient and submissive, were moved by a sense of determination, a pattern of sacrifice and conquest, a lifelong practiced tendency toward self-control and self-privation, all, of course, directed toward a higher purpose for the praise of God and toward eternal salvation. At the same time—and here we see again the similarities—each of these women underwent a personality crisis over autonomy. They struggled against feeling enslaved and exploited. They ensured that their food refusal was not merely seen as capriciousness but proved them to be the determined people they wished to be. St. Catherine of Siena, co-patron with Francis of Assisi of all Italy and a doctor of the church, had vowed to devote her life to the service of Christ (Bell 1988). She had made a contract with God that he would save not only her but her entire family if and only if she ate only the absolute necessary. Pressured by the family to marry her brother-in-law after an older, beloved sister died, she refused and fought for a solitary life of sacrifice in a convent, where, in spiritual community with Christ, she designed a life of privation as a relentless, physically torturing challenge, suffering and ultimately dying from chronic anorexia nervosa.

Now, let us return to the role of the personality. As mentioned, the person who develops the restricting form of anorexia nervosa differs from the one who tends to be bulimic. The first is typically shy, retiring, somewhat inhibited, and cautious but intellectually well organized, a thinker, and discreetly competitive. The second tends to be more emotional, more volatile and expressive, more socially adept, and endowed with a more lively fantasy life. These distinct characteristics observed during the illness have been confirmed by many investigators independently (Casper et al. 1980; Garfinkel et al. 1980; Strober et al. 1982).

We have recently completed a study that suggests that these traits endure (Casper 1990). Young women who had fully recovered from the restricting form of anorexia nervosa were found to differ in personality from their sisters and a control group of young women without eating problems. We included sisters as a control group because, during treatment, many patients asked at some point, Why did this illness befall me, why not my sister? Interestingly, when we turned to the patients for an answer, they described their sisters as different in temperament. So, when we planned a long-term follow-up study of all patients whom we had seen eight to ten years earlier, we asked their sisters to participate. It turned out that those young women who were well, who had recovered from the restricting form of anorexia nervosa, continued to differ in temperament when compared not only to their sisters but also to normal controls and to bulimic patients. They tended to be emotionally more reserved and showed greater self-discipline and a tendency toward perfectionism and conscientiousness, which served them well professionally. Sisters and control subjects tended to be more spontaneous, gregarious, and flexible; they also had more fun in life. Unexpectedly, we found that patients and their sisters shared strong beliefs in ethical and traditional values in contrast to control subjects. This suggests that there might be a familial element in the transmission of moral standards. The personalities of women with bulimic anorexia nervosa, or bulimia nervosa, were not much different from normal controls; at most, they showed a slightly greater tendency toward being more adventurous and took risks more easily. It comes as no surprise that a shy girl given to discipline and strong moral beliefs would be at greater risk for becoming a single-minded fanatic embracing a desired cause than a gregarious, self-confident girl.

In most contemporary anorexia nervosa cases, not eating is rarely used as controlled penance but tends to serve self-improvement. It is also unlike the manner in which suffragettes used food refusal around the turn of the last century to bring attention to their powerless status and to achieve voting rights. Anorexia nervosa patients tend to focus not on changing society but on bringing about changes in themselves through changes in their body size. Lacking other tools for self-assertion, which could not grow in a life of compliance (the "good upbringing," they were "good" children to their parents), one might say that patients use food rejection in a misguided struggle against feeling dominated by others to achieve individuality and independence.

In each case, instead of symbolizing nourishment and care, food eventually takes on harmful, intrusive connotations, and in rare cases the loathing includes the body, as in the case of Nadine described by Janet (1903). In medieval society, guided by religion, when the act of eating was thought to represent base physical urges and desires as a reflection of the corrupt life on earth, surfeit could kill the eternal soul. Without the representative power of religious beliefs, the refusal of food and "fat" nowadays more often represents freedom from inter-

nalized, oppressive, parental influences to save the self. This is sometimes the only escape and defense available if the person has no resources to understand and work through the vicissitudes of personal
relationships psychologically. The deprived body in the process of the
illness becomes the representation of the liberated self and embodies
independence and autonomy from outside influences. Such a restruc-
tured self, subject to its own value system, emotionally invested in
defending the heroic achievement, offers a formidable resistance to
treatment, which, of course, would mean change. Physiologically, as
in any case of sensory deprivation, the unsatisfied needs assert themselves, hence the preoccupation with food, the love to bake and cook
in anorexia nervosa.

To the parents, the process conveys a double message. On the one
hand, patients insist on being emotionally and physically self-
sufficient, on not needing anyone or anything. On the other hand, their
pitiful appearance draws attention to the fact that their lives have gone
terribly wrong, that not only their bodies but their souls need care.
Better than any description, three selected poems, written by two patients during treatment, will convey a trace of the inner struggle. The
two young women differed in the form their eating disorders took. The
differences in personality and temperament are conveyed in the poems
each wrote, as is the notion that therapy is a dialogue that takes many
forms. Both patients kindly gave me permission to have their poems
reprinted:

> Alone, I am,
> in a cage of thorns and dead roses.
> A few of the needles are poisoned,
>   and is the risk of encountering one
>   going to stop you?
> It is okay, I will understand.
> Besides, I am hungry for nothing
>   but starving for all.
>
> J.R.

> How can I believe what you say
> when my mind speaks the opposite?
> Unless I am confident about myself

nothing you tell me can lift me up
    off the ground.
I will never stand on my own
until I feel safe with myself,
because if you try to hold me up,
    but fall,
I too will fall down.
Your kind words assure me
and with that hope I can walk
farther into this dark tunnel
    of enlightenment.
But it is I that has to journey
    through it
and learn for myself that
what you say, I can believe.

               J.R.

Them that I love
    are into my world
        and they are cleaning
           what's good and old
               like my faded jeans.

Ignite the fire of my emotion
    of anger—
        expressed
        finally
in destruction
    of myself

Out! All of you
    Out!
and the emotions leave too,
    and I am empty.
        Guilty,
        sorry,
        done.

Come back
and fill me with love
and pleasure
and safety
and peace
  of mind
  soul
  body
is now filled
with food,
which is rejected
as the emotions.

  Empty.
  Again.

One by one
 the feelings
  check in for an hour
  and leave
   a vacancy
    sign,
which is a warning
that the pattern
    must change.

Filled up
   with what?
   God?
Maybe at the end
   with people?

Them that I'm scared of
who I'm not in control of
   yes, I'm learning
   just learning
yes
   there's
   Hope.

         S.H.

REFERENCES

American Psychiatric Association. 1987. *Diagnostic and Statistical Manual of Mental Disorders.* 3d ed., rev. Washington, D.C.: American Psychiatric Association.

Andersen, A. E. 1990. *Males with Eating Disorders.* New York: Brunner/Mazel.

Bell, R. 1988. *Holy Anorexia.* Chicago: University of Chicago Press.

Casper, R. C. 1983. On the emergence of bulimia nervosa as a syndrome: a historical view. *International Journal of Eating Disorders* 2:3–16.

Casper, R. C. 1990. Personality features of women with good outcome from restricting anorexia. *Psychosomatic Medicine* 52:156–170.

Casper, R. C., and Davis, J. M. 1977. On the course of anorexia nervosa. *American Journal of Psychiatry* 134:974–978.

Casper, R. C.; Eckert, E.; Halmi, K.; Goldberg, S. C.; and Davis, J. M. 1980. Bulimia: its incidence and clinical importance in patients with anorexia nervosa. *Archives of General Psychiatry* 37:1030–1035.

Casper, R. C., and Jabine, L. N. 1986. Psychological functioning in anorexia nervosa: a comparison between anorexia nervosa patients on follow-up and their sisters. In J. H. Lacey and D. A. Sturgeon, eds. *Proceedings of the 15th European Conference on Psychosomatic Research.* London and Paris: Libbey.

Casper, R. C., and Offer, D. 1990. Weight and dieting concerns in normal adolescents: fashion or symptom? *Pediatrics* 86:384–390.

Falstein, E. I.; Feinstein, S. C.; and Judas, I. 1956. Anorexia nervosa in the male child. *American Journal of Orthopsychiatry* 26:751–772.

Garfinkel, P. E.; Moldofsky, H.; and Garner, D. M. 1980. The heterogeneity of anorexia nervosa: bulimia as a distinct subgroup. *Archives of General Psychiatry* 37:1036–1040.

Grossman, S. P. 1984. Contemporary problems concerning our understanding of brain mechanisms that regulate food intake and body weight. In A. J. Stunkard and E. Stellar, eds. *Eating and Its Disorders.* New York: Raven.

Janet, P. 1903. *Obsessions et la psychasthénie.* 2 vols. Paris: Alcan.

Laurioux, B. 1985. Spices in the medieval diet: a new approach. *Food and Foodways* 1:43–76.

Richards, M. H.; Casper, R. C.; and Larson, R. 1990. Weight and eating concerns among preadolescent and young adolescent boys and girls. *Journal of Adolescent Health Care* 11:203–209.

Russell, G. 1979. Bulimia nervosa: an ominous variant of anorexia nervosa. *Psychological Medicine* 9:429–448.

Strober, M.; Salkin, B.; Burroughs, J.; and Morrell, W. 1982. Validity of the bulimia-restricter distinction in anorexia nervosa: parental personality characteristics and family psychiatric morbidity. *Journal of Nervous and Mental Diseases* 172:345–351.

VIVIAN M. RAKOFF

We had come back from a prize-awarding ceremony—a splendid occasion at a great university. In response to the invitation, we—Abraham, who had received the prize, his wife, Leonora, Bernard, Rufus, and I—had dressed formally. We all looked better groomed than we usually do. The glow of the evening was still with us, and we wanted it to go on. We decided to sit for a while in the Palm Court of the Plaza Hotel in New York City, though it is not quite the splendid place it once was. But it is still formal and elaborate, with its palms, grand Corinthian marble columns, candelabra, and the little orchestra playing Broadway show tunes in a sub-Viennese style.

We thought we would have coffee. No one was hungry after the celebratory banquet, but, when the waitress came to take the order, someone suggested we should have a bottle of champagne. None of us drink much, but the champagne seemed like a good idea. It was, I suppose, a ritual, a literary touch ("Champagne in the Palm Court") for the occasion. We all knew this coming together of old friends needed a private ceremony to complete the earlier public one, with its speeches of giving and acceptance among the pillars under the Roman dome of the library. "Who needs champagne?" Abraham protested, his hand covering his mouth in a characteristic gesture. His voice and his gesture were totally at variance with the articulate, clear utterance he had used to explain and guide us through the extraordinary accumulation of his scientific achievements when he had accepted the prize.

"Ah, come on," said Rufus. "How much did you win?" he teased. Shy and defensive, Abe said, "You can read in the paper how much."

For A, B, L, and R.

Bernie laughed. For a moment, he assumed his paternal, mocking distance from us "boys." He is, after all, the oldest of the group by two years, which is not much, now that we are all in our fifties. It was a significant gap in our twenties, when he was already halfway through medical school and the rest of us had just begun our studies. "Fifteen thousand," he laughed. "You won fifteen thousand, and you can't buy a bottle of champagne?" Lena joined in the affectionate punishment of our genius, our hero of this night, our dear friend, and added the subtle ambiguities of a long-tested marriage. "Champagne," she insisted, "*and* strawberries." For motives that do not matter here, I offered, "I'll buy the champagne—and the strawberries." "No," Lena insisted firmly, "it's Abe's party." "Champagne and strawberries," she told the waitress, who had been waiting with unusual patience. We were all much funnier to one another than, I suppose, any outsider might have found us.

Presently, the champagne and strawberries arrived, and we toasted one another, but the conversation was of the same kind of gentle backbiting I have just described. As we were sitting there in our formal clothes, drinking champagne, eating strawberries, and laughing a lot, I had one of those moments when one regards oneself and one's situation from a distance. I imagined myself looking at our group from across the room and saw a group of middle-aged, respectable people having a good time. We might even have had, for that brief moment, a polish of the kind that people like to call glamorous. But, inside the group, I was happily aware that we had reestablished and reevoked relationships that represented a different dimension of experience. We were all comfortably evoking our well-established choreography of relationships. Someone hearing our conversation might have thought of it as adolescent and silly (and they would have been right), but we were experiencing our mutual friendship. Even though we now lived on separate continents and in different cities, we could evoke enough of our shared past to recreate, almost instantaneously, old relationships. Now this in itself is fairly obvious. We were enjoying one another's company, we were comfortable with one another, and the content of the occasion was very simple. We were, of course, celebrating a shared history.

The evening was the end point of over thirty years of mutual support, shared good and bad times. However, at the instant of my imagined look at ourselves from across the room, I was very much aware that the moment, the relationships, the pleasure, and the affection we were experiencing were very valuable. It represented one of the currents that sustained me and my friends through trouble, struggle, displacement, and many intimate vicissitudes. One pauses for a moment and wonders if something quite simple is not being beaten into a significance beyond its actual content. Yet friendship is clearly one of the kinds of relationships vitally important for sustaining a connected, meaningful human existence.

Thinking about this afterward, I was aware that I had thought very little about the particular qualities that differentiate friendship from other kinds of supportive relationships. It has a character, emotion, and social contractual basis that differentiates it from family relationships, erotic relationships, love with a sexual component, and membership in formal and work groups. I was aware that the feeling I had for my good friends was different from the emotional tone of family relationships and close, loving, erotic relationships. There was a lightness, a pleasurable easiness in my sense of what went on between myself and good friends. This was not an attempt to exclude the ambiguities, the ups and downs, the coming closer, and the separating that affect the relationship of friendship as they do all other relationships but rather an attempt to sort out within myself, and from the description of others, the particular taste of friendship.

Background

By now, there are many studies devoted to examining the "networks" of patients with psychiatric difficulties. These range from relatively primitive counting of social contacts to more subtle attempts to differentiate between supportive and nonsupportive social contacts, to determine the difference in the nature of support people derive from spouses and family, neighbors and friends.

In a survey of social networks among psychiatric patients, Greenblatt, Becerra, and Serafetinides (1982) point to the variety of studies of and, at the same time, the curious lack of specificity in relationships that have been so far described and summed up in Caplan's (1974) succinct formulation, "Social networks provide emotional sustenance and instrumental aid." All discussions of loneliness since the turn of the century are anticipated by Durkheim's (1951) clear association of suicide with anomie and alienation. Short of dying for lack of attachments, there are the pains of loneliness, cataloged by Weiss (1974). These were articulated in more detail by Perlman and Peplau (1981) in connection with adolescents who came from families with "an absence of emotional nurturance, guidance or support." Lowenthal and Haven (1968) found that old people are "best able to survive traumatic social losses such as retirement or death of a spouse" if they have confidants (not necessarily spouses or lovers). Recently, Vachon, Sheldon, Lancee, Lyall, Rogers, and Freeman (1982), in a study of enduring distress patterns following bereavement, found that "deficits in social support" correlate, among other factors, with enduring "high distress." It is not, however, my intention here to reiterate the simple, terrible pain of loneliness or the fact that human beings, as social creatures, require what we now like to call "significant others" to maintain themselves through both the ordinary and the crisis-laden episodes of their lives. Rather, my attempt is to understand the particular phenomenology and nature of friendship in general and in adolescence in particular.

An immediate distinction must be made between the varieties of erotic attachment and involvement and friendship. Since we are implicitly or explicitly all heirs of the psychoanalytic intellectual hegemony, we are prone to accept as a primary given the importance of the erotic libido as the source of energy and emotional investment in interpersonal relationships. And the libido has been invoked as the primary engine driving diverse activities not manifestly erotic or con-connected with relationships, such as aesthetic productivity, athletic aggressiveness, the courage to explore, indeed optimism versus pessimism. While a formal defence of this assumption may now be rare, it hovers in the wings of our assumptions regarding relationships. The vagaries of the erotic life have become the metaphor, if not the operational description, of our descriptions of the ways people live together. In discussing the relationships of friendship, it would not be surprising if it were assumed that we are concerned with a subcategory of the erotic life. Yet it is a common finding that, when a sexual relationship comes to an end, it is very difficult for people to maintain friendly relations.

Friendship is clearly not a component of those intense sexual relationships marked by enmity, hatred, and contempt. In extreme cases, individuals may have totally ego-alien sexual needs. They may feel that they are the victims of socially reprehensible sexual proclivities. In spite of all the social disapproval or the threat of punishment and disgrace, they can be almost powerless to resist "acting out" such overwhelming sexual needs. (How far rape, masochism, faceless sexual encounters through toilet-stall partitions, wife beating, and pedophilia are from friendship!)

The distinction between sexuality and friendship was made in different terms by Aristotle (1980). He writes, "Love is ideally a sort of excess of friendship," and he recognizes that erotic satisfaction, which is a component of love between adults, is a kind of utilitarian good: the lover gets something, namely, sexual pleasure, from the beloved and, ideally, returns a similar kind of pleasure. But equality is not necessarily a characteristic of loving, and it is quite possible for there to be intense sexual yearning and loving felt for someone who does not return it. Whereas the essential nature of the friendship relationship is one of mutuality and equality without a utilitarian good being exchanged, it is quite possible for someone to be wildly in love—in the erotic sense—with someone who does not return that love at all. While one may have friendly feelings for someone who does not return similar feelings, one cannot claim such a person as a friend. Friendship is defined by the essential qualities of mutuality, equality, nonutilitarianism, positive regard, affection, and a sense of interdependency and connectedness that may survive distance and time. By contrast, the erotic relationship is utilitarian, sometimes ludicrously short lived, and it may imply very little mutual obligation. As Montaigne (1958) said, "In friendship there is a general and universal warmth, all gentleness and smoothness with no roughness or sting about it. What is more, in sexual love there is only a frantic desire for what eludes us." One is, of course, aware that sexuality and loving can also be thought of as separate, although related, entities, and there is a component of attachment or loving that is not bound to the erotic, which may be commonly shared between lovers and friends. But it is common experience that, once the erotic enters into a relationship, the nonerotic affectional component usually becomes hostage to the sexuality. There may even be a degree of distrust and difficulty in the erotic plus affectionate relationship that does not as characteristically torment and trouble friendship. The distrust, jealousy, misunderstanding, infidelity, anger, and disappointment that often accompany the love relationship, which combines the erotic with the affectional, is the material of endless fiction and drama. To put it aphoristically, one may discuss one's lovers with one's friends, but one rarely discusses one's friends with one's lovers.

Parent-child ties and relationships constitute the usual, accepted major category of affection without sexuality. Yet the strong, bonded attachments of family relationships are not the same as friendship. The obvious primary distinction is that family relationships (other than those between husband and wife, which are, optimally, strongly erotic as well as affectional and friendly) are involuntary. Powerful ethological forces somewhere between imprinting and learning shape the profound and involuntary relationships of parents to children and siblings to one another. One is fortunate if one's family members (brothers, cousins, uncles, aunts, etc.) are also seen as friends, but they are not necessarily so.[1] Family relationships may be emotionally inescapable, but they only too often lack the supportive characteristics of a true friendship. The important role of early family relationships in laying down the matrices of the future capacity for friendship and sexuality is well known and is not the topic of concern in this chapter.

Friendship and Adolescents

In the life history of the individual, the need for friends is most strongly felt during adolescence. The cultivation of a benign social network outside the family, a more or less voluntary association of supportive others, begins early in life. The infant, however, has no "friends," and the toddler indulges in parallel play that is hardly involved with companions. Between the ages of approximately five and puberty, there is increasingly intense involvement with friends, who help create a more or less solipsistic world in which the rules of parents and adult society are suspended. In those clubhouses, baseball teams, fishing expeditions, summer camps, "hanging out" between school and supper, the Eriksonian moratorium is prefigured. But, at this stage, the world of "chums" is very frail compared with the primary focus of family to which the child and pubertal adolescent returns almost daily. There are certainly group pressures, "best friends," "second best friends," rivalries, jockeying for position, and even the beginning of erotic play, but normatively there is still a considerable degree of parental control of association outside the home. At this stage, when, and if, the family moves, the children go along, with tears perhaps, and promises of undying love and the assurances of regular exchanges of letters and visits, all of which usually fade rapidly. The basis of these early friendships is often mere contiguity: the same school class, street team, summer bunk, with some degree of shared interest as a determining factor. However, it is clustering in an almost mechanical sense that fundamentally determines association.

In middle and late adolescence, an alternate and transitional family develops, the kind of fraternity/sorority aimed at in the slogan "Liberty, Equality, Fraternity." A society of friendly brothers or sisters emerges that will facilitate the essential move away from family into the society at large. In that society, the individual moves almost as if without parents. The adolescent must, in a sense, become an orphan in order to become an adult. If he is fortunate, the cohort of friends in which he has to establish his new self, a self that will continue for the rest of his life, will permit a secure sense of community in the nonfamilial world. Indeed, it is the ideal hope of humanist, political aspirations that society at large will have the characteristics of an ideal supportive family. Such a family provides security, a sense of personal value, without it having to be constantly earned and justified. As Aristotle said, "Of a perfect society friendship is the peak." This has not happened and, apart from small unifamily nomadic groups, probably never happened. The cohort—the group of young men and women that in some simple societies was the group of reference for puberty rites, induction into a tribally recognized adult identity, military service, and hunting bond—is now more tenuously represented by school graduating class, college roommates, fraternities, and army induction group and platoons. It is from this group that more intimate friends are selected. A historical irony is at work. Now that family, community, fixed values, places, and groups of reference are most needed, they are often attenuated to the point where their potential for support and for generating friendship is diminished.

At other times and other places, the reference group or cohort, while providing a nonfamilial social matrix, had a definite place in the total social fabric. It was essentially a time-bound group with which the individual moved in the relatively changeless pattern of the community. The youth or maiden could see himself or herself in the elders of the community since this is what they would eventually become. Their distance from their parents, grandparents, and younger siblings was the inescapable distance of being born at a different time. There was no radical difference of values and expectations. No doubt there are always subtle movements in mores in even relatively stable societies, but the movement with the cohort was often entirely predictable in preindustrial societies. Even in industrial societies, once the great discontinuity from rural to urban-industrial life had been accomplished, the strong (and often cruel) patterns of continuity were reestablished. The discontinuities were along lines of class rather than generations. Hoggart's (1957) moving photographs in *The Uses of Literacy* show working-class lads in the 1930s dressed like their fathers, prematurely (by our standards) middle aged. Their cohort did not generate separate values but essentially defined the group in which they would find their friends and, in the perennial fashion, nonincestuous sexual partners whom they would marry and with whom they would establish their own families. Certainly, friendships were always important and valued for the same reasons they are today, but the support they gave was more narrowly focused. They did not have to carry, in addition to the needs for nonerotic intimacy, a complex, shifting, poorly defined need for social orientation and expectation, as they now often have to do. There was more continuity than we sometimes believe. Nevertheless, in the post–World War II period in the industrialized West, the middle and late adolescent cohorts have been more or less a separate society and not only a distinct age group within a given society. It is possible to make too much of the generation gap, but it has some reality, and the notion of a discontinuity between our older and our younger has—as they say—a measure of face validity. The result is an added expectation of cohort support—more friendship and comradeship as well as a sharing of symbols and rallying points, while each of them is a focus for the consolidation of identity.

Comradeship and Friendship

Yet a further distinction has to be made between comradeship and friendship. The comradeship developed through membership in a cohort, such as the shared experience at college, in the army, or in camps, constitutes a genuine enough community of association, but within that community there can be only a few to whom one would give the label "friend." Montaigne (1958) has somewhat hyperbolically described why friendship, in its fully realized form, cannot be given to many: "In the friendship I speak of, they mix and blend one into the other in so perfect a union that the seam that has joined them is effaced and disappears. If I were pressed to say why I love him I feel that my only reply could be: because it was he, because it was I. . . .

Such a friendship has no model but itself and can only be compared to itself." Such friendships are rare and valuable, and most people have to be content with far lesser attachments, less rhapsodically perfect but, nevertheless, valuable and sustaining. In reality, most of us will settle for comradeship in the absence of the perfect association.

The identity of the individual adolescent is often confirmed and given external expression through the group of friends. They are of a kind and develop a shared language of reference and interests. The strong history of the group formed in adolescence is the stuff of later nostalgia and is a considerable source of literary inspiration. The film *Diner* is a prototypical example. It is clearly a memoir, a reminiscence, and many of us recognize the form, if not the specific content, of the relationships. Home, parents, family, hover in the wings, but the nexus of experience is in the meeting of the young men, all of them strongly differentiated, but their lives and careers still largely potential and unrealized. They have not yet discovered the elaborate consequences of the moves they make during this period of their late adolescence. The diner where they meet and eat is a safe "transitional" place where they are separated from direct reality.

If the adolescent is fortunate, the protofamily of friends is benign and affirms the normative and healthy aspects of the self. However, while friendship is valuable, not all friends are valuable. The strong relationships may direct the adolescent into the worst aspects of negative identity and provide group support for destructive or delinquent behavior.

Helen, at fifteen, was the daughter of upper-middle-class parents. They had separated when Helen was thirteen. She gradually, but definitely, transformed herself into a caricature of a street kid. At first, her rebellious yearning, which showed itself in her costume and her curious haircut, rough clothes, and sexy walk, could have been passed over as the normative experiments of middle adolescence. But her behavior was a clear signal for a kind of association not available in her home neighborhood, and, on her walks through downtown streets, her messages were received by other youngsters who dressed and felt as she did. She started disappearing from home for weekends and often returned home bruised and hungover. Most of the time, she attended school, but she often took days off. She cultivated a surly and suspicious manner, which she dropped with her therapist but assumed as soon as she was "on the street." When I last saw her, she was walking

112

along a downtown street. She was smoking, her hair was bizarrely brushed, and her costume was fully realized punk. She was with two other girls similarly costumed. I knew from her sessions that her friends had almost identical sad histories.

I include this short vignette as a reminder. Good friends and warm, affectionate relationships do not require much description or explanation, but the associations with "bad" friends highlight the power of the association to, and the entry into, society.

In North America, where there is a great deal of moving around, the word "friend" has lost its nuances and become diluted. It can cover mere acquaintance or association, occasionally it is a quasieuphemism for a lover, and of course it refers to the fully developed mutuality of true friendship. I believe that this wide, imprecise use of the word not only is a result of sloppy language but also reflects profound social and personal need. Excessive mobility, once every three to five years, huge urban conglomeration, and disruption of marriage all increase the need for voluntary, affectionate connectedness. At the same time, these forces work against the establishment of long-term association in which true mutuality may be explored and a shared history established.

Lewis, Gantz, and Wellman (see Wellman 1981) have described how the earlier supports of close neighbors and physical communal closeness have given way to the establishment of networks of association based on shared interests and sustained by forms of telassociation and communication. One is tempted to reject nostalgic notions of the warmth of small towns, fixed urban neighborhoods of a few decades ago, as visions through a rose-colored retrospective, but Fischer (1981) supports the notion that the big city, more than the small community, is genuinely inimical. He writes, "Research tends to show that various types of group conflict—racial disorders and major industrial disputes, for example—are disproportionately likely to occur in large communities." He cites in support of his statement Tilly's (1976) descriptions of urban chaos, Morgan and Clark's (1973) analyses of racial disorders, and Lincoln's (1978) examination of the relation of community structure to racial conflict.

This urban "world of strangers," as it has been called by Lofland (1973), is nevertheless the world where millions of people conduct "good enough" lives. They go about their ordinary affairs and see friends and family. Lofland (1973) admits that, while the city may be generally alienating, "it does not estrange individuals from familiar and similar people." Wellman (1981)—and others already referred to—have noted that, while mere numbers of contacts do little or nothing to sustain people in big cities, the tropism human beings have for one another smells out familiars. It seems to seep through the obstacles arising out of hypermobility, violence, and racial tension and bring people together. The new technologies are used as connecting cables, and the city continues to be livable—telephones against alienation! Most people live on some small island of a private archipelago in the shark-filled urban sea.

How appropriate it seems to blame the city as we know it for the disruption of community. Durkheim (1951), after all, wrote at the end of the nineteenth century, by which time capitalism had broken down the rural fixity and security of preindustrial Europe. Multitudes had been displaced to find themselves, at worst, in urban slums or, at best, rich but alienated in other ways. Anomie, it would seem, has been one of the worst by-products of the apparent liberation from earlier contexts. One is tempted to perceive our times as worse than any other—a kind of historical provincialism. It is easy enough to muster evidence for such a position over and above the sociological studies cited. In particular, suicide statistics in Canada vary directly with mobility and prosperity and inversely with lack of mobility and a sustaining local community. On the other hand, there is the dismal predatory anonymity of singles bars—places where the need for intimacy has undergone a pathological transformation—inappropriate sources for the satisfaction of a real but unidentified need.

Aristotle, who lived in a small community where the elite were fairly well known to one another and there was a profound identification of a free man with the city-state, recognized that, even within this tight community, friendship constituted a separate and essential mode of support. He wrote, "For without friends, no one would choose to live though he had all other goods; even rich men and those in possession of office and of dominating power are thought to need friends most of all; for what is the use of such prosperity without the opportunity of beneficence which is exercised chiefly and in its most laudable form towards friends? Or how can prosperity be guarded and preserved without friends?" He adds an unusual and uncontemporary note: "But it is not only necessary, but also noble." He also says wryly, "A wishful friendship may arise quickly, but friendship does not." He gives comfort to those of us who live in an excessively mobile world: "Distance does not break off the friendship absolutely, but only the activity of it." He recognizes, like Montaigne, that "one cannot be a friend to many people in the sense of having friendship of the perfect type with them, just as one cannot be in love with many people at once." In his own terms, he anticipates a contemporary preoccupation when he says that only those that are capable of self-love in the best sense of the word are capable of having full, true, equal, and affectionate friendships.

In preparing this chapter, I conducted a preliminary literature survey and found many references to the need all human beings have for community that, in itself, is not news but is now documented and "statistically valid" beyond common sense. While there were many references to friendship, little seemed written on the phenomenology of friendship itself. After having written the bulk of this short chapter, I turned (after being alerted by friends) to Aristotle and Montaigne and found in their essays descriptions that paralleled (more elegantly) my own stumbling toward definition. They emphasized the great value of friendship, its separation from sexual need, its relative rarity, its mutuality, and its virtue. One is touched by the unembarrassed largeness of their emotional descriptions of friendship, and one yearns for a contemporary vocabulary that can encompass such feelings without apology or feeling some sense of falseness.

It is a common contemporary experience to find that we do not have the words for perennial human experiences. We fumble, for example, with our vocabulary for death and mourning. The lack of vocabulary cannot deny the reality of the emotions and needs. By identifying need clearly, in this instance friendship, we restore it to its place as a central clinical concern. It is important for all age groups, but particularly for adolescents, who must make the crucial transition from the context of the family to wider, often inimical, turbulent, public context.

Conclusions

Friendship is a unique and specific form of relationship. It is characterized by affectionate regard without an erotic relationship, although an erotic relationship may accompany friendship. Between friends there is relative equality of feeling, and the relationship, when fully developed, appears to be sufficiently resilient to survive separation of space and time. Friendship has its own epigenetic developmental pattern. It is not a feature of infancy; it is poorly formed in early childhood, begins to develop in the latency period, but is most significant in middle and late adolescence. During that period, the society of peers and particularly a small group of friends allows the adolescent to move from the family of origin into the general society. Close friends formed through voluntary association in adolescence (as compared with the essentially nonvoluntary association of family membership) may remain vital and important throughout life. While friendship has always been valued, it is now particularly significant since many other social sources of security—organized religion, fixed social networks, and consistent family ties—have become attenuated or discredited. Networks of friends have, in many large cities, become protective and supportive islands in the large, anonymous, and sometimes inimical larger community.

NOTE

1. Montaigne (1958) cites Plutarch, who tried to reconcile two brothers and was told, "I do not value him any more highly for having come out of the same hole" (p. 92).

REFERENCES

Aristotle. 1980. *The Nicomachean Ethics.* Translated by David Ross. London: Oxford World's Classics.

Caplan, G. 1974. *Support Systems and Community Mental Health.* New York: Behavioral Publications.

Durkheim, E. 1951. *Suicide: A Study in Sociology.* New York: Free Press.

Fischer, C. S. 1981. The public and private worlds of city life. *American Sociological Review* 46:306–316.

Greenblatt, M.; Becerra, R. M.; and Serafetinides, E. A. 1982. Social networks and mental health: an overview. *American Journal of Psychiatry* 139(8): 977–984.

Hoggart, R. 1957. *The Uses of Literacy: Aspects of Working Class Life, with Special References to Publications and Entertainment.* London: Chatto & Windus.

Lincoln, H. R. 1978. Community structure and industrial conflict. *American Sociological Review* 43:199–219.

Lofland, L. 1973. *A World of Strangers*. New York: Basic.

Lowenthal, M. F., and Haven, C. 1968. Interaction and adaptation: intimacy as a critical variable. *American Sociological Review* 33:20–30.

Montaigne. 1958. *Essays*. Translated by J. M. Cohen. Harmondsworth: Penguin.

Morgan, W. R., and Clark, T. N. 1973. The causes of racial disorders. *American Sociological Review* 38:611–624.

Perlman, D., and Peplau, L. A. 1981. Toward a social psychology of loneliness. In R. Gilmour and S. Duck, eds. *Personal Relationships*. Vol. 3, *Personal Relationships in Disorder*. London: Academic.

Tilly, C. 1976. The chaos of the living city. In C. Tilley, ed. *An Urban World*. Boston: Little, Brown.

Vachon, M. L. S.; Sheldon, A. R.; Lancee, W. J.; Lyall, W. A. L.; Rogers, J.; and Freeman, S. J. J. 1982. Correlates of enduring distress patterns following bereavement: social network, life situation and personality. *Psychological Medicine* 12:783–788.

Weiss, R. S. 1974. *Loneliness: The Experience of Emotional and Social Isolation*. Cambridge, Mass.: MIT Press.

Wellman, B. 1979. The community question: the intimate networks of East Yorkers. *American Journal of Sociology* 84:1201–1231.

Wellman, B. 1981. Applying network analysis to the study of support: resource paper no. 3. In Benjamin H. Gotlieb, ed. *Social Network and Social Support*. Beverly Hills, Calif.: Sage.

8 THE ROLE OF HUMOR AS AN INTEGRATING FACTOR IN ADOLESCENT DEVELOPMENT

JOHN L. SCHIMEL

The subject is humor and its role as an integrating factor during adolescent development. Humor is part of larger cognitive and emotional capacities and is related to play, playfulness, laughter, and games and to the socialization process generally. The focus of this chapter will be on the development and function of humor as patterned behavior between and among individuals. Some rapprochement between developmental and modern game theory will be attempted, along with some observations regarding these matters in the therapeutic situation with an adolescent patient.

Freud's lifelong interest in humor is well known and was expressed in such works as *The Psychopathology of Everyday Life* (1901), *The Interpretation of Dreams* (1900–1901), and *Jokes and Their Relation to the Unconscious* (1905). He recognized wit as part of a social process that he greatly enjoyed. Some of the jokes he reported, old even in his time, are still making the rounds, for example, "Never to be born would be best for mortal man, but . . . hardly one man in a hundred thousand has this luck." Freud emphasized the role of pleasure in the use of humor, particularly, he thought, when the humor is a means of coping with the unpleasant or conflictual.

Generally speaking, humor refers to an amused attitude toward the human condition. Wit, in contrast to humor, utilizes pungent, sharp, incisive speech and may be unkind. On another level, wit can be seen to be a more or less socially acceptable way of communicating sexual and aggressive thoughts or impulses.

Where does humor begin? I do not believe that this can be answered completely at present. Laughter is, however, a capacity from earliest infancy. Black (1984) has noted that laughter is unique in that it is both a reflex and a psychosocial event. As a reflex, laughter can be elicited by tickling or, as a psychosocial event, by a pratfall. Bateson (1971) pointed out that laughter is one of the few convulsive behaviors of ordinary people, the others being grief, orgasm, and sneezing. Laughter can also be consciously engaged in or an expression of psychopathology. It may serve a hostile or a loving function; it may be a simple expression of pleasure or joy. For the psychoanalyst, laughter as a response to humor generally represents a situation in which the censor is bypassed because of the element of surprise, which permits the association of two ideas whose connection is usually forbidden.

Laughter in the infant has been explained by an arousal-safety model. Laughter is an expressive consequence resulting from unexpected stimuli that do not fit into the infant's schema. If the arousing stimulus is judged not to be dangerous, laughter is likely to result. If the initial arousal to the stimulus is high, the response is likely to be avoidance. If the arousal is only moderate, curiosity and attempts at problem solving or exploration may follow, rather than laughter. It is when a stimulus is relatively arousing and not judged to be dangerous that laughter results and achieves the function of dissipating tension.

Laughing, early on, becomes patterned. The infant comes to anticipate the laughter-provoking stimulus that the parent provides. The infant's laughter stimulates reciprocal smiling, laughing, or cooing behavior on the part of the parent. I did not see this reciprocal laughing process with infants of Mexican and Peruvian Indians or in a limited experience in China. In any event, beginning in earliest infancy, laughter can be seen to be the result of social activity in that it involves at least two individuals.

The social activity described falls under the general rubric of mutual play or games. Quiet humor, good humor, and laughter all occur in a social context and follow the patterns of play and games. A child fingering its toes, a child, all alone, mothering its doll, is engaged in activities that form the basis of games but are not games in themselves. Let the mother recite, as she or the baby touches each toe, "This little piggy went to market," and the social situation necessary for a game is met. "Peekaboo" meets the criteria for a game. A game is a drama. There are games in which there is no winner and no loser, but in most games a winner and a loser emerge, even in "This little piggy" and in "Peekaboo." And no one gets hurt. In general, at this level, a game is a plot worked out by the players during its course of action. The infant may initiate variations of games. However, no game is possible without rules, either tacitly or explicitly understood by the players. The infant can be observed to have learned the rules after very few repetitions. The sequences must be adhered to, or anxiety, rather than laughter, appears. Improvisation is admissible where necessary, but infants and children, as well as adults in adult games, tend to frown on such anarchic behavior.

Children's games have been extensively studied. The basic patterns for game playing can be seen to have been laid down in infancy for the fortunate child. Problems in this area appear at nursery school age or earlier. Patterned mutual behaviors, specifically those that result in laughter, have been assigned adaptive or even survival value by some authors. Early laughter games may foster two kinds of learning: (1) the development of general expectations and (2) the social experience of learning that one's actions can influence the actions of others, hence adaptive.

In his *Origin of Species* (1859), Darwin claimed that laughter developed because the long dependency in infancy required strong signals that reward caretaking by adults. Thus, laughter developed as a signal of well-being—a counterpart to crying, a signal of discomfort. Also, on a paleontological level, the genial aspect of laughter, it has been suggested, could derive from the banding together of companions, laughing in a mutual realization of safety. It has been suggested that social laughter is an expression of unity in group opinion. In his studies of primitive peoples, Lorenz (1971) noted that "shared laughter not only diverts aggression, but also produces a feeling of social unity"; that is, laughter developed as an obverse form of aggression. There is evidence that organized games existed from earliest antiquity.

The verbal aspect of games appears with the development of speech in the infant and earlier since infants respond to verbal cues prior to the appearance of their own speech. However, they are soon seen to be participating on a verbal level. They play with words as they do with the physical aspects of their environment. When does humor appear? I believe that it must appear as soon as the infant can play with ideas. Let me tell you about David's first joke. He is approximately eighteen months old, precocious, and bright. He is in his high chair eating some cereal. His mother is nearby. The telephone rings. Mother hears some bad news. Her face clouds over. She soon notes that David has stopped eating and looks worried. She assures him that her gloom has to do with the message she is receiving and has nothing to do with him. He resumes eating. Shortly, David announces, "Look at Mommy with the happy face." David has already mastered the form of wit that Freud (1958) referred to as following the rules of "representation through the opposite." One might suggest that, in this mastery, David has already progressed beyond mere laughter in his grasp of this particular form of word game. Note that, on this verbal level, there are rules, a winner, and a loser and that it is quintessentially a social situation.

Game theory in psychiatry has borrowed from mathematics, where it had to do with the relation of the ordering and sequences of numbers to the probability of outcome. It was later used to study sequences in human interactions. A great deal of useful work was based on these observational concepts by Bateson (1971), Watzlawick (1983), and others, leading to the concept of the double bind. Here, the player, the child or adolescent in a disturbed family, for example, was repeatedly led into a situation in which any response on his part had to lead to defeat and loss of self-esteem.

Some of this work was based on earlier observations by Sullivan (1953), whose transactional version of psychiatry focused on the sequences of events occurring between and among individuals. He advocated an explicit and phenomenological approach to human interactions. He always wanted to know who said what to whom and under what circumstances. One might say that he was trying to tease out the rules of the game that the patient was engaged in with parents, peers, authorities, and therapist. He wanted to know about these matters with great explicitness—not only the words, but also the tone and ambience. Perhaps one could say that he, and subsequently Bateson (1971), was attempting to divine the central games or basic plots of the patient's life with others in order to study their disjunctive effects. Repetitive sequences of behaviors with others can serve as either integrative or disjunctive factors in development. I believe there is a clue here, too, for both the conduct of the inquiry in exploring the problems of patients and the observation of the transferential and countertransferential aspects of the treatment situation with patients.

With the foregoing as preamble, let us leap into the adolescent situation. Our Davids are now adolescents. Have they developed or maintained some sense of humor as they confront the monumental tasks of coping with bodily changes, an insistent lust dynamism, the need for supportive peer relations, the evolution of hierarchical positions vis-à-vis parents, siblings, coaches, and teachers? What role does humor play during this stage? What is the role of the adolescent's knowledge of and mastery of the sequences of behaviors that go on among people, a mastery that tends to foster self-esteem? What of the adolescents whose interactions with others have developed along a disjunctive plane?

In disjunctive interactions, an essential ingredient is a lack of humor. Both protagonists must engage in ongoing interactions with great seriousness and as matters of grave consequences, no matter how trivial, otherwise the disjunctive interaction is over, perhaps to be replaced by a more congenial one. This is easily seen in angry young children, toward whom a good-humored response may lead to a congenial change while a serious or angry response tends to perpetuate the angry interchange (Schimel 1980). Let me remind you of the definition of (good) humor as an overall attitude toward the human condition in which a perspective broader than the immediate circumstances is brought to bear, along with a genuinely compassionate attitude. One might sum up that an adolescent who can laugh at himself has won half the battle.

Are there such adolescents? I believe there are. Perhaps all are, potentially at least. Are there such therapists? Winnicott (1982) suggested that, in the therapeutic situation, at least one of the participants, the therapist, must know how to play—and that, for progress in psychotherapy, therapist and patient must learn to play together.

Case Example

A nineteen-year-old college student at an initial session complained of depression, insomnia, and a general loss of interest in work. His parents were protective but really, he felt, quite unsympathetic. Antidepressants had been recommended by a consultant but resisted by the patient. These matters were presented in a perfunctory, listless manner. However, he did want to talk about an argument he had been having with his father for months. His father insisted that there was no unconditional love, that love had to be earned. The patient was angry. His father, he said, wanted him out of the house and had begun to talk about his leaving home since the patient was twelve. His former therapist, he believed, had taken his side and was quoted as saying that love was the most important thing in the world and made the most difficult things possible.

If we pause here, we can observe that the patient was reporting repetitive integrations with father and his previous therapist and was laying the groundwork for the ongoing patterning of a relationship with his new therapist. The argument with father was ancient, a family drama with its own rules, in which the previous therapist was seen and quoted as an ally by the patient. The integration with the previous therapist is perhaps more interesting and not as immediately comprehensible. One might presume the possibility that cautious professional statements, probably in response to the patient's importuning for support, made it possible for the patient to use the therapist as an auxiliary in the struggle with father. Where does humor fit in consideration of such matters? Where is its facilitating effect in the patient's life or therapy?

The patient turned to the therapist and demanded:

P. Where do you stand on the subject of unconditional love?
T. It sounds nice.
P. But do you believe it exists?
T. I remember Erich Fromm talking about it.
P. Don't you have a stand on it?
T. Well, I'm getting along in years.
P. I thought psychiatrists agreed on things.
T. Well, Erich Fromm believed it exists.
P. (Sighs with relief.)
T. He thought it probably existed during infancy with many mothers, not all, and less so with fathers. After that, he thought, it was conditional. You had to earn it.
P. I don't believe it. You seem to have different ideas than my former psychiatrist. I thought you'd all be alike.
T. Like homogenized?
P. (Begins to chuckle; leaves with a worried look.)

I suggest that the therapist has introduced a series of interactions that are novel to the patient, at least in the therapeutic setting. He has rebuffed the patient's attempt to make him an ally in the struggle with his father but without attacking the patient's self-esteem. The therapist's wry remarks are deliberately made in a slow and thoughtful manner, interrupting the patient's rapid-fire breakneck style of interacting, whether reporting or demanding answers. The rules are being changed toward a more reflective mode. The therapist's question, "Like homogenized?" introduces a note of playfulness and humor. The patient chuckles. He seems amused, although puzzled. A different kind of drama in the therapist's office is evolving for this patient. The patient left the initial hour puzzled. He promised to phone for another appointment as soon as he was settled in his new school. He calls shortly, stating that financial complications are causing him to postpone his treatment for about two months and that he would call then. He said he was eager to start. He called after two months. He had been puzzled by the previous session. He was surprised at how well he had felt on leaving but could not understand it. He had spent a lot of time mulling over the difference between his previous therapist and me, and it bothered him. In the meantime, however, his girlfriend had left him, and he really wanted to talk about that:

P. I'm so angry. She left me. I need sex. When I don't have it, I feel empty and unhappy. I think that I may never have another girlfriend who is as good sexually or so good looking. I'm very needy and very angry. I feel inadequate and unattractive. Maybe I'll never find another girl. I'm very angry with her.

T. She sounds irresponsible.

P. (Slowly.) Are you kidding?

T. No, considering your great needs, she certainly must be very irresponsible!

P. (Laughing hard.) You make the whole thing sound absurd. But I do have strong sexual needs.

T. Sex is not a need. It may be a strong urge. Eating, sleeping, breathing, defecating are needs.

P. That's funny. I had a date on Saturday night. We went to bed. It was easy. She said she had a strong sexual need. I guess it was OK. It's funny. I wish she had been prettier. It makes me feel good to be with pretty women. It makes me feel more attractive. What's it all about? My father resents my being at home. He tells me I should move out. He's been saying it since

I was twelve. My previous therapist said that some parents feel abandoned when their child leaves home so they reject the child first.

T. Your father probably wanted you to grow up.

P. That's what my girlfriend said when she left me. She said I was too dependent, too demanding, that I ought to grow up. Maybe she was right. She wasn't too happy with me.

The discussion illustrates some of the points made earlier. In neither session did the patient fit the criteria of someone needing medication, although his suffering had been real enough. It is true that his reporting tended to be listless, strident, and demanding. Yet he was able to respond to the therapist's input with curiosity and exploratory moves on his own and to experience pleasure and even to laugh during the encounters. A new patterning between himself and the therapist is emerging, I believe, that bodes well for treatment and for facilitating the developmental tasks of his adolescence as well as reworking the incompleted tasks of earlier stages of development. The next patient, who had encountered the young man in the waiting room, reported, "That young patient left with a big smile on his face. He was laughing and chuckling. He must have had a good time with you."

I hope that I have conveyed an intimation of the early patterning of human capacities that are indicated by such notions as humor, play, playfulness, and games and that these capacities can facilitate the socialization and developmental process. In the clinical vignette, one may see a patterning of the therapeutic situation that may recall the early play of mother and infant. Would it be too farfetched to think of psychotherapy as a later version of "Peekaboo" or even this little piggy? The patient's expressed puzzlement and chuckling in the first session was not too unlike the infant's first experience with a new laughter game. His delighted laughter in the second session could recall the delight of an infant comfortably at play with a trusted caretaker.

Conclusions

I believe that these matters are not new, although their negative counterparts are much more frequently attended to under such rubrics as hostility, narcissistic concerns, the negative transference, the repetition compulsion, and the like. Patients, I believe, are more regularly probed for their destructiveness or other evil psychic propensities, postulated in our theories, than for their capacities, no matter how latent, to respond good humoredly to others. One did not have to probe for the patient's hostility, narcissistic concerns, or destructiveness. They were all too apparent. I believe that it may have been a surprise to the audience to see that, in short order, this patient was also able to show a capacity for humor and even compassion.

REFERENCES

Bateson, G. 1971. *Steps to an Ecology of Mind.* San Francisco: Chandler.
Black, D. 1984. Laughter. *Journal of the American Medical Association* 252(21).
Freud, S. 1900–1901. The interpretation of dreams. *Standard Edition* 4:1–338, 5:339–686. London: Hogarth, 1958.
Freud, S. 1901. The psychopathology of everyday life. *Standard Edition* 6:1–279. London: Hogarth, 1960.
Freud, S. 1905. Jokes and their relation to the unconscious. *Standard Edition* 8:9–236. London: Hogarth, 1960.
Lorenz, K. 1971. *Studies in Animal and Human Behavior,* vols. 1, 2. Cambridge, Mass.: Harvard University Press.
Schimel, J. L. 1980. Some thoughts on the uses of wit and humor in the treatment of adolescents. *New Directions for Mental Health Services* 5:15–23.
Sullivan, H. S. 1953. *Conceptions of Modern Psychiatry.* New York: Norton, 1980.
Watzlawick, P. 1983. *The Situation Is Hopeless, but Not Serious.* New York: Norton.
Winnicott, D. W. 1982. *Playing and Reality.* London: Tavistock.

PART II

DEVELOPMENTAL ISSUES IN ADOLESCENT PSYCHIATRY

EDITOR'S INTRODUCTION

The failure to recognize adolescence as a separate stage of development did not occur by accident but has a long history related to marked discomfort about adolescent process and the emergence of sexual and aggressive impulses. What was seen as a natural change of status from dependency to semidependency to final independence and reflected a change in roles in the family must now be evaluated from an appraisal of the dynamic state of an adolescent's stage of separation-individuation and self-development. The imposition of weighty social expectations, such as school, ethical systems, and career choices, on a psychic system not yet ready to master the growth demanded of it can result in conflict owing to regressive aspects of change at the service of ego.

Max Sugar notes that late adolescence is somewhat ignored in reviews of adolescent development and treatment and presents an overview of the years eighteen to twenty-five. He discusses biological aspects of maturation, sociological views, and developmental tasks. In describing psychic structure in late adolescence, Sugar describes the ego, superego, and ego ideal differences in males and females and their separate pathways. The parents' contribution is viewed in light of their own residual oedipal conflicts, rearoused when their own children reach adolescence. Adolescent attitudes and behaviors are described in sexuality, education and vocational choice, psychiatric breakdowns, psychotherapy, and inpatient therapy.

Kimberly A. Schonert presents her study of the differences in the moral and cognitive development of severely emotionally disturbed (SED) male and female adolescents. Previous work was extended by comparing those boys and girls and by exploring the interrelations among IQ, moral reasoning, cognitive development, and age in this population. Thirteen males and twelve females were administered

Rest's Defining Issues Test and six Piagetian tasks. The findings revealed that males displayed more immature forms of moral reasoning than did females when IQ was statistically controlled. No sex differences in cognitive development emerged. Moral reasoning, cognitive development, and IQ were significantly related to one another. A number of interpretations for the findings are offered.

Hadas Wiseman and Amia Lieblich study the attainment of ego identity, as it implies a sense of meaning in relation to the social world, from the perspective of kibbutz-raised young adults. Most of the attitudes were represented by reaction to the kibbutz, others, and the self. Some of the attitudes were positive, and some were negative. The authors concluded that the need to establish distance from the family and community allows the emergence of the adult, individuated self.

A special section in this part on developmental issues is a monograph authored by Harvey Golombek and Peter Marton that reports the findings of the Toronto Adolescent Longitudinal Study.

9 LATE ADOLESCENT DEVELOPMENT AND TREATMENT

MAX SUGAR

Various psychiatric efforts are directed toward childhood, adolescence, geriatrics, and even infancy, but little attention is given to the late adolescent period as a particular entity. In this chapter I wish to address some selected aspects of this period with the current culture of the United States in mind.

Late adolescence appears to be thought of in a synecdochical manner, that is, taking one part or achievement as the whole. This seems to reflect the question of what maturity and adulthood really mean. Depending on the state, a driver's license is available at various ages. The right to drink alcohol publicly arrives at age eighteen or twenty-one. Auto insurance premiums are higher until age twenty-five for males, and a slightly younger age for females, than for older drivers. An officer in the military has to be twenty-one, but in wartime that may be reduced. Not too long ago, the right to vote was lowered from age twenty-one to age eighteen. There is a certain minimum age to become a congressman, a city councilor, an alderman, a mayor, a state representative, a member of Congress, and the president. Do these reflect the partial emotional and cognitive achievements of adolescence on the way to adulthood as way stations to maturity, or are these sociocultural reflections, some chronologic form of gauge, or a standard for attainment of these privileges?

Late adolescence varies, according to the youngster's personal situation, aside from whatever personal assets or liabilities that attend it from an emotional or physical standpoint. For instance, late adolescents involved in the work force have decreased dependency, learning opportunities, and capacity for self-observation, but they have an increase in consolidation of their character, a heightened sense of independence, increased autonomy, and decreased regression available to them in the service of any growth.

College youngsters experience a somewhat different situation. They have decreased character consolidation, more learning opportunities available, more regression in the service of growth, and a prolonged opportunity for trying out different identities. When we consider college students, we usually think of a certain age range and, as a culture, tolerate some limited regression. Even in older age groups who remain in a dependent position, such as in postdoctoral or residency training, there may be a tendency to exercise a certain amount of regression, even among those who may be making an income or having a family of their own. At this stage, they are not truly committed to their jobs since they are at a temporary step on the way to their ultimate goal. They have a continued commitment to learning and an opportunity for further identifications with their mentors, including additional tryouts in their ego ideal formation, while they have developed less autonomy in other areas.

Definition of Late Adolescence

Late adolescence is the final stage of the adolescent process and is most important in the resolution of that developmental period. "Adolescence," which is derived from the Latin *adolescens,* means the state of growing up. "Adult" comes from the Latin word *adultus,* which is the past participle of *adolescere,* "to grow up." As a noun, "adult" refers to one who has arrived at mature years or attained full size and strength. As an adjective, "adult" means fully developed and mature or pertaining to, befitting, or intended for mature persons (Whitney 1899). Thus, there is a similarity in roots for the words "adolescence" and "adult."

Late adolescence is variably defined chronologically as follows. According to the *Century Dictionary* (Whitney 1899), adolescence for males is fourteen to twenty-five and for females twelve to twenty-one. For Levinson, Darrow, Klein, Levinson, and McKee (1978), adolescence ends at twenty-two, and early adulthood is from seventeen to forty-five, with seventeen to twenty-two as the early adult transition.

Offer and Sabshin (1984) consider twenty-five as the end of young adulthood, while for Guntrip (1973) and Marshall (1973) it is thirty. Arnstein (1984) takes eighteen to twenty-five to be young adulthood, while Adatto (1958) classifies age eighteen to twenty-five as late adolescence. The interval to be used here for late adolescence is eighteen to twenty-five years.

As a historical aside, adolescence was not invented in the twentieth century. It was described by the emperor Constantine as ending in the twenty-first year. In the sixth century, "according to Isidore it lasts till twenty-eight—and it can go on till thirty-five.—Afterward follows youth, and this age lasts until forty-five according to Isidore, or until fifty according to others" (Aries 1962, p. 21). Perhaps late adolescence is best viewed as the stage of being on the road to maturity, which includes physical, emotional, social, and vocational aspects.

Adolescents make comments such as, "We go crazy until we're about sixteen, and then we start growing up," and, "Don't trust anyone over the age of thirty." Perhaps there is some wisdom in these folk sayings.

Biological Aspects

There is a large difference among adolescents in their rate of physical maturation. The male who matures early has been found to be "more sociable as an adult," while the girl who physically matures early is affected differently (Tanner 1978). She may be embarrassed about her precocious development since she is out of the mainstream that her peers are in, although she may have a sense of glory in this position. Despite this earlier development and readiness, such a girl has limits set by age, cognition, emotions, family, and culture that give her a longer period of frustration of her sex drives, frustration in her drive to independence, and time in establishing a vocation compared to her more slowly maturing peers. In this context, consider a girl who reaches menarche at eight and has obvious breast buds and rounding of the hips.

The brain develops at least until adolescence, but there is some question as to whether growth continues into adult life. Height is of great concern to adolescents and more so to males as a symbol of masculinity and strength. Girls have usually completed their linear growth by sixteen, but boys may continue for several years after. In

133

industrialized, temperate climates, tall females have a more successful reproductive history than short ones, but this does not hold true world-wide. In New Guinea and the Peruvian Andes, the shorter females are more successful in having more surviving offspring (Tanner 1978). Therefore, temperature and altitude are factors affecting late adolescent females, but not males, in their reproductive capacities.

With continuing advances in knowledge in the neurosciences, there may soon emerge finite indicators of the beginning and end of late adolescence. The new data may derive from sophisticated measures of neurotransmitters, the immune system, or hormone levels. It is clear that in adolescence the immune system functions more effectively than earlier since adolescence is a period in which there are fewer infections and other physical illnesses than in earlier periods of life. From clinical experience, this is not the case with borderline patients since they have frequent infections, accidents, and somatic complaints compared to other adolescents. Observations from a chart review by Shanok and Lewis (1981) that female delinquents through age twenty-one had significantly more hospital visits, accidents, and injuries appear to confirm this.

The termination of adolescence is a vague concept, although certain biological factors help define it anatomically. By age twenty-one, red blood cell formation is confined to the flat bones since the red marrow of the long bones changes to fat over the preceding seven years (Boyd 1943, p. 973). Closure of the epiphyses may serve as a variable end point. They close in some at twenty-two, yet in others closure is much earlier. They also close earlier for girls than for boys because of girls' earlier growth peak. Although limb growth stops with epiphyseal closure, the vertebral bodies may continue to grow at the rate of three to five millimeters a year until age thirty (Tanner 1978).

The last physical development for the male, which is chest hair, may not occur for some until the late twenties. Biology, therefore, does not provide a finite statement about the regular onset or end point of late adolescence.

At any age, physical changes bring many anxieties, and this is augmented in early adolescence with its numerous height, weight, contour, hormonal, cognitive, and emotional changes. The feelings about physical changes do not end with mid-adolescence, and they affect the body image.

Depending on their assessment of their physical development by the end of mid-adolescence, late adolescents may have feelings of pleasure and acceptance of, or inadequacy about, the body image. The boy with insufficient beard to shave, or a smaller than hoped for penis, or below-average height, may have a marked sense of inadequacy about his masculinity and attractiveness. Regardless of their actual pulchritude, most girls and women, according to colleagues in obstetrics and gynecology, will have some continuing displeasure and sense of unattractiveness about their weight and, more prominently, their breasts.

Adjustment to these conditions continues during late adolescence, and, for some, the passage of time takes care of them. For example, temporizing and reassurance is probably best for early adolescent boys with gynecomastia since the condition usually disappears after several years. For those youngsters who feel that they have disproportionately large noses, the further growth of the face changes the proportions so that by late adolescence the nose is not so prominent. If necessary, some may elect to have surgery.

Sociological Views

Modell, Furstenberg, and Hershberg (1976) listed five transition points to define the beginning of adulthood: exit from school, entrance into the work force, departure from the family of origin, marriage, and the establishment of a household of one's own. In comparing the age for achieving those markers, they found little difference between 1880 and 1970, although there was some narrowing of the age spread for the last three items in 1970.

Developmental Tasks in Late Adolescence

The tasks of late adolescent development are consolidation, separating from parents, identity formation, achieving genital primacy and a sexual identity, and the development of a time perspective (Buhler 1968; Neugarten 1969); commitment to a life goal and development of intimacy and friendships (Erikson 1959); and the further development and harmonizing of the ego, superego, and ego ideal.

While one of the developmental tasks of late adolescence is consolidation, there are issues to be reworked, refined, and harmonized from previous developmental stages. These are the preoedipal (dependency vs. autonomy; trust vs. distrust), the oedipal (with positive and negative features), and the latency periods (industry vs. inferiority). These are involved with the forward movement of the late adolescent stage—developing a sense of commitment and fidelity (Erikson 1950).

The significance of identity formation as a task in late adolescent development can be observed among a nonpatient group of youngsters. These are the adoptees, who, at this period, often begin openly to seek information about their biological parents to try to close up the emptiness they feel about themselves without knowledge of forebears.

The normal adolescent mourning process (Sugar 1968) has to do with giving up the infantile objects and the reactions to that, consisting of the separation-protest, disorganization, and reorganization phases. In the first phase, the separation-protest phase, the normative urge to separate is commingled with unconsciously determined, angry, rebellious behavior, which is a protest in an effort to restore the lost objects. In this period, there is some psychic disequilibrium as the youngster unconsciously vacillates between separation efforts and protests against this.

The disorganization phase follows when the futility of reunion with the infantile objects has been somewhat accepted unconsciously. In this phase, the adolescent may feel worthless, empty, and inadequate and may be restless, depressed, withdrawn, seeking new thrills, or isolated.

The next phase, that of reorganization, which occurs in late adolescence, is relatively calm but may also have some upheavals since it involves shifts back and forth to the disorganization phase. Involved here are wishes for freedom from parents' and other authorities' restrictions, the need for exploring and handling reactions in relation to persons of the same and the opposite sex, testing one's omnipotentiality, arriving at a sense of fidelity and commitment to self and object choice—with the superego still being in flux, amid the further adjustment and reorganization about the object loss.

Blos (1979) writes about separation-individuation in adolescence as a second stage of separation-individuation, the first being that of infancy and toddlerhood. Such individuation implies that the individual is taking increasing responsibility for what he or she is and does, rather than attributing it to parents or other adults. The end of adolescence is viewed by Blos (1979) as involving character formation and four developmental preconditions that have to be resolved in some fashion. These preconditions are the second individuation process, dealing with the residual traumata from childhood, developing ego continuity, and establishing a sexual identity. He refers to all these as being involved in the personality consolidation of this period.

Psychic Structure in Late Adolescence

THE EGO

Apropos of the second separation-individuation stage in adolescence, an accompanying issue is about developing autonomy. More autonomous functioning by the adolescent is not entirely related to being partly or wholly different from the parents. The youngsters can be aware of their efforts to be independent in some ways while they remain dependent on the same authorities against whom they rail and attempt to disqualify as standard-bearers of their values.

By mid-adolescence, the ego has had a mass of individuation experiences and has internalized these with a sense of distinctness and competence. The youngster has also been involved with peers, to whose values he religiously conforms and imitates in clothes, music, and behavior. The ego ideal of early and mid-adolescence can be compared to jello. At mid-adolescence, youngsters often question whether their ego ideals are the best models, and they frequently reject them to find new models. This shifting and searching is an effort that helps define, refine, and separate their own egos and values from those of their parents and friends.

Another aspect of autonomy involves youngsters with their own introjects. The most troublesome of these reside in the archaic, prohibitive superego. During latency, the ego is dominated by the superego with its rigid strictures. The child is very much involved with doing the right thing, listening to the teacher, and following the rules. In adolescence, this aspect of ego autonomy is an internal one—an effort to wrest controls from the superego, a large part of which is projected. Then the superego can be dealt with as something alien, something "not belonging to me," "something that authorities are putting on me," whether it is the parents or teachers or coaches. As a result, it is less threatening to self-esteem.

This reworking and restructuring goes on in the ego during this period and leads to a capacity to regulate self-esteem internally. This now involves the construction of a stable reality sense of self-

137

representation that can withstand the archaic guilt as well as the reality-related disapproval. For Blos (1962), the development of the self-critical ego at the onset of adolescence serves to complement and eventually supplant the self-valuing aspects of the superego.

THE SUPEREGO

With the presence of concrete thinking in latency, the superego beginnings are equivalently limited by rigidity and inexperience. The child often has an uncomfortable contrast between his own and the reality superego of the parents, along with experiences that confront and then modify the harshness of the latency superego. In adolescence, sexual fantasies and actions (masturbation) lead to secrets and guilt that challenge the superego. With further cognitive development, the attainment of abstract thinking (Piaget 1972) in adolescence, along with further reality experiences, the reality ego begins to decrease the power and rigidity of the superego.

Some of their introjects and values come from identifications with various adults, members of their family circle, or their environment. The sources of these identifications for boys and girls are partly from each parent, with a special emphasis on the identification with the same-sex parent. Also, identifications from others in the environment will become very important to them, whether teacher, coach, or whomever. These might be looked on as transference objects because they are representative of, but not the same as, parents.

After object removal begins in early adolescence, the ego feels depleted and does not have its usual source of support and dependency. The youngsters now look more to themselves to handle these issues, conflicts, feelings, and fears. But they feel unequal to the task and may, if projection is not predominant, turn to other authority figures and values for help. These others are used by adolescents as way stations toward becoming an adult. These identifications have contributed to the development of the superego in latency and continue to help modify its development in adolescence. Modifications occur in the superego in late adolescence as the youngsters' accrued experiences with, and expectations of, the world around them conform or conflict with their values and internal representations.

Some believe that a mature and reliable superego is not available until after age thirty (Pearson 1951, p. 63). In this context, we can return to the wisdom of adolescent folklore—"don't trust anybody over thirty." Past age thirty, there appears to be a different set of moral values, and people are in a steadier developmental state than before.

Pearson's (1951) statement appears to be confirmed by Gilligan (1982) and Rest, Davison, and Robbins (1978). Rest et al. (1978) studied cross-sectional, longitudinal, and sequential groups for the predominant use of principled thinking and found that it varied by age and education. The percentage of principled thinking rose from 2.5 percent in junior high, to 7.5 percent in senior high, to 45 percent in college, to 60 percent in seminarians, to 93 percent in doctoral students in political science and moral philosophy. They concluded that "adults in general seem to slow down in moral judgment development in their 20s and to plateau after leaving school" (p. 266).

From her studies of males and females in college and five years after college (about age twenty-seven), Gilligan (1982) summarized that, though both sexes move away from absolutes during this time, the absolutes differ for each sex. In women, there is a shift in morality from that of absolute care to a need for personal integrity and equality. For men, the absolutes of truth and fairness gave way to the realization of multiple truths and lead to generativity and care. "For both sexes, the existence of two contexts for moral decision makes judgment by definition contextually relative and leads to a new understanding of responsibility and choice."

There has been a question raised over the years whether the superego of females is different, deficient, or defective compared to that of males. The consensus today is that "the female superego is not defective but different" (Jacobson 1964, p. 113) from the male's, with the difference being only in the contents, not the function (Muslin 1979). Jacobson (1964, p. 113) believes that "the little girl develops the nucleus of a true ego ideal even earlier than the little boy." Further delineation of this is given later in the chapter.

THE EGO IDEAL

"That which he projects ahead of him as his ideal is merely a substitute for the lost narcissism of his childhood . . . the time when he was his own ideal" (Freud 1914, p. 94). Jacobson (1964, p. 96) adds that "the ego ideal, which is forged from ideal concepts of the self, and

139

from idealized features of the love objects, gratifies indeed the infantile longing of which we said that it is never fully relinquished: the desire to be one with the love object." With the passing of the oepidal phase and beginning development of a more definitive superego, the idealized future becomes part of the superego. "The superego is the inner representative of the ego's future" (Settlage 1972). Ritvo (1971) refers to the distinction Jacobson (1964) has made between the ego ideal and the wishful self-image as "the grandiose, glorified, heroic fantasy figure which may have elements of the ego-ideal in details of the contents but it is primarily the inflated self image cathected with the libido withdrawn from the parental object ties at a time when psychological independence from parental objects has not been established, and intolerable anxiety is easily aroused by the hazards of failure if the attempt is made." Ritvo points out that, by "the end of adolescence, these images tend to become increasingly ego dystonic and their persistence beyond their appropriate and useful time precipitates the crises of late adolescence." This may be the forerunner of some individuals seeking treatment because the two are dystonic.

SEPARATE PATHS FOR MALES AND FEMALES

Male and female adolescents have some similar normative sources of anxiety, with some significant differences throughout their development. For the boy, separation and performance needs and vocational choices become paramount in late adolescence, although fidelity and object choice are important.

For the girl in this stage, affiliative needs are in the ascendancy, and she has to concern herself with choices and anxiety about career and/ or family planning. In our culture now, there are more choices available to females beyond marriage and motherhood, except for those of lower socioeconomic status (SES). For the middle- and upper-class girls, there is now more freedom of vocational choice, about whether to get married, and, if married, whether to be a mother. But these girls also have more turmoil about delaying or making these choices in contrast to previous generations, when there was essentially only one choice—marriage and motherhood.

Separation-individuation for the girl in adolescence relates to the preoedipal ties to the mother, while for the male adolescent the focus is a reawakening of oedipal issues (Blos 1980b).

Ritvo (1976) writes that girls in adolescence have more shame, inferiority feelings, and guilt with the resurgence of anal and phallic-oedipal issues, especially with the onset of menses. The latter contributes feelings of helplessness and being soiled since there is no control over their menses, unlike sphincter control. Ritvo feels that the girl regresses to the pregenital stage in puberty, which is related to her body image, and reacts to menarche as uncontrollable soiling. These reactivate the preoedipal relationship to the mother. In adolescence, with the loosening of the tie to the mother, the girl loses the support and organization that she has had from having parental ego, superego, and ego ideal as auxiliaries to her own. Thus, beginning separation has more of an effect on the girl than the boy since she concomitantly has some regression to preoedipal issues and begins the separation from a closer relationship to the parents in latency than the boy.

Gilligan (1982) has described "a moment of resistance" occurring in girls around age eleven, when they have a sense of outspokenness and authority along with being very honest about relationships and things that hurt them. By age fifteen or sixteen, this resistance has gone underground, and girls say, "I don't know, I don't know," and start not knowing what they know. According to Gilligan, the change in girls comes about when they are confronted by the wall of Western culture and find that their clear-sightedness may be dangerous. Then they learn to hide and protect what they know to censor themselves and be able to think in ways that differ from what they really think.

She proposed two separate moral voices in women: one of these attends to abstract principles such as justice; the other is of human connection and care, which asks how moral decisions will hurt or help those involved. Gilligan also emphasizes collectivity in females as a higher development than that of individuation and autonomy, and, therefore, the ability to collaborate is viewed as a highly esteemed goal.

Long before a girl reaches late adolescence, she has usually become clearly aware that her sense of attractiveness is mixed with the threat, and fear, of rape as well as of unwanted pregnancy. She has repeatedly heard, "You know what men do," "You know what men are like." Unlike the boy, whose sense of masculinity does not have such threats, the girl's sense of femininity has this twofold cloud of physical vulnerability. Perhaps these factors are also related to the self-in-relation (Miller 1976) development by the girl since they would lead the girl to be involved with affiliative processes as a protective measure.

The change in the girl to be more passive in adolescence compared

141

to prepubescence, with decreased assertiveness, confidence, and decisiveness, is tied to the circulating hormones and may also be related to the normative adolescent mourning process (Sugar 1968). This process is different for girls than boys since, with the surge for separation-individuation, the boy is supported by the culture as well as the parents while girls are still given less positives for such endeavors by parents and society.

Erikson (1959) stressed the importance of intimacy and friendships for both males and females in late adolescence, and this has been validated by Vaillant's (1977) long-term research in males. But this is different still from the affiliative and collaborative pursuits in females.

Currently, many women in the United States who are in late adolescence and older prefer not to feel dependent on a male and marriage for the sake of a continuing reciprocal relationship and instead choose to have serial monogamy by living with a man for variable periods of time. If they marry, many woman choose to continue with a career whether they choose to have children or not.

Miller (1976) stated that for many women the threatened disruption of a relationship is perceived not just as a loss of the relationship but almost as a "total loss of self." Freidin (1986) elaborates on this, the self-in-relation theory of female development (Miller 1976), and emphasizes the female's wish to maintain empathic connections with others in order to validate her capacities as a person and the need to feel valued for her nurturing role. She feels that women inhibit anger and aggression, fearing that they will disrupt important relationships.

Generally, males have more difficulty with intimacy, while females have difficulty with separations. A female's sense of self-esteem is achieved through an active role in affiliating, and her sense of self is attained through continued empathy in relationships, not by separateness, as in males. This reliance on the need to maintain relationships and threat of loss of self (Miller 1976) makes females more vulnerable to depression and explains its greater frequency in females (Freidin 1986). This is already apparent in late adolescent females.

The Parents' Contribution

Since parents usually have aspects of their own residual oedipal conflicts rekindled when their offspring reenter the same arena in adolescence, the two generations then resonate to similar issues at that time. Often fathers withdraw emotionally from their daughters, while sons and daughters withdraw from their mothers. The frequent upsurge of hostility between parents and their adolescent youngsters is derived not just from the adolescent's rebellious, separation-individuation needs or as a defense against fears of fusion or incestuous wishes but is also partly initiated and maintained by the parents as a defense against their unconscious incestuous wishes toward their offspring. Parents in mid-life have much unconscious envy and jealousy of their offspring. This is reflected in their overconcern about power and control (Sugar 1990), which is also often involved in their hostile defense against their incestuous wishes.

Adolescents and their parents are in transition and have to adapt to shifts in their social situation. The cohesiveness of their separate groups is less defined, which increases separation anxiety for both generations. Meanwhile, the parents may have experienced a death, retirement, or relocation of their own parents, extended kin, and close friends. There also may have been marked changes in interests, vocational and avocational, in the parents.

In today's society, male adolescents are still given more support and freedom to be autonomous and individuate by both parents, but especially by the father. Both parents still expect more, especially in performance in school and work, from the adolescent boy through all stages.

For the girl, the task of individuating is compounded by her own needs for affiliating, for collaborating, for not sundering relationships, and for caring; the father's distancing himself while continuing to generally be more indulgent toward her dependency needs; and the mother's continuing wish for an involved, mutual, caring relationship. While hoping for maturation and personal fulfillment for the girl, the mother continues to be available for her passive-dependent needs through late adolescence and on into adulthood.

The adolescent may have made a shift from close ties with parents and grade school friends to another set of friends or a rapidly changing grouping of new friends as part of trying out new ideas and interests. The parents may be having troubled reactions to their teenager's sexuality stemming from envy and jealousy as well as displaced feelings about the youngster separating from them. The youngsters have questions about their value in relation to the opposite sex, how to establish themselves vocationally, or what they will do with their lives. The

143

youngster has to develop and mature, drop off unnecessary baggage, and accommodate to feelings of potentially being able to achieve heretofore hidden or forbidden wishes. The ego has to mediate between these and the available resources for achieving such goals. The teen's superego has to reorganize in the face of these inner and outer needs. What was formerly forbidden is now becoming a subtle demand on the part of adults urging him, at times unflatteringly, to get his act together.

Sexuality

Sarrel and Sarrel (1990) pointed out that even college students with very high SAT scores have misinformed notions and much anxiety about sexual functioning. This lack of knowledge enables youngsters to use denial instead of protecting themselves against an unwanted pregnancy.

A recent study (Grace, Emans, and Woods 1989) found that 26 percent of heterosexual AIDS patients were women, one-third of whom may have been exposed to HIV during adolescence. Ninety-four percent of the nineteen to twenty-five-year-old women were sexually active. Among their sexual partners, only 28 percent used condoms, and the women had no perceived need for the use of condoms in spite of the AIDS issue. This again highlights the use of denial in sexual functioning.

Currently, about 50 percent of all adolescent females have had sexual intercourse by age nineteen. Adolescents are less likely to seek medical treatment when early signs of sexually transmitted diseases are present (Sanfilippo 1990). Pelvic inflammatory disease (PID) is ten times more likely to occur in adolescent females than in twenty-four-year-olds, and about one in eight sexually active adolescent girls will contract PID. Among a group of hospitalized teenagers with PID, of whom 20 percent had a pelvic abscess, Cromer, Brandstaetter, Fischer, and Brown (1990) found that those with a tubo-ovarian abscess had more than two months of abdominal pain while those with PID had the pain for less than two weeks before hospitalization. These observations again emphasize the significant denial utilized by adolescents in health care and sexuality, which may relate to their sense of omnipotence.

Education and Vocation

Among the educational issues is the question of the adequacy of the preparation for a vocation and the youngsters' alacrity in choosing an educational or vocational path. Education may be prolonged for some to avoid the issue of independence, commitment to an ideal, military service (in times of national crisis), or as part of their late adolescent omnipotentiality (Pumpian-Mindlin 1965).

In late adolescence, there are also anxieties about really being independent and self-sufficient. Along with this come the attendant concerns about actual ability, self-esteem, making the correct vocational choice, and preparation for the long term. The accompanying emotions are a fear of failure and rejection.

Incidence of Psychiatric Difficulties

Despite appearing well emotionally, about 10 percent of late adolescents are not acceptable for induction into military service. Seven to ten percent of the inductees are discharged in recruit training, and 5–10 percent are discharged after completing recruit training. Even so, a large number, perhaps 7–10 percent, are later discharged because of various psychiatric diagnoses. Many of these eventually become Veteran's Administration patients, helping make that system the largest in the country.

In most four-year colleges and in many junior colleges, there are psychiatric outpatient services available to the students. This has come about especially in the past three or four decades. Since 1980, at the McLean Hospital, 30 percent of the patients seen were between the ages of twenty and thirty. This is the largest group of any by a single decade age span (Grob and Eisen 1989).

According to Regier, Boyd, Burke, et al. (1988), the current one-month prevalence rate of mental disorders in the United States for the age group eighteen to twenty-four, inclusive, was abundantly represented. Except for ages eighteen to twenty-four, men and women had the same total rates of mental disorder, with 16.5 and 17.3 percent, respectively. These statistics are higher than the generally accepted figure that 15 percent of youths need psychiatric treatment. Substance abuse rates for this age group were 9.3 percent in males and 4.5 percent in females. The rate of affective disorders in this group was 5.1 percent for females and 4.5 percent for males. Again, it is obvious that young adults, or late adolescents, constitute a large population requiring psychiatric care.

Psychotherapy Aspects

In psychiatric training programs, the older adolescent group of patients is usually seen during general psychiatry training. Even in programs where residents rotate through college mental health services, the patients aged eighteen to twenty-five are generally not seen by the child-adolescent trainees. This serves to obfuscate this group as having special developmental and emotional characteristics and thereby requiring some particular consideration for their treatment needs.

In the psychiatric assessment of a young adult, developmental status has to be considered along with the biological. Is growth continuing? Are there reactions connected with body image and physical changes, hormonal aspects, and emotional issues? What are the family relations? What is the educational status? Is there a learning disability? What are the vocational pursuits and goals? What is going on in terms of reactions to losses and changes? How much separation anxiety is there behind some of these phenomena? Is the youngster pregnant? Is all this normative, or is this an adjustment reaction related to some special stress? Those are some of the many important issues to be considered on first meeting the late adolescent.

In treatment, or even during the evaluation stage, there may be shifts from the initial position, and pain and regression may show up. For example, the youngster may feel comfortable in the first session, but in the second there may be some unanticipated reaction because he or she had been at a higher level of functioning the previous day. Now there has been a shift to some earlier level of functioning, which raises the question as to whether the youngster is sicker than the initial impression or more open to seeking help.

Excessive weight may be given erroneously to an adolescent's poor judgment in a particular piece of behavior as evidence of a severe psychiatric disorder. However, the deficient judgment should be clarified for the situation since it may not be global and routine but due to such factors as inexperience, inability to understand the consequences, impulsivity, drug effects, or denial, and it should not be used alone as the basis for a diagnosis.

It is always necessary to assess the possibility of substance abuse. For this, clarification is required about the amount relied on to make it through each day, whether usage is experimental or a long-standing pattern of behavior, and whether it is a means of self-medicating for schizophrenia, bipolar disorder, an eating disorder, severe character pathology, or borderline personality disorder.

Separation anxiety reactions are encountered when youngsters leave home to go to college, work, or the military. Many of these are mild and self-limited reactions and remit in short order. However, with some, the symptoms may be the first manifestation of more serious psychiatric disorders. Older adolescents begin to implement decisions that may have been made or were in the making years before. Marked delay in taking these steps, such as choosing long-term goals, career, and friends, may signify an underlying identity disorder. The presence of this diagnosis in DSM-III-R (American Psychiatric Association 1989) indicates a broader awareness on the part of the psychiatric profession of such adolescent difficulties and affirms Erikson's (1959) view that identity diffusion reflects a failure in development, that is, pathology.

Ritvo (1976) said that the older adolescent who comes in for analysis usually has had a prolonged, difficult struggle over developing psychological independence from his parents. This dynamic will play a central theme in the transference from the outset. It will also become a major focus for resistance, whereby the adolescent will be shunning or denying any dependence on the analyst, at the same time seeing the analyst as a new and more powerful ally than his parents in his search for independence. According to recent developments in the theory of female development (Miller 1976; Freidin 1986), I would suggest that Ritvo's remarks would apply even more to the girl than the boy, and we see more late adolescent girls than boys with this as a major feature of their complaints.

Freidin (1986) suggests that, with depressed females, the issues of helplessness and dependency needs should be viewed as resistance and worked through, but additionally the therapist needs to validate the woman's wish to care for others. This involves validating the woman's capacities and wishes to do for others and reassurance that the "relational ties will not necessarily be broken by the achievement of action or pleasure." The therapist also needs to support the woman's wish to remain single or have no children if she desires.

Most writings on the treatment of adolescents do not distinguish the early, middle, or late stages from one another. The late adolescent should be treated as an adult with a similar diagnosis, but the therapist must keep in mind that adolescent development is still incomplete. Even if this development is nonconflicted, it may contribute to difficulties in treatment unless the therapist is prepared to see some regression (or even major regression during the session) and dependency vacillation with less consolidation of object relations, values, and character than with adults. By contrasting this state with the expectations in treating an early or mid-adolescent, the therapist will be better able to appreciate the late adolescent's proximity to adulthood.

Although the tasks of this stage are commitment and fidelity (Erikson 1950), these are not accomplished in lockstep fashion by a particular age. If these attainments are viewed as a process with variations that include delay, inhibition, or avoidance, the therapist may have a more suitable perspective than if the absence of a commitment is always taken for granted as pathology (Pumpian-Mindlin 1965).

When there is a shift of influence from the superego to the ego, the ego reacts more intensely to the dystonic elements with anxiety symptoms and worries about the future. Often this is the starting point for the late adolescent coming into treatment. Late adolescents, even with parents paying the fee, usually come in for treatment on their own, unless they are so disorganized that they have to be brought in by others. Even with their newfound legal status, the request for help is based on their giving up some of their omnipotence (which is difficult) and then asking the parents to pay for it. The following case illustrates some issues related to this.

CASE EXAMPLE 1

A college student who felt that his father (who paid for the therapy) was intrusive and controlling (with detailed inquiries about his daily activities, although a thousand miles away) related the father's request to meet me to discuss the treatment (cause of illness, progress, etc.). His therapy was stalemated as he ambivalently avoided providing me with the necessary authorization to relate anything to, or meet with, his father but worried that father would carry out his threat not to pay the fees unless he could speak with me. Meanwhile, he avoided and resisted in treatment since he feared any disclosure would be revealed to the father. Eventually, he decided not to grant authorization to discuss anything with his father and continued in treatment by developing a resourceful program to pay his own fees. Thus, he did not compromise his therapy and was able to maintain autonomy.

The late adolescent, although much more advanced in psychic structure and function than he was in the preceding stages, may shift abruptly from being engaged in therapy to feeling "it's a waste" or becoming silent. In many situations, the therapist is viewed as a real object, unlike the parents.

Positive and negative transference manifestations occur often and unexpectedly during therapy with this age group, but attitudes are not as clear or involved as they are with adult patients. Feelings toward the therapist may shift abruptly, particularly due to the fear of fusion, incestuous ties, or loss of impulse control. These features may make it difficult to identify the issue as transference. Although late adolescents have a transference situation somewhat similar to that of adults (Sklansky 1972), they typically are, "for long stretches of time, only intermittently involved in the analytic process via transference" (Blos 1980a). Transference interpretations should therefore be utilized cautiously, to avoid therapeutic blocking resistance.

The ability of most youths to free associate is limited since such efforts may lead them to feel a loss of emotional control. Thus, their talk, which may be lengthy and free, will not be of the same quality as adult free associations. This is particularly the case with dream material. Although acting out has usually diminished by young adulthood, it is still encountered and is best viewed as an adolescent phase-specific form of communication rather than just drive discharge (Blos 1980a). Most therapy with late adolescents will be more psychoanalytically oriented and less intensive than classic psychoanalysis, with much of the material focused on the immediate situation, but the principles mentioned may serve the therapist well in the endeavor.

Those youngsters who leave therapy on moving to an out-of-town college often have an immediate upsurge of separation anxiety and seek treatment soon after arriving at college. However, the initial treatment efforts may need to deal with the anxiety about separation from the previous therapist rather than the parents. If this is overlooked and not interpreted, the patient may feel misunderstood and change therapists abruptly.

The typical college schedule, with summer and other holidays, often limits the treatment to intermittent working periods. Once a therapeutic alliance is established, these interruptions may lead to a great deal of emphasis on separation issues. These need attention but should not obscure other treatment issues.

In treating late adolescents, the relationship of the therapist with the family is a variable. Depending on the degree of disorganization present, the parents may be involved in the history taking, family therapy, compliance with medication, or commitment, as indicated. Where the youngster is at the neurotic end of the spectrum, the parents may have only phone contact with the psychiatrist, and the treatment may proceed satisfactorily without their direct involvement.

Inpatient Treatment

Grob and Eisen (1989) presented nine variables that were predictors of good outcome in the treatment of late adolescents in hospitals. These include the quality of the educational level of the patient, a diagnosis of bipolar disorder rather than schizophrenia, alliance with the therapist on admission, the patient's level of work functioning prior to admission, and the patient's family's alliance with treatment early in hospitalization. Negative predictors were history of suicide attempt by the mother, a second diagnosis from Axis I, the early onset of psychiatric symptoms, and a diagnosis of personality disorder.

The importance of the family alliance in the treatment program is worth emphasizing. If there is an Axis I diagnosis, the patient may need regular parental involvement with the parents included in family therapy, as the following case illustrates.

CASE EXAMPLE 2

Following the accidental death of a close friend, a college student became depressed, angry, and disorganized and threatened violence. Initially, this appeared to be a reaction to the loss of his friend since the targets of his anger were the individual who caused the death and the authorities, who were perceived as not punishing this person properly. After the patient was hospitalized and diagnosed as having a manic disorder, he refused pharmacotherapy. However, with repeated limit setting, reassurance, and support from his parents, he accepted medication and improved. The parents continued to be regularly involved with his treatment after discharge because his variable compliance with medication required their monitoring his lithium intake, arranging for the routine blood levels, and continuing with family therapy. The omnipotence of a manic patient was combined here with that of adolescence and his wish for autonomy to interfere in therapy. Without the parents' partially compromising his autonomy, therapy probably would not have been initiated or, if initiated, successful.

Optimally, the inpatient treatment of the late adolescent should be on a unit separate from the early and mid-adolescent owing to disparate developmental and functional levels. This need has led to the development of a special unit at some hospitals for those age eighteen to twenty-five. Here they may attend school at their own level and have their own program in recreation, activities, and outings that can be totally different from those of the younger adolescents or adults, with more focus in their group meetings on their particular developmental issues.

CASE EXAMPLE 3

After an almost lethal suicide attempt, a substance-abusing college freshman who was admitted to a psychiatric hospital of the family's choice was discovered to continue abusing substances (which were easily available) on the unit. Since the unit, geared to adults for short-term stays, was nonsupportive of his developmental and therapeutic needs, the patient was transferred to another hospital with a suitable unit for young adults. Limit setting then ended his substance abuse in the hospital, and he became more involved in individual, family, and milieu therapy and also considered further academic pursuits. With the assistance provided by the hospital teaching staff, he was able to resume his studies, and on discharge he was not behind in his classwork.

On the other hand, does a patient who turns eighteen in the hospital remain on the adolescent unit or transfer to the young adult unit? One such patient remained in the adolescent unit because she had been there for a while before her eighteenth birthday and she was now in the termination phase of her hospital therapy. As she progressed toward discharge, she enjoyed her status doubly—as a terminating patient and as a healthier big sister who could be genuinely helpful and offer support to the other patients. Her successful discharge was aided by the added self-esteem gained from her supportive efforts.

Conclusions

This chapter focuses on selected aspects of late adolescence in an attempt to provide some cohesion in addressing these patients' needs. The separate of late adolescence from adulthood and mid-adolescence is beset with difficulties from the biological beginning and end points, as well as the sociological views. An emphasis on the developmental tasks and changes in psychic structure in late adolescence provides a more cogent presentation of the youngster's status. The difference in paths for the female and the male are highlighted. The period may best be conceptualized as being on the road to maturity.

The parents' contribution to the adolescent's progress is stressed. The large number of late adolescents requiring psychiatric assessment and treatment are cataloged. Some particular considerations in approaches to their assessment and treatment needs are suggested for outpatients and inpatients.

REFERENCES

Adatto, C. 1958. Ego integration observed in analysis of late adolescents. *International Journal of Psycho-Analysis* 39:172–177.

American Psychiatric Association. 1987. *Diagnostic and Statistical Manual of Mental Disorders.* 3d ed., rev. Washington, D.C.: American Psychiatric Press.

Aries, P. 1962. *Centuries of Childhood.* New York: Knopf.

Arnstein, R. L. 1984. Young adulthood: stages of maturity. In D. Offer and M. Sabshin, eds. *Normality and the Life Cycle.* New York: Basic.

Blos, P. 1962. *On Adolescence: A Psychoanalytic Interpretation.* New York: Free Press.

Blos, P. 1979. *The Adolescent Passage.* New York: International Universities Press.

Blos, P. 1980a. The life cycle as indicated by the nature of the transference in the psychoanalysis of adolescents. *International Journal of Psycho-Analysis* 61:145–151.

Blos, P. 1980b. Modifications in the traditional psychoanalytic theory of female adolescent development. *Adolescent Psychiatry* 8:8–24.

Boyd, W. W. 1943. *Textbook of Pathology*. Philadelphia: Lea & Febiger.

Buhler, C. 1968. The course of human life as psychological problem. *Human Development* 11:184–200.

Cromer, B. A.; Brandstaetter, L. A.; Fischer, R. A.; and Brown, R. T. 1990. Tubo-ovarian abscess in adolescents. *Adolescent and Pediatric Gynecology* 3:21–24.

Erikson, E. H. 1950. *Childhood and Society*. New York: Norton.

Erikson, E. H. 1959. *Identity and the Life Cycle*. New York: International Universities Press.

Freidin, M. 1986. Depression in women. Paper presented at Mount Auburn Hospital, Cambridge, Mass., May 6.

Freud, S. 1914. On narcissism: an introduction. *Standard Edition* 14:73–102. London: Hogarth, 1968.

Gilligan, C. 1982. *In a Different Voice: Psychological Theory and Women's Development*. New York: Harper & Row.

Grace, E.; Emans, S. J.; and Woods, E. R. 1989. The impact of AIDS awareness on the adolescent female. *Adolescent and Pediatric Gynecology* 2:40–42.

Grob, M. C., and Eisen, S. V. 1989. Most likely to succeed: correlates of good versus poor hospital outcome in young adult inpatients. *Psychiatric Hospital* 20:23–30.

Guntrip, H. A. 1973. Young adult: 18 to 30 years—personality. In R. R. Sears and S. S. Feldman, eds. *The Seven Ages of Man*. Los Altos, Calif.: Kaufman.

Jacobson, E. 1964. *The Self and the Object World*. New York: International Universities Press.

Levinson, D. J.; Darrow, C. N.; Klein, E. B.; Levinson, M. A.; and McKee, B. 1978. *The Seasons of a Man's Life*. New York: Ballantine.

Marshall, W. A. 1973. Young adult: 18 to 30 years—the body. In R. R. Sears and S. S. Feldman, eds. *The Seven Ages of Man*. Los Altos, Calif.: Kaufman.

Miller, J. B. 1976. *Toward a New Psychology of Women.* Boston: Beacon.

Modell, J.; Furstenberg, F. F.; and Hershberg, T. 1976. Social change and transitions to adulthood in historical perspective. *Journal of Family History* 1:7–34.

Muslin, H. 1979. The superego in the adolescent female. In M. Sugar, ed. *Female Adolescent Development.* New York: Brunner/Mazel.

Neugarten, B. L. 1969. Continuities and discontinuities of psychological issues in adult life. *Human Development* 12:121–130.

Offer, D., and Sabshin, M. 1984. *Normality and the Life Cycle.* New York: Basic.

Pearson, G. H. J. 1951. *Emotional Disorders of Children.* London: Allen & Unwin.

Piaget, J. 1972. Intellectual evolution from adolescence to adulthood. *Human Development* 15:1–12.

Pumpian-Mindlin, E. 1965. Omnipotentiality, youth, and commitment. *Journal of the American Academy of Child Psychiatry* 4:1–18.

Regier, D. A.; Boyd, J. H.; Burke, J. D.; Rae, D. S.; Myers, J. K.; Kramer, M.; Robins, L. N.; George, L. K.; Karno, M.; and Locke, B. Z. 1988. One-month prevalence of mental disorders in the United States. *Archives of General Psychiatry* 45:977–986.

Rest, J. D.; Davison, M. L.; and Robbins, S. 1978. Age trends in judging moral issues: a review of cross-sectional studies of the defining issues test. *Child Development* 49:263–279.

Ritvo, S. 1971. Late adolescence. *Psychoanalytic Study of the Child* 26:241–263.

Ritvo, S. 1976. Adolescent to woman. *Journal of the American Psychoanalytic Association* 24(suppl.): 127–137.

Sanfilippo, J. S. 1990. Editors workshop. *Adolescent and Pediatric Gynecology* 3:1–2.

Sarrel, L. J., and Sarrel, P. M. 1990. Sexual unfolding in adolescents. In M. Sugar, ed. *Atypical Adolescence and Sexuality.* New York: Norton.

Settlage, C. 1972. Cultural values of the superego in late adolescence. *Journal of the American Psychoanalytic Association* 27:74–92.

Shanok, S. S., and Lewis, D. O. 1981. Medical histories of female delinquents. *Archives of General Psychiatry* 38:211–213.

Sklansky, M. A. 1972. Indications and contraindications for the psychoanalysis of the adolescent: panel report. *Journal of the American Psychoanalytic Association* 20:134–144.

Sugar, M. 1968. Normal adolescent mourning. *American Journal of Psychotherapy* 22:258–269.

Sugar, M. 1990. Developmental anxieties in adolescence. *Adolescent Psychiatry* 17:385–403.

Tanner, J. M. 1978. *Fetus into Man*. Cambridge, Mass.: Harvard University Press.

Vaillant, G. 1977. *Adaptation to Life*. Boston: Little, Brown.

Whitney, D. W., ed. 1899. *The Century Dictionary*. New York: Century Co.

10 INDIVIDUATION IN A COLLECTIVE COMMUNITY

HADAS WISEMAN AND AMIA LIEBLICH

The attainment of ego identity, according to Erikson (1968), implies a sense of meaning in relation to the social world. Thus, identity must be based on an implicit mutual contract between the individual and society. The mutuality between self and society may take on a special meaning in the context of communal life.

The Israeli kibbutz being, at present, one of the most established and well-documented forms of communal life (see Bettelheim 1969; Blasi 1978; Lieblich 1981; Rabin and Beit-Hallahmi 1982; Rosner 1981; Spiro 1958, 1972; Talmon-Garber 1972), it provides a unique setting to study the process of identity formation. Founded in Israel in the beginning of the century, the kibbutz is a rural collective of several hundred members, based on the principles of full equality and cooperation. All income-producing branches are owned jointly by the collective, which, in return for the member's work, provides total care to the individual, for example, common eating facilities as well as all other personal services, health, and education. The oldest kibbutzim (plural of "kibbutz") now have four generations of members and a long, accumulated experience in communal child raising, which has probably been the most innovative feature of the kibbutz life-style.

We would like to thank Dr. Michael Nathan of the Institute of Research on Kibbutz Education, Oranim, for facilitating this research; the Institute for Study and Research of the Kibbutz and Cooperative Idea, University of Haifa, and the kibbutzim that participated, for their cooperation; and the Sturman Centre for Human Development, Hebrew University of Jerusalem, for financial support. Thanks also go to Idit Michaeli, who meticulously transcribed the interview tapes. Finally, special thanks to the interviewees themselves, who so freely talked about their experiences.

Both social science reports and personal accounts indicate that the kibbutz of the late 1980s is at a crossroads (Shner 1986). The ideological aspect of life in the kibbutz and its social-political mission have lost much of their clarity and determination in the eyes both of its own members and of society at large. Many kibbutzim, which have been used to a high standard of living, now suffer from economic hardships, having accumulated large debts, and some are on the verge of financial crisis. While the kibbutz is grappling with various programs and attempts to implement structural changes, more than ever before many young kibbutz-born adults are choosing to leave and are making their way into urban life in Israel or abroad (Lieblich 1989a). While the mere fact of growing up in a collective justifies a study of the process of individuation of the kibbutz-raised individuals in its own right, the recent tendency to move out of the kibbutz at the transition to adulthood has raised additional interest in the process. At the core of the transition to adulthood we find the formation of identity, separation-individuation from family of origin, and attempts or choices concerning intimacy and career (see, e.g., Levinson, Darrow, Klein, Levinson, and McKee 1978). Some of the students in this field underline the importance of cultural context for this major transition (Lieblich 1989b), while others stress gender differences in the process (Josselson 1988a).

The present chapter explores specific features of the transition to adulthood in the context of the kibbutz. It attempts to present and understand the process of identity formation as it occurs in kibbutz-born and -raised young adults. However, the developmental process of the kibbutz child and adolescent is shaped not only by the system of the kibbutz but also by specific features of Israeli society around it. While the analysis of these combined influences is beyond the scope of the present work, one aspect of Israeli society in general is important to note, namely, that kibbutz-raised adolescents (like all other Israelis) are obliged to serve in the military between the ages of eighteen and twenty-one (Lieblich 1989b; Lieblich and Perlow 1988). A normative delay in the progression of the process of transition to adulthood therefore takes place. As a result, most Israelis in their twenties are dealing with dilemmas known to occupy late adolescents elsewhere. At the transition to adulthood, after completing his or her military service and the psychological process entailed, the kibbutz-raised young adult faces a major dilemma—whether to stay a member of the kibbutz or to start the path toward adulthood independently outside it. This decision-making process—which usually continues into the late twenties or early thirties, until the individual achieves full social adulthood—influences decisions about long-term occupational, familial, and communal roles, which unfold through a relatively fixed time schedule (see Dar 1989). However, only preliminary reports are presently available on the developmental process of the relevant age group in the kibbutz (Avrahami 1988; Zamir 1988). In this chapter, we set out to portray the mental world of kibbutz-raised young adults as they face this major decision and make their first steps toward its realization.

Two theoretical concepts seem relevant to our attempt to capture the essence of the transition to adulthood of the kibbutz-raised individual under the circumstances outlined, namely, the formation of identity (Erickson 1950, 1968) and separation-individuation (Blos 1967; Mahler, Pine, and Bergman 1975). According to Erikson's theory, the formation of identity occurs both in the core of the individual and in his or her communal culture. Since identity is concerned with values and beliefs, among other components, the ideological structure of one's environment becomes essential for the ego, and the stage of identity formation is one in which the individual is closest to his or her "historical day" (Erikson 1968). Similarly, the sociological conception of youth portrays this life stage as the time of maximal exposure of the individual to the myths and values of his or her culture (Eisenstadt 1962). For the kibbutz-raised individual, acceptance or rejection of the basic values of the commune is an essential aspect of identity formation. Since, for social-historical reasons, the ideology of the kibbutz has lost much of its stamina and clarity, and since the parents' generation is ambivalent about the kibbutz as a way of life, identity formation of kibbutz-raised young adults is complicated by the contradictions and conflicts of their social environment. Generally, if identity must be experienced in a social context in that it represents the individual's sense of what he or she stands for in the world (Josselson 1988b), the development of identity of kibbutz-raised young adults cannot be viewed out of the context of the kibbutz. How the individual views the kibbutz and its members, after being raised in the common education system and living in the collective for twenty years or more, becomes an integral part of his or her definition of the self at the transition to adulthood.

As the process of identity formation takes place, the young adult is involved with separation from the family of origin with the aim of emerging from the process as an autonomous person. Although this happens gradually, according to Blos (1967), the adolescent sharpens the boundaries of self as distinct from others, taking on responsibilities previously assumed by parents and other adults. On gaining autonomy from parents, a revision of the former relationship within the family takes place. This process, too, is different for kibbutz-raised youths. While children raised in regular urban families have strong ties with their family of origin as the major system in which the process of individuation takes place, children of the kibbutz have a completely different experience. Since biological parents and siblings do not live together in one home and parents do not provide all the daily care for infants or children, relationships within the family may be considered as relatively weaker or less significant for the growing child (Bettelheim 1969; Rabin 1965; Spiro 1958).[1] Growing up in a small commune, where all children are housed with their peers and families are responsible for fewer of the socialization tasks than are Western urban families, the kibbutz child develops within a system in which boundaries between the self and nonfamily others (peers) on the one hand and between the family (parents and siblings) and the total community on the other hand are blurred. Deep, meaningful relationships of kibbutz children encompass their peer group and caretakers, who may be viewed as a large, surrogate family, and the community, which is, as a whole, conceived of as "home." If attachment and separation are major developmental tasks, the kibbutz child, adolescent, and young adult have the whole community to attach to and separate from. A clarification of this process is meaningful both because of its unique psychological features and as a possible explanation for why so many young people at present choose to leave the kibbutz.

Method

SUBJECTS

The sample for this study consisted of forty-eight (twenty-four men and twenty-four women) kibbutz-born young adults. All interviewees were single and ranged in age from twenty to thirty (the mean age for men was 25.75, and for women it was 23.75). Of the forty-eight interviewees, twenty-two were "kibbutzniks" living in the kibbutz at the time of the interviews, and twenty-six were "leavers" living outside the kibbutz, whether formally still kibbutz members or not. The group of kibbutzniks consisted of two subgroups: thirteen interviewees were living in the kibbutz following their army service and before going out on leave of absence,[2] and the remaining nine were living in the kibbutz after having returned from a leave of absence. The mean age for the group of kibbutzniks was 25.36 for men and 22.19 for women. The group of leavers consisted of three subgroups: five were interviewees on leave of absence (in Israel), fifteen were students, and the remaining six were leavers (formally) working in the city. The mean age for the leavers group was 26.03 for men and 24.46 for women. All the interviewees were raised in the communal living arrangement. The kibbutzniks in the sample came from four different kibbutzim. Half the sample of leavers came from the sample kibbutzim, and the remaining half were from thirteen different kibbutzim across the country. According to their proportion in the total kibbutz population, about two-thirds of the total sample were interviewees born and raised in kibbutzim of the United Kibbutz Movement, and the remaining third were from the Kubbutz H'artzi.[3]

PROCEDURE

Semistructured interviews were conducted by a clinical psychologist (Wiseman). The interview focused on social networks and interpersonal relations of kibbutz-born, single young adults, a topic that will be presented separately. Some of the questions posed to the interviewees were as follows. (*a*) Please describe your network of friends? Who are your friends? Are they also kibbutzniks? How intimate are you with them? (*b*) When you were growing up, did you have a best friend? Do you have one now? (*c*) In time of crisis or distress, who would you turn to? (*d*) Could you tell me about periods in your life when you have felt lonely? Has your experience of loneliness in the kibbutz been different than in the city? Attitudes toward the kibbutz and perceptions of self and others were expressed more or less spontaneously throughout the interviews and provided the data for the present chapter.

The interviews with the kibbutzniks ($N = 22$) were all conducted in their kibbutzim. Leavers from these kibbutzim ($N = 13$) were contacted by mail, and those who responded were interviewed in their homes in the city. Additional leavers, all of whom were students ($N = 13$), were recruited by an announcement posted in the Hebrew University student newspaper and bulletin boards and were interviewed on campus. All interviewees signed a consent form.

The interviews were tape-recorded and later transcribed verbatim. All statements regarding the kibbutz were extracted, reviewed, and organized according to their contents. Recurring themes were pulled together, as agreed on by two judges. The findings will be presented in a qualitative manner, demonstrating the prevalent responses rather than counting utterances. Terms like "equal," "more," "less," "minority," and "majority" are used to indicate salient trends in the relative frequency of the different categories.

Results of the Content Analysis

Interviewees' statements regarding themselves vis-à-vis the kibbutz were categorized into three broad topics: their perceptions of the kibbutz community in which they were raised, of the adult members that belonged to the community, and of themselves. Statements about and attitudes toward the total community reflect the individual's conception or representation of the kibbutz as a physical-social environment. Clearly, the young adults who were interviewed could not refer to themselves without providing the background of the kibbutz, and this "background" permeates all their utterances on the different subjects that the interview dealt with. A second large unit in this inner representation is the members who inhabited the kibbutz. The interviewees seem to have generalized their experience of the individual members of the community into a stereotype of the adult kibbutz member, with the help of which, or against which, they characterize their own identity. Finally, the individual describes himself or herself along dimensions that relate or differentiate between the self and the kibbutz at large on the one hand and the stereotype of the members on the other hand. Following is a description of this tripartite representation, phrased, as much as possible, in the words and the styles of the statements that appeared repeatedly in the interviews.

The Tripartite Representation

1. ATTRIBUTES OF THE KIBBUTZ
AS AN ENVIRONMENT

Four characteristics of the kibbutz as a social ecology stand out from the interviews and appear repeatedly in the young adults' accounts. Security is seen predominantly as a positive attribute, control leans toward the negative, while ideology and opportunities are areas that give rise to mixed and ambivalent attitudes.

IDEOLOGY

Young adults characterize the kibbutz as a community with unique values and ideals, for example, communality of property and services and equality of members. Their position vis-à-vis the kibbutz idealism varies, however, a great deal. Some of the interviewees say, as did the previous generations of kibbutz members, that the kibbutz is a way and a belief that provides a system of values acceptable to them. Others are concerned with the process of change in which the ideals have been altered or disregarded in reality and are questioning the present values of the kibbutz and their relevance to either the needs of society or their individual goals. They say that the present aims of the kibbutz are not as clear cut as they used to be in the past or that there is a lack of continuity between the former ideals and life in the kibbutz as it is nowadays. At the other extreme are people who argue that the old-time ideology of the kibbutz has become meaningless, that the kibbutz of today is as materialistic as any capitalistic way of life, and that it is not a great honor to belong to a kibbutz anymore.

SECURITY

The kibbutz is considered by many of the kibbutz-raised young adults as providing them abundantly with security of different kinds. They say that the kibbutz is their home, and as such it is well organized, pretty, quiet, clean, healthy, and in harmony with nature. They feel that, whatever happens to a member, the kibbutz will take care of him or her. A member is sure to receive a place to live in, a job, and the best health care and can live without any financial worry.

There is no crime and no danger for children. Holidays are celebrated in a beautiful manner together by all.

Yet, within this representation of the kibbutz as a big, good, providing family, a minority of the interviewees said that the kibbutz is too big to enable personal warmth simultaneously with the satisfaction of basic needs. Some are even more extreme in saying that the kibbutz uses the individual members to fulfill collective needs, disregarding their own wishes, or even that it mistreated and abused them in various ways.

CONTROL

All kibbutz-raised young adults describe the kibbutz as exerting a great deal of control over the individual. Control is employed either formally or informally, intentionally or unintentionally. Having clear rules and regulations for every right and obligation of the kibbutz members produces a system of formal control, which is applied and sanctioned via the general assembly or the different committees of the kibbutz. One needs approval for every step, from taking a car on outside visits to applying for a study program at the university. Young adults describe the kibbutz as "square," heavy to move, difficult to change, rigid, and bureaucratic. Enforcing its rules and demands, the kibbutz makes a member take on many obligations for the fulfillment of its collective goals.

Informal control is applied through public opinion of the community, which the interviewees present as having too much weight. The kibbutz is described as lacking in privacy, a place where everybody knows everything about everyone. Gossip serves to reinforce public opinion and limit one's privacy. Pettiness is another feature of the system, keeping everybody well in line. Public opinion also functions by categorizing people and assigning them, from a very young age, an image that is almost impossible to change.

The outcome of all these devices of control, according to a consensus of the interviewees, is that total conformity is enforced and individual deviation from the norm punished. Yet, from the perspective of a minority of the respondents, control also has some positive aspects: everybody shares in an individual's happiness, in time of disaster one gets maximal support, and one may receive a lot of attention.

OPPORTUNITIES

The kibbutz is depicted by the respondents as providing or withholding opportunities for their growth, development, and actualization. On
a general level, the interviews include statements that present the kibbutz as challenging—or not challenging—as a life-style and a community, whether for all or particularly for the young generation. A few of
the interviewees make a distinction between their own kibbutz, which
is well established, "too big," and relatively old, thus depriving the
young of a sense of a new creation or of having an effect on it, and a
young kibbutz that they prefer because it may provide more opportunities for them. Some say that they can actualize themselves in their
kibbutz or in a kibbutz in general; however, the opposite claim is more
prevalent. On the negative side, one finds references to the routine
and boredom of kibbutz life, to the fact that nothing new seems to
happen in this small community and that life is prearranged for the
next twenty years or more.

More specifically, the interviewees refer to several areas of opportunities. In the work sphere, they say that the kibbutz cannot fulfill the
occupational aspirations of all its members because there will always
be a need for many workers to do simple services and maintenance
work. On the other hand, a small number of men report that they could
not have advanced as quickly and successfully at work in a larger
and more complex community. Concerning educational opportunities,
many individuals praise the kibbutz for the education it provides children, while several criticize it for encouraging conformity and mediocrity. Since it is an affluent society, they say that the kibbutz can support any study program and that its provides the opportunity to
combine studies, work, and family life. Several of the women interviewed depicted the kibbutz as not providing equal opportunities for
women, offering them a small number of occupational paths, especially
in education and services to the community. Finally, in the social area,
many young adults describe the kibbutz as offering too little for their
needs. The community is small, and one has few chances to meet new
people. Furthermore, it is a closed system, where all social circles
overlap: the people you grow up with are your only friends, and later
on your neighbors, the people you work with, raise your children with,
etc. Even when one is dissatisfied, one cannot move to a different
social circle. Unpopular children can never escape their role or place

in the children's society. One cannot avoid being with the same people all the time.

2. A STEREOTYPE OF THE KIBBUTZ MEMBER

General statements concerning the character of a kibbutz member appear frequently in the young adults' interviews. These so-called kibbutznik's traits taken together may be considered as a stereotype of the adult in the kibbutz from the point of view of the interviewed sample. It consists of two general areas: the kibbutz member is extremely familistic on the one hand and characterized by lack of self-actualization on the other.

FAMILY ORIENTEDNESS

The typical adult kibbutz member is seen as married and is a parent. Most of the respondents who were single at the time of the interview see the kibbutz as a community of families and believe that one cannot live there happily without a partner. Being single, or looking for a spouse, is the most common reason for leaving the kibbutz. On the other hand, many of the singles claim that they may consider returning to the kibbutz when married, given that their partners will agree. They believe the kibbutz is good for raising children.

FRUSTRATION

Kibbutz members who belong to the parents' generation are depicted as frustrated because they did not have the chance to develop their potential to its maximum. (In that, they differ from the grandparents' generation, whose creation of the kibbutz itself is conceived as a great act of self-actualization.) The kibbutz makes members give up many of their personal strivings for the sake of the collective goals. Moreover, it does not reward people differently according to their contribution to the kibbutz. Some work very hard, and all they get for it is more work and responsibility, while others are "parasites."

MEDIOCRITY AND NARROW-MINDEDNESS

The kibbutz is considered by many of the respondents as a retreat for mediocre people, people who could not make it in the free, competitive world outside. The ones who left admit that they feel superior to those who decided to remain in the kibbutz. The kibbutz member is depicted as "square," narrow-minded, and boring, a person who gives top priority to work and does not invest any energy in other interests or studies. He or she tries not to stand out in any way. The education provided by the kibbutz encourages mediocrity and produces individuals who do not strive for achievements, in spite of the fact that the kibbutz could have supported them in their pursuits.

INHIBITION

Kibbutz members, both children and adults, are described as inhibited by the collective system in both emotional expression and intellectual development. Emotionally, they are considered to be people who lack security and spontaneity, restricted in the expression of their inner feelings, lacking trust for each other, and afraid to change or go out of the kibbutz. They are socially closed, do not form deep friendships, and do not let newcomers join their social network. They are ascetic in their ways and do not tolerate too much happiness or contentment. Cognitively, they are described as anti-intellectuals, people who despise pure intellectual pursuits, do not develop any hobbies or strong interests, and lack original, critical, or independent thinking.

INDIFFERENCE AND PASSIVITY

People in the kibbutz, according to this perception, care not for each other but only for themselves. A member of the kibbutz can live in it with minimal efforts, without any struggle. People in the kibbutz think that they deserve to get everything from the collective.

3. CHARACTERIZATION OF SELF

The self-image presented is portrayed against the communal picture on the one hand and the stereotype of the members on the other. It is described mostly as rebelling against or accepting the setting of the group and differentiating oneself from the nonself as summarized in the members' stereotype. Following are the major features of the depicted self-image.

ATTACHMENT VERUS RESENTMENT

Most of the interviewees described themselves as attached to or resentful of the kibbutz. Many say that they love the kibbutz, that they feel good there or feel a great pain at having decided to leave it. On the other hand, about the same number of people say that they feel bad in the kibbutz, that they dislike or resent the kibbutz and its society, and that it does not fit their personality. Most extreme are individuals who claim that their kibbutz is bad or that they do not mind if it disappears. A few admit to having ambivalent feelings, both love and resentment toward the kibbutz.

NEED FOR SEPARATION

Many of the interviewees relate the fact that a large number of their peers have already left the kibbutz or plan to leave, that they are presently lonely in the kibutz, and that therefore they feel they should go elsewhere too. Some say that leaving the kibbutz is the present norm for the young; they therefore plan to leave or have left. Some justify their step by saying that most young people tend to move out of their homes into different places or societies. They claim that they experienced too much family pressure in the kibbutz and felt the need to separate from their family.

NEED FOR EXPERIMENTATION

Several people reported that the kibbutz pushed them into responsible positions too early, before they were ready to settle down. They preferred more stimulation and challenges than were offered by the kibbutz. They loved the "action" in the city. A great number of respondents said that they simply want to try different life-styles.

NEED FOR AUTONOMY

People tended to describe how oppressed and suffocated they felt in the kibbutz, owing to the pressure, control, and constant criticism. They want freedom, rather than being told what to do all the time. They refuse to accept the fact that their life would be run by people less worthy than themselves or that they are expected to work every day. They strive for independence, making their own decisions, making money, and spending it as they wish. They strive to buy things, to own a car, a home of their own. They want to have entertainment, travel, or studies according to their own plans and earnings.

GUILT

Guilt feelings in the context of the values of the kibbutz, the general community, and most often the family are the major factors mentioned in preventing one from leaving the kibbutz. Several of the interviewees said that they feel guilty for leaving the kibbutz and feel like traitors when they come back to visit. Others seem to have recovered from this feeling and claim that they are presently free of guilt regarding their decision to live outside the kibbutz.

Case Example

Following is an excerpt from one of the interviews that is rather typical and in which the tripartite representation (i.e., kibbutz environment, stereotype of the kibbutznik, and self) is depicted.

INTERVIEWEE 8

The interviewee was a kibbutz-born male, age twenty-six. After one year of volunteering, he was an officer in the army and served for four and a half years. He returned to his kibbutz for about a year, went abroad for close to two years, and during this extended stay abroad officially left the kibbutz. He returned to Israel and is currently studying in Jerusalem:

I love my kibbutz very much, I adore the beauty of the place, and I feel good there. Despite that, I think that right now it is not the place for me. I feel connected to every cotton field and to every piece of landscape, but, on the other hand, when I was there after the army, not as a child, and lived more the real life of the kibbutz, I felt it was very heavy for me and very predictable. When I came back from the army, I had a real fall in the ideological area. What I took in the past for ideology I suddenly saw as pettiness, and I began to feel repelled by it. The idea that in the kibbutz I can say today what I will be doing in the next twenty years and who, more or less, are the people that I will know and that I cannot expect anything new—that really scared me. So I said to myself that I want to go to study immediately after I return from abroad so as not to feel an obligation toward the kibbutz that might interfere with my ability to choose freely.

In New York, I came to the conclusion that I am not a country mouse but more of a city mouse. I loved the endless stimulation of the people and the challenges, the cultural richness and variety. I enjoyed the fact that you cannot know what the next day will bring, the freedom—I decide for myself, I'm my own master. I have lived with many slogans in life—Zionism and socialism. I was sure it was all part of me. When I lived in the kibbutz, I took these things for granted and didn't examine them in depth. When I was in New York, I changed my views on many things and came to the conclusion that the basic question is what is good for me. The main justification in life should be people's happiness rather than big words like Zionism or kibbutz. When I was in the kibbutz I was at the opposite extreme—it was clear to me that I would compromise my own needs rather than those of the collective. Today I think that I lost a lot of things because of that. For example, I didn't develop any hobbies because I wanted to be with my peers. Playing the piano means being alone, but it's not worth it, and so I played basketball instead. I regret that now because I think I was capable and I'm musically talented.

In the future, I may return to the kibbutz; it will depend on what my partner may want. But I'm afraid to be in the position in which I'll feel that I returned because of failure, because the kibbutz is a very secure system. It may so happen that, if reality hits me in the face and I see that what I aspire for isn't working out, I may actually want the security that the kibbutz provides. As I see things now, I will return to the kibbutz only if I don't succeed in actualizing my aspirations in the economic and social sense. It happens to a lot of people that they realize that their fantasies were just fantasies and reality is different. Right now, I don't know where I will live in the future. It is good, yet perhaps somewhat unsettling.

I think people should live where they feel good. But, if the end of my kibbutz will come, it will be very painful for me to see the

169

place falling apart. The kibbutz needs to change—to provide more place for individualism. There is a sense of a certain mediocrity in the kibbutz, as if those who stay are the ones with fewer personal aspirations. I personally don't feel any superiority over those who stay, but there is something of that.

Aside from that, people of my age who stay in the kibbutz are all married; all the singles left. Singles are afraid to stay in the kibbutz with such a scarcity of social opportunities, so they leave.

Comparison between Kibbutzniks and Leavers

Following the content analysis of the total sample of the interviewees' statements, the next step was to review the statements regarding the tripartite representation by subgroups. Two comparisons were made, namely, kibbutzniks versus leavers and men versus women.

Regarding the kibbutz as an environment, kibbutzniks and leavers share a similar perception, with a few interesting differences. In referring to ideology, there are more kibbutzniks who say that the kibbutz is a way of life and a belief, that it provides a system of values that they accept. Yet many kibbutzniks, no less than leavers, view the ideology as meaningless today and share the view that the kibbutz is not what it used to be or that the kibbutz is too materialistic. More kibbutzniks mentioned that the kibbutz was pretty, calm, and part of nature, but they were also concerned by the kibbutz being too big. Probably owing to their exposure to city life, only leavers, with the exception of one kibbutznik who had already experienced city life, indicated the lack of economic difficulties that the individual in a kibbutz enjoys as an important aspect of the security offered by life in the kibbutz. In the area of control, both the kibbutzniks and the leavers seem to be occupied by the formal as well as the informal aspects of control and are particularly concerned with the lack of privacy. The leavers and those who have already been outside the kibbutz seem to express their criticism over the informal control in more extreme words, such as the statement that the kibbutz demands total conformity and will kick you out if you are different. Further, the leavers and a few of the kibbutzniks, after leaves of absence, state that the kibbutz imposes a label on you that is impossible to change. As we shall see later, this opinion is related to their greater concern with issues of separation and autonomy.

With regard to the stereotype of the kibbutz member, again the kibbutzniks and the leavers had rather similar views. Interviewees from both groups viewed the kibbutz as family oriented, but more leavers emphasized that one could not live in the kibbutz without a partner. The negative characteristics of frustration, indifference, and passivity were also mentioned equally often by kibbutzniks and leavers. The kibbutzniks, however, were more concerned by frustration in the area of work due to the lack of different reinforcement. Two negative attributes that were much more predominant in the leavers' statements referred to inhibition and mediocrity. Interestingly, only leavers, and a few interviewees from the kibbutz after a leave of absence, raised the issue of inhibition in emotional expression and in intellectual development. Although kibbutzniks shared the criticism of leavers that kibbutz education encourages mediocrity, more leavers referred to this characteristic; they made harsh statements such as, "A kibbutz is a retreat for mediocre people," and they viewed members as "square, narrow-minded, and boring." Also, as one might expect, only leavers made statements to the effect of feeling superior to the members who stayed and view leavers who return to the kibbutz as failures.

The topic that most differentiates the kibbutzniks from the leavers is that of characterization of self. First, regarding attachment versus resentment, as could be expected, kibbutzniks are the ones who state that they feel good in the kibbutz and love the place. In contrast, the leavers dislike the kibbutz and are the ones who feel that it does not fit their personality. However, just as many kibbutzniks as leavers stated that they dislike kibbutz members and are bothered by the inability to select the people they need to live with. With regard to the need for separation, although both kibbutzniks and leavers talked about the influence of peers leaving the kibbutz, only leavers expressed the strong need to separate from their family. The need to experiment and try different life-styles was expressed more by those living in the kibbutz. This was stated by kibbutzniks who were waiting to go out on leave of absence but also by kibbutzniks who had already experimented with life outside the kibbutz; apparently, they still felt that they had not exhausted this desire and had not yet unequivocally chosen the kibbutz as their way of life. Both kibbutzniks and leavers expressed a strong need for autonomy, but statements in this area were more often made by leavers and were more explicit. Leavers stated with great conviction that their independence is important to them and that they need freedom. Some described the feeling that the kibbutz was suffocating them.

Gender Differences

Examining the statements of the young men and women on the attributes of the kibbutz environment by gender, an interesting difference emerged. While more men made statements concerning ideology, more women referred to the dimension of security. Attitudes concerning control did not differentiate the genders, but, on the issue of opportunities, more women stated that the kibbutz could not fulfill the occupational aspirations of all its members. A related statement made only by women stressed the lack of equal opportunities for women in the kibbutz.

The stereotype of the kibbutz member was viewed in a very similar way by both genders. There were only a few subtle differences. More women viewed kibbutz members as personally frustrated. This might possibly be related to women's greater concern over lack of occupational opportunities and lack of gender equality. Second, only women stated that people are emotionally closed and that subgroups did not let you join in. Finally, more men raised the issue of the passivity of kibbutz life in that you could live in the kibbutz without any struggle.

The depicted self-image of the young men and women was remarkably similar. They did not differ in the expression of their need for separation or in their need to try different life-styles. Consistent with the lack of gender differences in viewing the kibbutz environment as controlling is the finding that, remarkably, both men and women expressed a strong need for autonomy. There was a tendency, however, for women to express this through their experience of pressure and criticism, while men expressed this need more in terms of not wanting to be told what to do. Although both male and female leavers admit feeling like a traitor, a clear expression of guilt feelings over leaving, or the possibility of leaving, was indicated only by women.

Discussion

The process of transition to adulthood can be viewed either from the perspective of the individual and his or her needs or from the point of view of the kibbutz, with its present-day dilemmas, and its place in and effect on the individual process. In what follows, we attempt to discuss the developmental stage in the context of the cultural-historical moment.

Most of the respondents' statements concerning their place in the kibbutz were represented by the tripartite division of kibbutz, others, and self. The kibbutz provides the cultural, social, and historical context for the development of the individual. It is characterized by the young adult as a way of life having—or lacking—a system of values that provides a degree of security and opportunities to its members and controls them, according to its historical ideology and structure. Some of the attributes of the kibbutz environment are positive, and some are negative, but its most outstanding feature seems to be its explicit, well-defined nature as a background for the growth and individuation process of its children. The interviews abound with references to the kibbutz as an ideological-social framework in which the individual's development takes place, providing values to adopt or rebel against. Thus, our data demonstrate Erikson's (1968) conviction that the communal culture and the individual identity are inseparably intertwined.

A generalized concept of others in the kibbutz appeared at the second head of the tripartite model. This common image, or stereotype, of the adult kibbutznik is, apparently, the most negative of the three parts of the total picture depicted here. The parental generation, which is referred to as adult members of the kibbutz, is presented as mediocre, narrow-minded, inhibited, and frustrated. Its only nonnegative characteristic is its family orientation, which can be interpreted as expressing warmth and nurturance on the one hand or as defense against extreme isolation and alienation of the kibbutz life-style on the other.

Why are the young so critical in their perception of their parents' generation—a rebellion much more common than in American youths today (Offer, Ostrov, and Howard 1981). Several explanations may be offered, but the most relevant one proposes that, since the kibbutz in its nature and structure controls many aspects of the individual's life, with obscure boundaries between self, peers, family, and the collective, young people need to invest extreme effort in separating from their psychological environment, to create a nonself against which they may define their own self. This argument is supported by the fact that the most outstanding self-characteristic from the perspective of the young kibbutz-raised adult is the need for autonomy and experimentation, indicating an active struggle to achieve freedom and private space. At an older age, after the formation of clearer personal boundaries and the creation of a new family unit, some of the negative aspects of the adults' stereotype may, therefore, change or even vanish.

The last part of the tripartite representation is the perception of the self, with its central dilemma of belonging and attachment on the one hand and individuation-separation on the other. A definition of self or identity seems to be the major concern of the young interviewees. One is amazed at Bettelheim's (1969) conclusion from his kibbutz research of twenty years ago: "Indeed, no further psychosocial crises are necessary beyond Erikson's fourth, that of industry versus inferiority. Since the fifth struggle, the one for a personal identity, would almost have to take the adolescent caught up in it away from the kibbutz, it is not pertinent for those who will stay. Nor can this crisis really develop. Those who fit into kibbutz life have no need to struggle for identity of a personal nature, since the community so largely defines it for them" (pp. 279–280). However, the kibbutz of the 1980s, with its greater permissiveness and flexibility as exemplified by the institutionalized year of absence, and with its own ambivalence about basic collective values, provides a fertile ground for the struggle toward identity.

The ingredients for the evolving identity of the young are taken from positive as well as negative instances and experiences of their lives in the kibbutz. Amazingly, young people who have decided to live in the kibbutz or to leave it resemble each other in many ways when referring to the description of the kibbutz, of others, and of themselves. The uniformity of statements regarding self and how different it is from the other adult kibbutz members reminds one of Erikson's (1968) observation that "the display [of youth] is really a declaration insisting on some positive identity not primarily based on the parental type of conformism or pretension. That such nonconformism, in turn, is a plea for fraternal confirmation and thus acquires a new ritualized character that is part of the paradox of all rebellious identity formation" (p. 28). While each one of the kibbutz youths interviewed is searching for identity in his or her individual manner, according to particular given life circumstances and potentials, the similarity of their background and upbringing provides a strong common denominator to the process.

As outlined, there are only a few differences between subgroups of kibbutz-raised individuals in their responses to the interview. People seem to be in different phases of the same process of testing and experimentation, and all care deeply for their autonomy. Indeed, even those who hope to live in the kibbutz emphasize the importance of making a free and informed choice about it rather than staying in the community out of no choice or inertia. Differences were found in that younger individuals have less elaborate opinions as compared to the relatively older respondents. People who have already spent a year of absence outside the kibbutz, whether in the city or abroad, develop more critical and complex attitudes and views. Thus, people who were interviewed while living in the kibbutz after some time outside resemble in many ways "leavers" rather than "members." In addition, the articulate responses of the students in the sample show that, as in other areas (Perry 1968), higher education seems to lend sophistication and depth to the elicited responses.

The central aspects, which were found to differentiate the kibbutzniks from the leavers, were focused around the self, indicating that the latter were more concerned with separation-individuation than the former, and this has probably determined their preference to live outside the kibbutz. On the other hand, the major difference between genders was found in describing the kibbutz as an environment by pointing to women's greater awareness of issues of security and men's more pronounced interest in ideology. This seems to be generally in line with the current theories about differences in men and women's self or identity (e.g., Gilligan 1982). However, gender differences were smaller than one might expect, taking into account the large research literature discussing the problematic status of kibbutz women. The fact that about the same ratio of women and men expressed their need for autonomy and freedom may be interpreted as an indication that, despite women's higher tendency to conform and greater need for security, the urge for separation-individuation that kibbutz-raised women experience in the transition to adulthood is so strong that it overshadows the more commonly found gender differences.

As mentioned earlier, kibbutz leaders are concerned with future membership of the third or fourth generation of the kibbutz born. In our sample, about half the interviewees were currently living out of the kibbutz, some with the intention of returning. On the other hand, of the people who were interviewed while living in the kibbutz, many were entertaining thoughts of leaving it temporarily or permanently in the near future. Only two of the total sample, both of them approaching thirty, declared convincingly that they saw their future in the kibbutz. As observed by other researchers too (Dar 1989), the twenty- to thirty-year-olds in the kibbutz seem, therefore, to be at a fluid state regarding their final decision to stay or not to stay in the kibbutz. Consequently, the mere fact of being now in the kibbutz was not found to be very significant in terms of the mental representation of self, others, and the community, only in the intensity or frequency of certain statements. This fluid state may be particularly characteristic of the singles (which was by definition the status of our sample). Many of the interviewees stated frankly that their future decision about life in or out of the kibbutz depended on the preference of their partner and the common agreement achieved by the couple unit. Interestingly for theories that claim that intimacy determines women's choices more than men's (Josselson 1988a; Miller 1976), the intention to postpone future decision until the establishment of a couple relationship appeared as frequently in the self-descriptions of women and men in our sample. While a study of married, kibbutz-raised individuals of similar ages may have resulted in a different picture, it is apparent, at least for the group under study, that the stage of moratorium (Erikson 1968), namely, of experimentation and nondecision, is prolonged well into the late twenties.

Our interview data strongly indicate that one of the major components of the conflict regarding future life in the kibbutz is the need to establish distance from the family and the community and to create private space so as to allow for the emergence of the adult, individuated self. In other words, we believe that the process of arriving at successful individuation under the circumstances of kibbutz socialization often demands physical separation from the family and the kibbutz community, at least for the critical period of the transition to adulthood (see also Zamir 1988). Separation from the nuclear family, which is the norm in other cultures, does not suffice in a collective community. This may explain the high rate of young leaving the kibbutz.

One may ask why this process did not occur as prominently before, namely, in the second generation. Historically, when the second generation of kibbutz members was brought up by their parents, the founders of the large and important kibbutzim (Lieblich 1981), the ideology of the kibbutz as a way of life and its mission for Israeli society were both very clear, thus counteracting the individual need to experiment in different life-styles and separate from home. However, social-historical developments have blurred the conviction in the kibbutz ideology and mission. In comparing the second-generation kibbutzniks to the third generation, Zamir reports that the latter identify with their parents' ideals to a much smaller extent than the former. In fact, her interviewees—as do some of ours—complain that their parents conveyed mixed messages, on the one hand wanting them to continue their way of life and on the other hand wishing them to have it easier than they had. Moreover, parents imply that perhaps today they would not have chosen the kibbutz way of life. Similar intergenerational processes would probably take place in groups or cultures undergoing secularization, liberalization, or other declines of well-defined ideological systems.

NOTES

1. Most kibbutzim have switched to family housing instead of the common sleeping arrangement, thus increasing physical closeness of the nuclear family and returning more functions of daily caretaking of children to their parents. However, all our interviewees were raised in the communal sleeping arrangement.

2. The opportunity to take a year's leave of absence from the kibbutz after at least a year of stay in the kibbutz following the return from the army has been legitimized by the kibbutz movement. The leave of absence most often includes travel abroad. Dar (1989) notes that, while in the more distant past few kibbutz youths opted for the leave of absence, in recent years it has become the general trend, and many kibbutz youths extend their leave to two or more years.

3. The United Kibbutz Movement (Takam) is the center kibbutz movement, closely aligned with the Israeli Labor Party (Ma'arach). The Kibbutz Ha-artzi is the left-wing kibbutz movement, closely aligned with the left-wing Mapam Party, and is considered more strict than the United Kibbutz Movement in its application of collective norms (e.g., the communal sleeping arrangement for children).

REFERENCES

Avrahami, A. 1988. The year of volunteering in kibbutz movement activities: A chapter in the socialization of the kibbutz-raised (in Hebrew). Preliminary report. Ramat Efal: Yad Tabenkin.

Bettelheim, B. 1969. *The Children of a Dream: Communal Childrearing and Its Implications for Society.* New York: Macmillan.

Blasi, J. 1978. *The Communal Future: The Kibbutz and the Utopian Dilemma.* Norwood, Pa.: Norwood.

Blos, P. 1967. The second individuation process of adolescence. *Psychoanalytic Study of the Child* 22:162–186.

Dar, Y. 1989. Youth in the kibbutz: the prolonged transition to adulthood. Hebrew University of Jerusalem. Typescript.

Eisenstadt, S. N. 1962. Archetypal patterns of youth. *Daedalus* 91(1): 28–46.

Erikson, E. H. 1950. *Childhood and Society.* New York: Norton.

Erikson, E. H. 1968. *Identity: Youth and Crisis.* New York: Norton.

Gilligan, C. 1982. *In a Different Voice: Psychological Theory and Women's Development.* Cambridge, Mass.: Harvard University Press.

Josselson, R. 1988a. *Finding Herself: Pathways to Identity Development in Women.* San Francisco: Jossey-Bass.

Josselson, R. 1988b. The embedded self: I and thou revisited. In D. Lapsley and C. Purcer, eds. *Self, Ego and Identity.* New York: Springer.

Levinson, D. J.; Darrow, C. N.; Klein, E. B.; Levinson, M. H.; and McKee, B. 1978. *The Seasons of a Man's Life.* New York: Knopf.

Lieblich, A. 1981. *Kibbutz Makom.* New York: Pantheon.

Lieblich, A. 1989a. Kibbutz Makom revisited (in Hebrew). *Davar,* May 9.

Lieblich, A. 1989b *Transition to Adulthood during Military Service: The Israeli Case.* Albany: State University of New York Press.

Lieblich, A., and Perlow, M. 1988. Transition to adulthood during military service. *Jerusalem Quarterly* 47:42–76.

Mahler, M. S.; Pine, F.; and Bergman, A. 1975. *The Psychological Birth of the Human Infant: Symbiosis and Individuation.* New York: Basic.

Miller, J. B. 1976. *Toward a New Psychology of Women.* Boston: Beacon.

Offer, D.; Ostrov, E.; and Howard, K. I. 1981. *The Adolescent: A Psychological Self-Portrait.* New York: Basic.

Perry, W. G., Jr. 1968. *Forms of Intellectual and Ethical Development in the College Years: A Scheme.* New York: Holt, Rinehart & Winston.

Rabin, A. I. 1965. *Growing Up in the Kibbutz*. New York: Springer.

Rabin, A. I., and Beit-Hallahmi, B. 1982. *Twenty Years Later: Kibbutz Children Grow Up*. New York: Springer.

Rosner, M. 1981. *The Changing Kibbutz Society: Recent Sociological Research, 1970–1980*. Cambridge, Mass.: Institute for Cooperative Community.

Shner, M. 1986. The kibbutz in transition from humanism to human totalitarism (in Hebrew). *Shdemot* 96:25–36.

Spiro, M. E. 1958. *Children of the Kibbutz*. Cambridge, Mass.: Harvard University Press.

Spiro, M. E. 1972. *Kibbutz: Venture in Utopia*. New York: Schocken.

Talmon-Garber, Y. 1972. *Family and Community in the Kibbutz*. Cambridge, Mass.: Harvard University Press.

Zamir, A. 1988. The development of leadership in kibbutz-raised and their involvement in activities (in Hebrew). Interim report. Ramat Efal: Yad Tabenkin.

11   BOARDING SCHOOL CONSULTATION: PSYCHOANALYTIC PERSPECTIVES

RICHARD M. GOTTLIEB

This chapter is primarily about boarding school and adolescence. In it I rely heavily on a single clinical illustration of psychotherapeutic work carried out in the boarding school setting. Since the boarding school experience has hardly been written about from a psychiatric perspective, I hope to convey the following two points. First, attendance at a boarding school can be profoundly important in an adolescent's life, and, should an adult patient have attended boarding school, the recovery of that experience in therapy may be quite important. Second, the decision as to the advisability of boarding school placement for a particular teenager is a complex one requiring careful assessment.

Let me state at the outset that I am an analyst and that I have approached this subject from a primarily psychoanalytic perspective. Necessarily, other points of view would emphasize other aspects of the subject.

Review and Synthesis of the Psychoanalytic Literature

Psychoanalysts have not written much about boarding school. In fact, I was not able to find anything that has been written that specifically and deliberately addresses the issue. "Boarding school" is not listed in any of the major psychoanalytic indices; with but two exceptions it does not appear in the contents of any of the great psychoana-

The author wishes to thank Drs. Eleanor Galenson, Aaron Esman, and the participants in Conference 408 of the New York Psychoanalytic Institute for their thoughtful comments on earlier versions of this manuscript.

lytic works on adolescence. Excepting one listing in a single issue of *The Psychoanalytic Study of the Child*, none of the major psychoanalytic journals includes "boarding school" in its contents or index.

Yet this is not apparently the case for analysts in their day-to-day clinical work. In conversation and correspondence (e.g., F. Baudry, 1989, personal communication; E. Galenson, 1986, personal communication), several have discussed boarding school with me and have indicated that they know of other analysts experienced with this clinical issue. The only written sources of clinical data, therefore, have come from reports of analytic work with adult patients who had attended boarding school as adolescents.

I believe that I have identified the first such report. This is a case of Freud's discussed in *The Interpretation of Dreams* (1900). Freud's patient was a young woman at the time of her analysis whose experiences at boarding school are not the main focus of his report. In fact, reading Strachey's English translation of this material, one would not suspect that the woman had ever attended a boarding school. Freud used her dreams and associations to illustrate his contention that the dream work makes use of so-called indifferent and innocent material to disguise deeper-lying sexual fantasies.

I found these little-cited pages worth dwelling on. Not only do they deal with the patient's boarding school experiences, but, notably, they also illustrate Freud's early awareness of important aspects of adolescent development. The analytic material, including the patient's manifest and latent dream thoughts, made repeated reference to the importance of her difficult adolescent development and to her boarding school experience, especially in relation to her then-evolving experience of her newly sexually mature body. Freud made clear his understanding of the importance of this developmental period in determining the dream's latent content. He wrote that "the interpretation of . . . [her] dream led us back at once to the time of her physical development at puberty, when she had begun to be dissatisfied by her figure" (1900, p. 186). It turned out that her dream of the broken candle was founded on recollections of her adolescence and of masturbation associated with her experience at boarding school.

The inference I draw from the analytic report is that this patient had been sexually assaulted during her early childhood. Her reactions to that experience had included a repudiation of her body—perhaps especially her genitalia—as "ugly" and "disgusting." Later, during her adolescence, she was again inclined to repudiate her sexually mature body, to fear repeated sexual assaults by men (as she did later on as an adult in her transference relationship to Freud), and to experience heightened conflicts over masturbation and other of her sexual urges.

Freud stressed that her adolescent development was a way station between her childhood trauma and her adult pathology, adumbrating what he was later to elaborate in the third section of the *Three Essays* (Freud 1905).

There is a handful of subsequent analytic reports in which boarding school experiences are mentioned, mostly in passing. A careful reading of these can convey the impression of an unacknowledged and unintended controversy (see, e.g., Biven 1977; Evans 1948, 1953; Kafka 1989; Kleban 1988; Kubie 1967; Stern 1968; and Weinshel 1977)—namely, does boarding school promote favorable adolescent development, or does it contribute to the vulnerability to breakdown? This question is one form of a question frequently asked of psychiatrists who treat adolescents, Would you recommend that our child attend a boarding school?

For example, in 1962, Peter Blos wrote that "boarding school placement of an adolescent can forestall deviate development caused by continuous noxious overstimulation by one or both of the parents" (p. 210). A few years later, Kubie (1967) published a case report that seemed in this respect to conform to Blos's observation. He described the analysis of a young man whose familial situation had handicapped his development. His relationships with his parents and his two siblings had contributed to his living "in shame and terror" during his early childhood. He feared growing up because of the dangers to which this would expose him. Kubie wrote that, "at a critical point, because of illness in the family, he was sent away to school. This almost accidental good fortune saved him temporarily, because once he was out from under the destructive forces in his home, he emerged as an outstanding scholar and athlete" (pp. 631–633).

The clinical reports of some other authors illustrate that boarding school placement can have a traumatic effect or that it may represent the continuation of a pathogenic influence in their patient's life.

Stern (1968), for example, described the analysis of a very disturbed thirty-eight-year-old man. He was plagued by multiple symptoms, and he required perverse fantasies in order to achieve sexual gratification. Stern wrote that "his childhood was replete with traumas." He had been repeatedly abandoned by his parents, who preferred traveling around the world without him. They gave him away in custody for the first time when he was six months old. Later, he was brought up in a boarding school. Stern viewed his patient's boarding school experience as part of a series of pathogenic experiences resulting from parental neglect.

A case discussed at some length by Moses and Eglé Laufer, whom they call "Paul" (Laufer 1976; Laufer and Laufer 1984), was analyzed as a young adult. Paul had attempted suicide while at boarding school. During his treatment, he would at times fear his analyst "as the person who might make him remember the most terrible time in his life" (referring to both the time when he first went to boarding school and the time in his adolescence when he felt he was becoming a pervert; worst of all was the feeling that nobody cared what happened to him at either time [Laufer and Laufer 1984, p. 18]).

The Laufers wrote further:

At the boarding school he had begun to feel that something was wrong with his thoughts. The only thing that could comfort him during his periods of despair and emptiness was his teddy bear, which he had had since early childhood. He still had it, and it remained important to him. At the school and later he would hug it close to him, and this would help to remove the empty hole he felt existed inside his chest. At school he had begun to feel that anything was better than to have nobody to love him, and he still believed that it was this that made him think that a homosexual relationship was at least a way of being held and cared for.

He had a close relationship with one boy of his own age; they masturbated each other, and Paul let his anus be investigated, "but that was all." He recalled it as something he did not like much, "but it was better than crying." [Laufer and Laufer 1984, pp. 15–16]

On the other hand, the Laufers report that Paul was able to find some comfort and reassurance at the boarding school because he slept with other roommates in his room. They noted:

He told the analyst that as a child he was terrified of the dark and needed his mother to be with him when he went to bed. When she left the room he would have to hug his teddy bear; otherwise he was frightened that something might happen to him. At boarding school this was easier to cope with because there were other boys in the room and he could feel safe with them, but he still needed his teddy bear in bed. [Laufer and Laufer 1984, p. 16]

In the face of such diversity of experience, the complexity of predicting whether boarding school will be helpful or harmful for an adolescent's development is great indeed. Concerned with our ability to make meaningful recommendations regarding boarding school (among other issues), Anna Freud (1965) essentially took the position that broad generalization was not possible. She believed that the result would depend on the particular psychology of the particular child involved. She argued that prediction in this instance required (1) a careful evaluation of the developmental state of the particular teenager and (2) an assessment of "the psychological meaning of the experience . . . in terms of [that child's] psychic reality, *i.e.*, according to the phase-adequate complexes, affects, anxieties, and fantasies which are aroused by [it]" (p. 58).

My own experience echoes Miss Freud's. On the one hand, there appear to be many children who benefit from the boarding school experience, from its enforced geographic distance from familial objects, its increased emphasis on relationships within the peer group, its (frequent) emphasis on religious precepts, its attenuation of conflict over incestuous libidinal and aggressive impulses, and its emphasis on athletic activities, sportsmanship, and the outdoor life. In contrast, there appears to be a significant group for whom the boarding school experience may trigger pathological developments or exacerbate preexisting symptomatic trends, as my review of the analytic literature confirms.

My clinical experience, limited as it necessarily is to pathological cases, cannot enlighten a comparison between these two groups. Nonetheless, my case material is illustrative of the effect that boarding school placement and the boarding school setting may have. Let me proceed, then, to such an illustrative discussion.

From a practical point of view, let me say a few things by way of introduction. On the whole, my boarding school cases are rarely self-referred. Referrals are usually made by the headmasters, assistant headmasters, deans, and the school personnel responsible for disciplinary matters. Less often, a family or psychiatrist who knows me may request my intervention.

No matter in which way a therapeutic situation has been initiated, the privacy of a boarding school student's psychotherapy is always compromised. This compromise is unavoidable. It derives from the closely knit nature of the boarding school community, the usually excellent supervision provided these youngsters, and the nature of the transportation and other arrangements required for an appointment to take place. Unfortunately and unavoidably, therefore, the fact of a student's psychiatric treatment is almost always a highly visible event on the boarding school campus. This fact often results in severe exacerbations of a teenage patient's feelings of shame, humiliation, and sense of defectiveness. I need not overemphasize that these are feelings for which adolescents as a group bear an exquisite sensitivity. Often, an otherwise viable treatment situation may be rendered impossible by the student's experience of repeated public exposure of a vulnerability. Occasional insensitive announcements of upcoming appointments made by faculty members, as, for example, in the community dining room, can at times destroy a treatment on the spot.

Finally, I must mention the fact that, unlike their counterparts living at home, boarding students live, eat, sleep, bathe, toilet themselves, and conduct their sexual activities in collective situations. The adults (e.g., teachers, athletic coaches, advisers, etc.) who inevitably become important to them are not—as at home—their parents. Rather, they are extrafamilial objects who represent, at one and the same time, important alternatives to early love objects and potential targets for transference-like involvements. Here, too, one may see the potential for certain kinds of intrapsychic interaction between the boarding school experience and the normal (or deviant) adolescent process.

Most often, beginning at around age fourteen,[1] these teenagers no longer live at home. Because most go on to attend boarding colleges, it is the usual case that they never live at home again. Therefore, these students experience a definitive separation from their families several years and a full developmental epoch earlier than is customary.

Broadly speaking, the implications for adolescent development of this radical and early separation are profound. Boarding school brings about an early separation from the "real" parental objects (as contrasted with their intrapsychic representations). This separation is sometimes experienced as akin to those losses brought about by divorce, the death of one or both parents, illness, or other circumstances. Like these events, the boarding school separation may powerfully reactivate—as my clinical illustration will show—earlier experiences of separation and object loss.

For all too many boarding school students, a particularly unfortunate confluence of events may occur. Not only may boarding school placement be experienced as emotionally similar to circumstances such as divorce, the death of a parent, illness, etc., but—and this is a crucial point—the decision for boarding school placement may itself have been brought about by these very circumstances. Such teenagers may be subject to a kind of "dual traumatization," having to accommodate themselves to both going away to school and, say, the parents' divorce.[2] Here, the potential for the complication of the adolescent process rises exponentially.

Whether or not such a dual traumatization takes place, these losses, and their consequences for adolescent development, will in any case present complications to the "normal" adolescent process. The nature of these complications may become particularly evident when viewed from the perspective of adolescence as the "second individuation process" (Blos 1967; Mahler 1963).

It has been my own experience that, for those individuals vulnerable to breakdown, the fact of the boarding student's separation from home is of an overarching psychological importance. I will now proceed directly to a presentation of illustrative clinical material, saving my theoretical observations for afterward.

Clinical Case Illustration

The case of Bob, like any case description, is necessarily abstracted and abbreviated. I intend it to illustrate some of the ways in which boarding school can function as a setting, background, and contributing cause of developmental breakdown while, at the same time, providing some of the raw material (language, if you will) for its expression.

Bob's case reveals, among other influences, the constantly operating pressure of his separation from home and of his consequent longing, seeking, and searching for object ties, especially for replacements for his two lost fathers. This pressure existed within the eye of a developmental storm, the outward expressions of which contributed to many of the familiar features of adolescence. Prominent among these was a series of urgent and rapid shifts among seemingly superficial and narcissistically colored identifications and transient identities.

As is so often the case in adolescent psychotherapy, the treatment was ultimately too brief and, paradoxically, too helpful to Bob to have allowed for a complete exploration of his pathogenic conflicts. This shortcoming notwithstanding, it will be apparent that, for Bob, boarding school had the capacity powerfully to revive thoughts and yearnings concerning his earliest separation due to his adoption and his quest for fantasied forms of lost objects. The therapeutic transference became the primary vehicle for the expression of these yearnings.

Bob had been adopted at a few days of age. He knew nothing about his biological father other than that he had been sent as a soldier to fight in Viet Nam and probably never returned home. Bob himself had evolved a fantasy—all too real to him—that, in part, equated his own having been sent to boarding school with having been sent as a soldier to combat in a remote battleground.

During my initial meeting with him, I strongly suspected that his psychopathology was quite serious. I reasoned that, if I were going to work with him at school, there would exist the potential for emergency developments, possibly dangerous ones. I decided, therefore, that I would need the headmaster's help[3] to monitor Bob's clinical status.

Bob was sixteen and in his junior year when his headmaster first suggested that he consult with me owing to his rapidly deteriorating academic performance, his increasing social isolation, and a quality of "oddness" about him that had become apparent to some of the faculty. Bob seemed preoccupied, "attending to a different drummer," they said. He seemed at times involved in a life of fantasy that drew him away from his schoolwork and peers.

In addition, although a "superb athlete," he had declined to participate in competitive sports for reasons that he had kept to himself. The headmaster reported that Bob had become surly, irritable, and apt to provoke confrontations with authority figures. At the time of my initial consultation with him, there was serious doubt about his ability to remain at school for very much longer.

In our first meeting, Bob was panicky. He seemed afraid for his sanity, and he described to me an array of altered states of consciousness and peculiar perceptions, particularly in the visual and tactile spheres.

The visual distortions, he said, were in fact occurring in the consulting room with me, right then and there, as they had often occurred in the past. This would happen when he found himself alone with a man in a position of authority. He called these distortions "the bigs and littles," a name he had devised in childhood for these illusions. I became larger than I was in fact, then I became small again, and finally smaller than I had been at the beginning.[4] I arranged to meet with his parents as soon as possible and to see Bob again in two days.

Here, I made a crucial decision, one to which not all psychiatrists in my situation would subscribe. I decided to try to maintain Bob at school. Frequently, the first decision to be made in a boarding school case is whether the child should be sent home. Sometimes this decision may be complicated by the fact that no home, in any ordinary sense, exists for the child other than the boarding school. Death, divorce, neglect, illness, or other catastrophic circumstance, having contributed to the need for boarding school placement in the first place, may eliminate home as an option. An informed decision, therefore, requires a careful assessment of the clinical status of the patient, of the home situation, and of the capacity of a particular boarding school to make the necessary accommodations to sustain the patient in that environment. This last consideration is unique to boarding school consultation, and schools vary greatly with respect to their ability to make such accommodations. Sometimes, with some schools, the referral to the psychiatrist represents merely the final step toward a medical suspension or discharge. In such cases, by the time I have been consulted the decision has already been made that the particular child can no longer be tolerated. Other schools, such as the one Bob was attending, have been able to work with me in supporting a student in some degree of crisis in the school context.

To Bob himself, I said that it seemed to me that he was having some difficulty recently and some recurrence of difficulties he had had in the past ("the bigs and littles"). I said that I thought the situation was serious but that he and I could arrange to talk some more and clarify just what was happening. In that way, I continued, I thought he would feel better able to remain at school if he wanted to. Bob was glad that I was not as worried as he, and he agreed to meet again in two days.

During the course of the next several months of twice weekly treatment, Bob's associations with me were organized around a central transference fantasy having to do with his being the devoted pupil of a man of heroic strength, canniness, and fierce retaliatory resourcefulness. It was in this transference environment that Bob first told me about M., a former Green Beret who now ran a private training facility for mercenaries. He had read about the training camp in *Soldier of Fortune* magazine, the contents of which he regularly devoured. He told me he was planning to spend his upcoming summer vacation at the camp learning guerrilla techniques. He had spent part of his previous summer vacation there. His parents had paid the tuition. He had learned, he said, to rappel from a helicopter, and he had watched as the trainees turned live automatic weapons fire on some game poachers. Bob said he idolized M., and he hoped that he might be fully trained by him and sent to Central America or some other "trouble spot."

Bob wore combat fatigues to my office and around campus during this period, and he would frequently make "jokes" when in groups of students that there were Viet Cong lurking in the forest that surrounded the school. For the faculty, these "jokes" had become alarming.

In a course on contemporary history, Bob had become unusually animated during a period when the class was studying the war in Viet Nam. However, given the intensity of his interest, his knowledge of the subject seemed to the teacher to be shallow and confused. He had said to me that he regretted terribly that the Viet Nam War had ended, that he would have been proud to serve in it, and that he longed to kill.

He insistently recommended that I see the movie *Rambo, First Blood, Part Two*. It concerns the heroic quest of Johnny Rambo (Sylvester Stallone) to rescue Americans missing in action in Viet Nam many years after the war's end. Of particular interest in relation to Bob is the fact that the American politicians and other corrupt authorities in the movie have repeatedly denied the existence of these missing soldiers, insisting that they have long been dead. Bob idolized Johnny Rambo, and he was especially enraged by Rambo's having been betrayed by his superior officers and the politicians.

During these early weeks of our psychotherapy, he told me that he had written two novels and that he was working on a third. When I questioned him about these projects, he agreed to let me read one of his manuscripts. It emerged that he had produced hundreds on hundreds of handwritten pages. These were all-consuming projects, and they lent additional substance to the faculty's observations that Bob seemed withdrawn and attending to a "different drummer."

The "novel" itself was a repetitive, poorly organized series of adventures of a male hero, a warrior who was, alternately, wronged, abused, menaced, betrayed, or captured. His keen intelligence and titanic strength, however, always led to the same result; he escaped and, in the course of a bloodbath, gained the upper hand, routing those of his enemies whom he had not already killed.

Having been adopted so young, Bob knew nothing about his "real" father other than that he had been sent to fight in Viet Nam and that this fact was somehow connected with the need that Bob's biological mother had to put him up for adoption. Perhaps, he thought, his real father had been captured by the Viet Cong and not returned. Maybe he had been killed. Maybe he had returned home alive. Bob had often wondered.

Bob had never met his "real" mother either. It later emerged that his adoptive mother had been frequently hospitalized for brief periods. My efforts to understand the nature of her illness were met with obfuscation and talk about vitamin deficiencies. From this and other information, I suspected that alcoholism was the cause.

Over the next several months of our psychoanalytically informed supportive psychotherapy, Bob seemed to have been supported and maintained by a particular transference fantasy. Part of the fantasy was that he was my student and apprentice. He had said that he was in awe of the number of years that I had attended school, and in the fourth month of the treatment he signed up for an elective course in psychology. I had become for Bob a kind of god-like soldier-wizard.

With respect to my technical approach, let me say that I made no effort to interpret aspects of this transference structure to Bob. He clung rather desperately to his ideas of my wisdom and omnipotence, displacing his rage states toward me in the direction of one or two of his teachers. When I judged that these rages were escalating dangerously, I would advise him on the "tactics" of how to stay out of disciplinary trouble and to remain at school. Consciously, he wanted very much to remain at school, as he viewed the possibility of dismissal as a potential defeat and humiliation. If he were able to prevent himself from being provoked at the moment by his teachers (enemies, jailers), then he and I could talk later; we could work out what was making him so very angry, and he would be able to "keep his cool" and stay at school.

Bob's idealization of me included paranoid elements, elements of unreality, and experiences of the uncanny. When feeling this way, he would experience the drive to my office as a journey to another world. (Was it Southeast Asia?) He spoke of the isolation and remoteness of my office, of the fact that he was there alone with me, and of his feeling that I was a weird doctor and this was my kingdom. He joked that there were Viet Cong lurking in the woods that surround my office.

Bob experienced sudden and far-reaching shifts in his own identity. During the earliest weeks of treatment, he was "Johnny Rambo." After several months, abruptly, and for the next several weeks, he declared himself a "Dead Head," that is, a fanatical devotee of the rock group the Grateful Dead. Bob now wanted nothing more out of his life than, he said, "to follow 'the Dead' " wherever they went.

My initial work with Bob, including frequent contact with his parents and with the headmaster, helped enable him to complete the academic year.

Some days before Bob was to return to school following the summer vacation, he was mailed his dormitory assignment. The day before school was to resume, he told his parents that he refused to go back. He was adamant. He objected violently to his dormitory assignment. "Who needs to look at naked boys?!" he had shouted cryptically at his mother. Bob insisted that he would not return to school if he had to live in that particular dormitory.

A flurry of telephone calls began to entangle me in the issue. A faculty member called me, stating his belief that he had thought all along that there was something "strange about this boy," intimating that Bob had homosexual leanings. He felt that the school could not and should not cater to such a demand. Bob's mother called me for advice. Without explicitly saying so, she expressed her hope that I influence the school officials to change their minds about assigning Bob to a dormitory more acceptable to him.

I judged it impossible not to take an action that would in all likelihood be understood by Bob to be the work of an all-powerful but weird soldier-wizard. I elected to telephone the headmaster. In conferring with him, I stressed my confident opinion that Bob was neither weird nor perverted. I emphasized my understanding that it was his severe anxiety connected to returning again to school that had caused him to be concerned about the dormitory. I said that, above all, I expected that his anxious state would subside after a short time, as it had in the past.

Bob was reassigned to a dormitory with a private shower. Feeling protected by me, he began what turned out to be a very successful senior year. His psychotherapy continued on a once and twice weekly basis until his graduation. He returned to full participation in competitive sports and gave several outstanding performances. He had his first relationship with a girl, a classmate, for a few months during the second half of the year. His academic work improved as well.

Bob's case illustrates the capacity of the boarding school separation to contribute powerfully to the reanimation of early object relations and of infantile ego states. Bob's breakdown at boarding school was organized around the regressive revival of fantasies concerning the loss of his biological parents very early in his life. He had lost his father, an all-powerful soldier-wizard whose presence would protect him from further dangers. Bob's biological mother, he thought, would never have sent him away had his father remained with her. This organization of fantasy also closely reflected Bob's experience in his adoptive family, an important aspect of this case. Bob's "solutions" to this central problem of his life were varied and in flux. In one of these, he became Rambo, the returner of missing soldiers. In another, he himself was the missing soldier. In another, he authored stories about combat that had a happier outcome. In another, a solution decisive for the favorable outcome of his psychotherapy, he became the apprentice to an omnipotent soldier-therapist. In the end, his only wish was "to follow the Dead," wherever they were.

Discussion

When the adolescent psychiatrist is asked for an opinion regarding the advisability of boarding school for a particular teenager, he is being asked for his views on how this particular external event will translate into internal experience for his patient.

Anna Freud (1965) wrote that the assessment of "the pros and cons concerning day or boarding school" and the companion assessment of when might be a "specific moment during the adolescent process when it is helpful for the young person to remove himself bodily from home" were important areas of preventive psychiatric work with adolescents (pp. 56–57). She felt that the task of the psychiatrist here was twofold: first, the job required a careful evaluation of the developmental state of the particular teenager; second, the job consists of "assessing the psychological meaning of the experience . . . to which the parents intend to subject the child." She continued that, "while the parents may view their plans in the light of reason, logic, and practical necessity, the child experiences them in terms of his psychic reality, i.e., according to the phase-adequate complexes, affects, anxieties, and fantasies which are aroused by them" (p. 58).

These are difficult tasks, yet as adolescent psychiatrists we are indeed expected to make these potentially decisive predictions. Most often retrospect becomes our most reliable way of knowing whether we were right or wrong. My clinical case presentation represents just such a retrospective view. It is, as it were, an individual outcome study of the results of one specific decision in favor of boarding school placement.

How can we best conceptualize what we observed? Here, I believe that Blos's (1967) contribution, in which he conceptualized the adolescent process as a "second individuation process," can help us. It is beyond a doubt that, even for the most psychologically healthy adolescent, boarding school represents a significant, though not necessarily pathogenic, complication of this second individuation. I will focus here, as I have in my clinical material, on the experience of separation.

Blos stressed the multifaceted mutual interactions between the process of progressive *separation* from familial objects and that of progressive maturation. The second individuation, he wrote, is preceded by "the shedding of family dependencies, the loosening of infantile object ties in order to become a member of society at large or, simply, of the adult world" (1967, p. 157).

In the course of the separation, Blos wrote, one observes as well varying degrees of regression, symptom formation, and a necessary reanimation of infantile emotional involvements and ego states (1967, p. 175). These shifts in intrapsychic conflict and compromise formations accompany a complex remodeling of the psychic structures, drives, and defensive patterning as well as far-reaching revisions of earlier identifications.

Bob had experienced multiple separations, both real and fantasied, which played organizing roles in his psychic conflicts. The abandonments that became highlighted during his boarding school experience and during his psychotherapy were related to his adoption. His story of his adoption and of the circumstances that brought it about are probably best viewed as a compelling and organizing set of fantasies that lent coherence and meaning to a great many other experiences of Bob's childhood. The boarding school separation revived resonances of his having been abandoned by his first mother. Bob's idea was that all this would not have happened had his father never left home and died or become missing in Viet Nam. The full story is, of course, much more complex. We knew, for example, that Bob's adoptive father, also a military man, had repeatedly abandoned him (for reasons having to do with his business obligations). He abandoned Bob to an adoptive mother who herself repeatedly abandoned him (for reasons related to her alcoholism). Nonetheless, Bob's near delusional preoccupations first with Viet Nam and later with following the Dead wherever they went reflected his quest for reunion with his earliest love objects. We saw in Bob an extreme and pathologically distorted form of the rapidly shifting, highly narcissistic identifications common in adolescence. He became Rambo; I became Rambo; he became me. The reanimation of early ego states became evident in his experiences of depersonalization, sensory and perceptual distortions, and compromised reality testing.

Conclusions

Because it seems intuitively obvious that boarding school experience may complicate the adolescent process, it is remarkable that psychiatrists and psychoanalysts have written very little about this subject. In this chapter, I have approached the subject of boarding school experience from the point of view of adolescence as a "second individuation process." For many teenagers (perhaps the majority), boarding schools offer unique opportunities for educational, athletic, religious, and outdoor experiences as well as for the establishment of rich networks of relationships with peers and faculty. However, for other, vulnerable teenagers, the experience of boarding school may represent a profound complication of the adolescent process and may result in severe symptomatic eruptions, character deformations, or other developmental difficulties. These considerations highlight the fact that the decision for or against boarding school placement may be momentous, even fateful for the individual involved. They also emphasize the importance of the reconstruction of boarding school experiences in psychotherapeutic work with adults.

I have presented in some detail a report of my psychotherapeutic work with a particular teenager, "Bob," while he was attending a boarding school. Although my report invites comment from many points of view, I have emphasized the effect of boarding school on his experiences of object loss and especially on the processes of the remodeling of his identifications. Bob's boarding school experience generated within him an overpowering object hunger, one especially connected with his two fathers. He experienced his having been sent away to boarding school as like being sent away to a remote battlefield, Viet Nam, from which his biological father had never returned. The psychological consequences for Bob were serious, resulting in transient psychotic states.

Although my case report cannot answer the important question of how best to decide if a particular teenager should attend boarding or day school, I believe that it does provide a vivid illustration of certain of the issues involved. In Bob's case, aspects of his history were known in advance that should have suggested that, if he were to attend boarding school, psychotherapy ought to be provided. In my experience, however, this course is all too rarely followed, often because parents are loath to reveal such a need to admissions personnel. However, under optimal circumstances all available data need to be taken into account in an effort to predict the effect of the boarding school experience. The most important of these data will be assessments of the particular developmental state of the teenager, together with assessments of the potential meaning of boarding school experiences to him or her.

NOTES

1. In considering the literature about boarding school, one must bear in mind that different nationalities use the term "boarding school" in connection with different age groups. For example, references in the English psychological literature to "boarding school" refer to institutions for children in the seven- to twelve-year age range. Other differences arise as potential sources of confusion, but the context usually clarifies which age group is under consideration.

2. Baudry (1989, personal communication) put the same issue slightly differently. He noted that the circumstances leading to boarding school placement have been, in his experience, as important as boarding school itself.

3. The question of confidentiality is an especially delicate one in this age group and in this setting, where the school functions for the most part in loco parentis. I have found that my decisions with respect to the frequently occurring necessity for breaches of the principle of absolute confidentiality have had to be made on a highly individualized and ad hoc basis. Perhaps the leading factor in these decisions is my assessment of a particular headmaster's (or assistant headmaster, dean, etc.) attitude toward the emotional needs of the student body and especially toward the need for psychological treatment. Through my years of experience with Bob's headmaster, I learned that he was uniquely equipped to deal productively with the kind of information about Bob's state that I shared with him. In addition, I thought that I might not be able to treat Bob at school without the headmaster's input. I have found, however, that one can make mistaken judgments in this very sensitive area, with resultant ill effects on the treatment.

4. A subsequent neurological examination and a sleep electroencephalogram done at my recommendation by a pediatric neurologist were found to be normal.

REFERENCES

Biven, B. M. 1977. A violent solution: the role of skin in a severe adolescent regression. *Psychoanalytic Study of the Child* 32:327–352.

Blos, P. 1962. *On Adolescence: A Psychoanalytic Interpretation*. New York: Free Press.

Blos, P. 1967. The second individuation process. *Psychoanalytic Study of the Child* 22:162–186.

Evans, W. N. 1948. The passing of the gentleman—a psychoanalytic commentary on the cultural ideal of the English. *Psychoanalytic Quarterly* 28:19–43.

Evans, W. N. 1953. Evasive speech as a form of resistance. *Psychoanalytic Quarterly* 22:548–560.

Freud, A. 1965. *Normality and Pathology in Childhood: Assessments of Development*. New York: International Universities Press.

Freud, S. 1900. The interpretation of dreams. *Standard Edition* 4:183–188. London: Hogarth, 1953.

Freud, S. 1905. Three essays on the theory of sexuality. *Standard Edition* 7:207–243. London: Hogarth, 1953.

Kafka, E. 1989. The superego: too much? too little? wrong notion? Paper presented to the New York Psychoanalytic Society, January 10.

Kleban, C. H. 1988. Transference manifestations as changing compromise formations throughout the course of an analysis. Paper presented to Colloquium 408 of the New York Psychoanalytic Institute, December 7.

Kubie, L. S. 1967. The relation of psychotic disorganization to the neurotic process. *Journal of the American Psychoanalytic Association* 15(3): 626–640.

Laufer, M. 1976. The central masturbation fantasy, the final sexual organization, and adolescence. *Psychoanalytic Study of the Child* 31:297–316.

Laufer, M., and Laufer, M. E. 1984. *Adolescence and Developmental Breakdown: A Psychoanalytic View.* New Haven, Conn.: Yale University Press.

Mahler, M. S. 1963. Thoughts about development and individuation. *Psychoanalytic Study of the Child* 8:307–324.

Stern, M. M. 1968. Fear of death and neurosis. *Journal of the American Psychoanalytic Association* 16:3–31.

Weinshel, E. M. 1977. "I didn't mean it": negation as a character trait. *Psychoanalytic Study of the Child* 32:387–419.

12   SEX DIFFERENCES IN MORAL REASONING AMONG EMOTIONALLY DISTURBED ADOLESCENTS

KIMBERLY A. SCHONERT

Although sex differences in the moral development of nondisturbed youths have been extensively examined (for reviews, see Thoma 1986; and Walker 1984), no research exists that has investigated sex differences in moral development among youths designated as severely emotionally disturbed (SED). Moreover, while researchers have made great strides in applying Piagetian and Kohlbergian theories to classroom settings, little effort has been made to apply these social cognitive theories to clinical settings. The goals of this study, therefore, were twofold. First, given the paucity of research investigating sex differences in the moral and cognitive development of SED adolescents, this study examined differences in the moral and cognitive development of SED adolescent boys and girls in residential treatment. Second, this study sought to explore the interrelations among moral development, cognitive development, IQ, and age in this clinical population. An investigation into the moral and cognitive development of SED boys and girls may shed some light on the manner in which

This chapter was prepared while the author was a postdoctoral fellow in the Clinical Research Training Program in Adolescence, jointly sponsored by Northwestern University (Department of Psychiatry) and the Committee on Human Development at the University of Chicago, funded by an institutional training grant from the National Institute of Mental Health (5T32 MH14668-14). Appreciation is expressed to Jacqui Sanders for constructive suggestions at various phases of the study and to the children and adolescents at the Sonia Shankman Orthogenic School for their participation in this project.

psychopathology interacts with these indices of social cognitive development.

Although Piagetian and Kohlbergian theories have been applied to normal populations, little exists in the application of these theories to developmental psychopathology. As Noam, Hauser, Santostefano, Garrison, Jacobson, Powers, and Mead (1984) state, "Developmental psychology has advanced considerably in the last decade, but few investigators have applied their theories and findings to the study of psychopathology. This is particularly true in the case of developmental research in the Piagetian cognitive-developmental tradition" (p. 184).

Background Research

Kohlberg, inspired by Dewey (1964) and Piaget (1932), delineated a six-stage sequence of moral growth. As with Piaget's stages of cognitive development, Kohlberg's (1958) moral development stages are both hierarchical and invariant. This means that, as individuals evolve, they progress toward higher levels of development. There is a move from an egocentric orientation of "what is in it for me" in stages 1 and 2 to, eventually, "compassion for mankind" in stage 6.

The belief that cognitive development underlies all growth in childhood morality is common to the theories of both Piaget and Kohlberg. Kohlberg (1969) proposed the hypothesis that cognitive development is a necessary but not sufficient condition for moral development. Support has been obtained for Kohlberg's postulate that moral structures emerge from and are dependent on the more basic logical reasoning structures described by Piaget (Kohn, Langer, Kohlberg, and Haan 1977; Lee 1971; Tomlinson-Keasy and Keasy 1974).

Nevertheless, we cannot assume that this relation between cognitive and moral development exists within emotionally disturbed populations. For example, research conducted by Selman (1976) indicated that SED children had a greater segregation of level of performance across logicophysical and social domains, with the logicophysical performance coming closest to the level of nondisturbed peers and the interpersonal and moral stages lagging farthest behind. Other research on psychiatric populations has suggested that functional abnormalities exist in logical reasoning (Ajuriaguerra, Inhelder, Jaeggi, Roth, and Stirlin 1970; Schmid-Kitsikis 1969, 1973).

Sociocognitive skills play a central role in normal socialization (e.g.,

Muuss 1982; Shantz 1975), and deficits in such abilities during childhood lead to unsuccessful adjustment in adulthood (Kohlberg, LaCrosse, and Ricks 1972). Unfortunately, applications of sociocognitive theory to the study of psychopathology have neglected examining sex differences. Although it is generally well accepted that deviant youths possess deficits in moral reasoning ability, the majority of existing studies examining the moral reasoning of disturbed youths either have included only males in their samples (Campagna and Harter 1975; Hains and Miller 1980; Lee and Prentice 1988; Selman, 1976) or have not examined sex differences (Sigman and Erdynast 1988; Sigman, Ungerer, and Russell 1983). Thus, it is difficult to determine if differences in moral and cognitive reasoning exist among emotionally disturbed boys and girls.

Females have been excluded from the majority of this past research because researchers have focused primarily on examining moral development among male delinquents, with the hope of elucidating the link between moral reasoning and behavior (Hains and Miller 1980; Jurkovic and Prentice 1977; Lee and Prentice 1988). One study that did examine sex differences in a deviant population (DeWolfe, Jackson, and Winterberger 1988) found incarcerated, adult female felons to be lower in moral reasoning than incarcerated, adult male felons. Nevertheless, we do not know to what extent this previous research can generalize to adolescent SED boys and girls. Scarce research exists examining the link between psychopathology and various indices of social-cognitive development.

From an intervention perspective, given the deleterious consequences (i.e., poor adult adjustment), it is important that clinical investigators turn their attention to the study of social-cognitive development in SED adolescents so that appropriate and successful interventions can be designed and implemented. Specifically, research investigating the moral and cognitive development of SED boys and girls will be able to improve the precision of intervention efforts. This information would also be particularly important for those concerned with stimulating moral development. In summary, prior to the creation of effective strategies aimed at helping SED children and adolescents, it is necessary for researchers and clinicians first to become cognizant of their moral reasoning abilities.

Disturbed adolescent boys and girls differ in the types of psychiatric symptoms they manifest. Adolescent girls express their disturbance through inwardly turned psychiatric symptomatology (e.g., depression, anxiety), whereas adolescent boys express their disturbance through externally turned psychiatric symptomatology (e.g., acting out, aggression) (Ostrov, Offer, and Howard 1989). Recently, internalizing and externalizing symptoms have been linked with social-cognitive development. For example, in the realm of ego development, Noam et al. (1984) found that externalizing symptoms were significantly related to lower levels of ego development. In addition, researchers investigating moral and cognitive development in a group of psychiatrically hospitalized adolescents (Noam, Didisheim, and Recklitis 1985) found that externalizing symptoms were associated with lower levels of moral and cognitive development while internalizing symptoms were associated with more advanced stages of moral and cognitive development. Thus, it appears that sex may mediate the relation between psychiatric symptoms and moral and cognitive development.

As mentioned, the current study was undertaken to examine sex differences in the moral and cognitive development of SED adolescents as well as to explore the interrelations among moral development, cognitive development, and IQ in this population. On the basis of the literature reviewed, it was predicted that moral development, cognitive development, and IQ would correlate positively with one another. No hypotheses with regard to sex differences in moral and cognitive development among SED adolescents were made.

Method

SUBJECTS

Twenty-five adolescents (thirteen male, twelve female) from a residential treatment center for SED adolescents participated. The sample was predominantly Caucasian, with the exception of two black subjects (one boy and one girl) and one Asian subject (a boy). The patients, in the majority of cases, had diagnoses of conduct disorder, depression, or anxiety disorders. The philosophy of the residential treatment center is based on psychoanalytic ego psychology theory implementing a "therapeutic milieu." The school admits those children and adolescents with average or above average intelligence and a history of personal, social, and emotional problems severe enough

TABLE 1
MEANS AND STANDARD DEVIATIONS FOR AGE, IQ, AND MONTHS IN TREATMENT

Variable	Females (N = 12), M (SD)	Males (N = 13), M (SD)	t
Age	16.43	15.55	.92
	(2.23)	(2.58)	
IQ	105.27	110.38	.81
	(18.22)*	(12.50)	
Months in treatment	40.75	48.84	.52
	(34.76)	(43.11)	

* N = 11.

to render them incapable of meeting the demands of living at home. Children who possess any organic pathology are not admitted. The socioeconomic and educational backgrounds of the adolescents were mixed, although the majority came from middle- to upper-middle-class backgrounds. Data from two subjects (one boy and one girl) were not included in the analyses because their performance on the moral reasoning measure did not pass a consistency check described by the test manual (Rest 1986).[1]

Sample characteristics are presented in table 1. *T*-tests demonstrated that the disturbed males and females did not differ significantly in age (t = .92, df = 23, p > .05), IQ (t = .81, df = 22, p > .05), or length of time in residential treatment (t = .52, df = 23, p > .05).

MEASURES

ASSESSMENT OF MORAL REASONING

The Defining Issues Test (DIT; Rest, Cooper, Coder, Masanz, and Anderson 1974)—a multiple-choice test derived from Kohlberg's evaluative approach—was employed to assess students' level of moral reasoning. Six moral dilemmas are presented in the administration of this form. For each moral dilemma, the subject evaluates the importance of each of twelve issues in deciding how to resolve the dilemmas by rating the issues on a Likert-type scale of importance ("great," "much," "some," "little," "no"). In addition, the subject ranks what he or she considers to be the four most important issues. For these ratings, a P score ranging from zero to ninety-five was calculated for each student that measures the relative importance attributed to principled (i.e., stage 5 and 6) considerations. The P score represents the sum of the subject's weighted rankings given to stage 5 and 6 items and is expressed as a percentage. The DIT has the most extensive data base yet collected with respect to any single measure of moral development. Also, no other measure of moral judgment exists that has repeatedly demonstrated such high reliability and validity. The DIT is an objectively scored measure of moral development that minimizes scorer error. Its stability, as assessed via test-retest correlation (two weeks), is relatively high ($r = .80$) when use is made of the P score (Rest 1986). In addition, because the DIT is a recognition task rather than a production task, it places fewer demands on verbal expressiveness than Kohlberg's Moral Judgment Interview (McColgan, Rest, and Pruitt 1983).

ASSESSMENT OF COGNITIVE DEVELOPMENT

Each subject was administered six Piagetian tasks. Tasks 1 and 2 were included to establish that the subject was concrete operational. The interview format and scoring system were derived from Renner, Stafford, Lawson, McKinnon, First, and Kellogg (1976). Two raters were presented with a four-point scale that provided a theoretical rationale and behavioral description of responses exemplifying concrete-operational substages IIA and IIB and formal-operational substages IIIA and IIIB. A description of each of the Piagetian tasks that were included in the present study follows.

Task 1: The conservation of solid amount. The student is presented with two balls of clay and allowed to work with them until he or she is convinced that each ball contains the same amount. The interviewer then distorts one of the clay balls into a pancake shape. The student is then asked whether the distorted clay or the clay ball contains more clay or whether each contains the same amount.

Task 2: The conservation of weight. The student is given two balls of clay and allowed to work with them until he or she believes the weights are the same. The interviewer then distorts one of the clay balls by shaping it into a hotdog. Next, the student is asked to indicate, without picking up the clay, if the portions of clay weigh differently or the same.

Task 3: The conservation of volume. The student is presented with two identical containers that contain equal amounts of water and is allowed to work with the volumes until he or she is convinced that the amounts of water are equal. The student is then asked whether the distorted clay (from task 2 above) would push the water level up more, whether the nondistorted ball would push the level up more, or whether the two amounts of clay would push the levels up equally.

Task 4: The conservation of volume using two identically shaped plastic containers of different weights. This task involves objects of the same size but different weights. In this task, the student is given two plastic bottles of exactly the same size but with an obvious difference in weight (i.e., one bottle is filled with water, and the other bottle is empty). All the foregoing properties of the bottles are pointed out to the student. The student is next presented with two identical containers partly filled with water and is allowed to adjust the levels until he or she is convinced that each container contains exactly the same amount of water. The student is then asked whether the heavy bottle would push the level up more, whether the lighter weight bottle would push the level up more, or whether the bottles would push the levels up the same amounts.

Task 5: The elimination of contradictions. The student is presented with a container of water and a selection of objects—a paperclip, a key, a cork, a penny, and two glass bottles partly filled with water. The student is then asked to classify the objects as floating or sinking and then test his or her hypotheses.

Task 6: The exclusion of irrelevant variables. The pendulum task requires that the student exclude variables by isolating various factors (i.e., length, weight, force, or release point) in order to determine which factor causes the pendulum to swing quickly. Following the procedure of Inhelder and Piaget (1958), the student is presented with twenty-gram, fifty-gram, and 100-gram lead weights that can be interchangeably attached to a string suspended from a small scaffold on a wooden stand. The string can be adjusted to varying lengths, ranging from five to sixteen inches.

Scores range from zero to sixteen, with a higher score indicating a higher level of cognitive development (for detailed scoring procedures, see Renner et al. 1976). In the present investigation, reliability for rating total task scores was 92 percent agreement between two raters.

PROCEDURES

Two sessions were used in the study. During the first session, the students were administered the DIT in small groups consisting of four or five students in their classrooms during school hours. All testing conditions were uniform across groups. The same female investigator administered the measure to all the groups. The administration took approximately twenty to thirty minutes. Specific instructions were given by reading aloud the information on the first page of the DIT to the students and carefully going through the illustrated example of the DIT format with them. Emphasis was placed on the idea that opinions were being sought and that there were no right or wrong answers. Communication among students was not allowed.

In the second session, which followed a day or two later, the six Piagetian measures were administered. Each student was seen individually in a classroom at the school apart from his or her regular classroom. Students' responses for each task were recorded verbatim. This session lasted approximately fifteen to twenty minutes.

IQ scores (Wechsler Intelligence Scale for Children–Revised; WISC-R) and length of time in residential treatment were taken from individual students' school records.

Results

SEX DIFFERENCES IN MORAL AND COGNITIVE DEVELOPMENT

The mean moral reasoning P score for girls ($M = 33.98$) was higher than that for boys ($M = 23.94$). Because moral reasoning correlated significantly with IQ ($r = .54$, $p < .05$), a one-way analysis of covariance was conducted. When IQ was statistically removed, the difference between the groups was statistically significant, $F(1,23) = 12.26$, $p = .002$. Comparisons between group means with regard to cognitive development indicated that disturbed boys and girls did not differ significantly from each other, $t(23) = .31$, $p > .05$. Indeed, the mean cognitive score for girls ($M = 13.50$) was almost identical to the mean score for boys ($M = 13.31$).

It is also worthy of note that the SED girls' moral reasoning P scores

TABLE 2
INTERCORRELATIONS OF AGE, IQ, P SCORE, AND COGNITIVE SCORE ($N = 25$)

Variable	1	2	3	4
1. Age	...	−.06	.33	.39*
2. IQ		...	.54**	.58**
3. P score			...	.65**
4. Cognitive score				...

* $p < .05$.
** $p < .01$.

are similar to the high school–aged norm scores ($M = 31.8$) presented by Rest (1986) in the DIT manual, whereas the SED boys' moral reasoning P scores are much lower than the norms.

INTERRELATIONS AMONG MORAL DEVELOPMENT, COGNITIVE DEVELOPMENT, IQ, AND AGE

Table 2 presents the intercorrelations among moral development, cognitive development, IQ, and age. Consistent with the findings of previous research, a significant correlation between moral reasoning and cognitive development was evidenced, $r = .65$, $p < .01$. In addition, both moral reasoning and cognitive development were positively correlated with IQ.

Discussion

The finding that females score higher than males on moral reasoning when use is made of the DIT is in consonance with findings from previous research (Thoma 1986). In a meta-analysis of studies employing the DIT, Thoma found that nondisturbed females scored significantly higher than nondisturbed males at every age/educational level. Three possible reasons are offered for this finding indicating that SED females are higher in level of moral reasoning than SED males.

First, the direction of the sex difference in moral reasoning is congruent with findings from other research related to social development, which indicates that females score higher in domains theoretically related to moral development, such as empathy (Hoffman 1977), altruism (Krebs 1975), and the decoding of visual and auditory cues (Hall 1978).

The present investigation points to a female advantage with regard to moral development among disturbed adolescents.

Second, previous research has indicated that differences exist between sex and symptomatology (Ostrov et al. 1989), with males displaying more externalizing symptoms and females displaying more internalizing symptoms. The observed sex differences may, therefore, be a reflection of these differences in symptomatology and how these, in turn, affect moral development.

In their study investigating the link between psychiatric symptoms and moral development, Noam et al. (1985) found that externalizing symptoms were related to lower levels of moral development whereas internalizing symptoms were associated with higher levels of moral development. Although the present investigation did not specifically examine symptomatology, it was noted that the majority of the SED girls were diagnosed with internalizing disorders whereas the majority of the SED boys were diagnosed with externalizing disorders. More specifically, the largest percentage of girls had diagnoses of depression (56 percent), and the largest percentage of boys had diagnoses of conduct disorder (69 percent). This suggests that perhaps the manner in which psychopathology is manifested has an effect on the development of moral reasoning.

Third, it may be that disturbed girls are able to benefit from the types of social experiences that facilitate moral growth whereas disturbed boys are not. Social experiences that allow a person to role take are necessary for facilitating movement to higher stages of moral reasoning. According to Kohlberg (1969), social interactions with peers facilitate moral reasoning development because these interactions provide opportunities for role taking. This ability to take another's perspective allows for the growth of mutual respect and appreciation of reciprocity and justice. On the one hand, it may be that the SED girls in the present study were still able successfully to interact with their peers and obtain the types of experiences, such as role taking, that are conducive to moral growth. On the other hand, perhaps the SED boys were unable to role take and successfully interact with their peers in order to obtain the necessary experiences for moral development.

Kohlberg (1969) has postulated that a specific level of Piagetian cognitive development is necessary but not sufficient for a corresponding level of Selman's (1980) social perspective taking (i.e., role taking), which, in turn, is necessary but not sufficient for attaining levels of moral development. That is, role-taking skills mediate the relation between cognitive development and moral development. The data in the current study indicate that, although the boys and the girls were equal in level of Piagetian cognitive development, girls were superior with regard to level of moral development, suggesting that it is the area of role taking in which the boys experience deficiencies.

Previous research indicates that normal adolescent boys and girls differ in the quality of their peer relationships. Girls report greater intimacy and emotional investment in their friendships than boys (Douvan and Adelson 1966; Hallinan 1980), whereas boys are more aggressive in their relationships (Maccoby and Jacklin 1978). In addition, disturbed adolescent girls are more likely to seek help from their female friends than disturbed adolescent boys are (Elmen and Offer, in press). This latter finding lends support for the contention that disturbed adolescent girls may be better able to engage in successful peer interactions despite their disturbance.

The finding indicating a positive relation between moral and cognitive development is in accord with findings from previous research linking Piagetian cognitive development to moral reasoning development in normal populations (Kuhn et al. 1977; Lee 1971; Selman 1976). In addition, the finding indicating that Piagetian cognitive development was more strongly related to moral reasoning than was IQ is in concert with Kohlberg's (1969) hypothesis that cognitive development underlies moral reasoning.

One unexpected finding was the lack of a relation between age and moral reasoning. It may be that development of moral reasoning during adolescence is slight and that changes may be evinced only over a larger time span. Furthermore, the small sample size in this study limits the generalizability of these findings. Indeed, a larger sample size would be needed to permit a firm conclusion that age is unrelated to moral reasoning among SED adolescents.

The original impetus for this study was to shed light on the moral and cognitive development of adolescents classified as severely emotionally disturbed. Although emotional disturbance does not appear to interfere with normal cognitive development, it appears to interfere with the development of moral reasoning in boys. The specific mechanisms by which sex differences in the moral reasoning of emotionally disturbed adolescents emerge remains unclear; however, those concerned with designing and implementing programs for disturbed adolescents should become cognizant of the sex differences that do exist.

Conclusions

To what practical use can these findings be applied? Because deficits in moral reasoning ability are related to adult adjustment difficulties and problems in moral conduct (Kohlberg et al. 1972), interventions to improve the moral reasoning of SED boys should be designed and implemented. There is suggestive evidence that it is possible to elevate the moral reasoning of disturbed youths. Specifically, the Moral Discussion Group (MDG), which was developed by Blatt and Kohlberg (1975), has been successful in increasing level of moral development. This approach gives youths the opportunity to be exposed to levels of moral reasoning higher than their own and thus experience the cognitive conflict necessary for moral growth to occur. Perhaps future interventions designed to promote the moral reasoning of SED youths should include both boys and girls so that the boys have the opportunity to be exposed to the higher levels of moral reasoning of the girls. Prior to the implementation of moral reasoning interventions for SED boys, however, we need first to assess whether SED boys possess the prerequisite skills (e.g., role-taking ability) necessary for moral development. The investigation of social cognitive development within clinical populations is an important direction for further research.

NOTE

1. The consistency check determines the usefulness of each subject's protocol by checking if the subject was taking the test seriously and filling out the test according to directions.

REFERENCES

Ajuriaguerra, J. de; Inhelder, B.; Jaeggi, A.; Roth, S.; and Sterlin, M. 1970. Troubles de l'organisation et desorganisation intellectual chez les enfants psychotiques. *La Psychiatre de l'Enfant* 12:2.

Blatt, M., and Kohlberg, L. 1975. The effects of classroom moral discussion upon children's level of moral judgment. *Journal of Moral Education* 4:129–161.

Campagna, A. F., and Harter, S. 1975. Moral judgment in sociopathic and normal children. *Journal of Personality and Social Psychology* 31:199–205.

Dewey, J. 1964. The need for a philosophy of science. In R. Archambault, ed. *John Dewey on Education: Selected Writings*. New York: Random House.

DeWolfe, T. E.; Jackson, L. A.; and Winterberger, P. 1988. A comparison of moral reasoning and moral character in male and female incarcerated felons. *Sex Roles* 18:583–593.

Douvan, E., and Adelson, J. 1966. *The Adolescent Experience*. New York: Wiley.

Elmen, J., and Offer, D. In press. Adolescent turmoil: implications of research for clinical practice. In P. Tolan and B. Cohler, eds. *The Handbook of Clinical Research and Practice with Adolescents*. New York: Wiley.

Hains, A. A., and Miller, D. J. 1980. Moral and cognitive development in delinquent and non-delinquent children and adolescents. *Journal of Genetic Psychology* 37:21–35.

Hall, J. A. 1978. Gender effects in decoding nonverbal cues. *Psychological Bulletin* 85:845–858.

Hallinan, M. T. 1980. Patterns of cliquing among youth. In. H. C. Foote, J. J. Chapman, and J. R. Smith, eds. *Friendship and Social Relations in Children*. New York: Wiley.

Hoffman, M. L. 1977. Sex differences in empathy and related behaviors. *Psychological Bulletin* 84:712–722.

Inhelder, B., and Piaget, J. 1958. *The Growth of Logical Thinking*. New York: Basic.

Jurkovic, G. J., and Prentice, N. M. 1977. Relation of moral and cognitive development to dimensions of juvenile delinquency. *Journal of Abnormal Psychology* 86:414–420.

Kohlberg, L. 1958. The development of modes of moral choice in the years ten to sixteen. Ph.D. diss., University of Chicago.

Kohlberg, L. 1969. Stage and sequence: the cognitive-developmental approach to socialization. In D. A. Goslin, ed. *Handbook of Socialization Theory and Research*. Chicago: Rand McNally.

Kohlberg, L.; LaCrosse, J.; and Ricks, D. 1972. The predictability of adult mental health from childhood behavior. In B. B. Wolman, ed. *Handbook of Socialization Theory and Research*. New York: McGraw-Hill.

Krebs, D. 1975. Empathy and altruism. *Journal of Personality and Social Psychology* 32:1124–1146.

Kuhn, D.; Langer, J.; Kohlberg, L.; and Haan, N. S. 1977. The development of formal operations in logical and moral development. *Genetic Psychology Monographs* 95:97–188.

Lee, L. C. 1971. The concomitant development of cognitive and moral modes of thought: a test of selected deductions from Piaget's theory. *Genetic Psychology Monographs* 83:93–146.

Lee, M., and Prentice, N. M. 1988. Interrelations of empathy, cognition, and moral reasoning with dimensions of juvenile delinquency. *Journal of Abnormal Child Psychology* 16:127–139.

Maccoby, E., and Jacklin, C. 1978. *The Psychology of Sex Differences*. Stanford, Calif.: Stanford University Press.

McColgan, E. B.; Rest, J. R.; and Pruitt, D. B. 1983. Moral judgment and antisocial behavior in early adolescence. *Journal of Applied Developmental Psychology* 4:189–199.

Muuss, R. E. 1982. Social cognition: Robert Selman's theory of role-taking. *Adolescence* 17:499–525.

Noam, G. G.; Didisheim, D.; and Recklitis, C. J. 1985. Cognitive and moral development in relationship to symptoms in a group of adolescent patients. Paper presented at the eighth biennial meeting of the International Society for the Study of Behavioral Development, Tours, France, July.

Noam, G. G.; Hauser, S. T.; Santostefano, S.; Garrison, W.; Jacobson, A. M.; Powers, S. I.; and Mead, M. 1984. Ego development and psychopathology: a study of hospitalized adolescents. *Child Development* 55:184–194.

Ostrov, E.; Offer, D.; and Howard, K. I. 1989. Gender differences in adolescent symptomatology: a normative study. *Journal of the American Academy of Child and Adolescent Psychiatry* 28:394–398.

Piaget, J. 1932. *The Moral Judgment of the Child*. New York: Free Press, 1965.

Renner, J. W.; Stafford, D. G.; Lawson, A. E.; McKinnon, J. W.; First, E. F.; and Kellogg, D. H. 1976. *Research, Teaching, and Learning with the Piaget Model*. Norman: University of Oklahoma Press.

Rest, J. R. 1986. *Manual for the Defining Issues Test*. MMRP Technical Report. Minneapolis: University of Minnesota Press.

Rest, J. R.; Cooper, D.; Coder, R.; Masanz, J.; and Anderson, D. 1974. Judging the important issues in moral dilemmas. *Developmental Psychology* 10:491–501.

Schmid-Kitsikis, E. 1969. *L'Examen des operations de l'intelligence-*

psychopathologie de l'enfant. Nechater, Switzerland: Lelacaux & Niestle.

Schmid-Kitsikis, E. 1973. Piagetian theory and its approach to psychopathology. *American Journal of Mental Deficiency* 77:694–705.

Selman, R. 1976. Toward a structural analysis of developing interpersonal relations concepts: research with normal and disturbed preadolescent boys. In A. D. Pick, ed. *Minnesota Symposia on Child Psychology*, 10:156–200. Minneapolis: University of Minnesota Press.

Selman, R. L. 1980. *The Growth of Interpersonal Understanding: Developmental and Clinical Analysis*. New York: Academic.

Shantz, C. U. 1975. The development of social cognition. In E. M. Hetherington, ed. *Review of Child Development Research*, 5:257–323. Chicago: University of Chicago Press.

Sigman, M., and Erdynast, A. 1988. Interpersonal understanding and moral judgment in adolescents with emotional and cognitive disorders. *Child Psychiatry and Human Development* 19:36–44.

Sigman, M.; Ungerer, J. A.; and Russell, A. 1983. Moral judgment in relation to behavioral and cognitive disorders in adolescents. *Journal of Abnormal Child Psychology* 9:503–512.

Thoma, S. J. 1986. Estimating gender differences in the comprehension and preference of moral issues. *Developmental Review* 6:165–180.

Tomlinson-Keasy, C., and Keasy, C. B. 1974. The mediating role of cognitive development in moral judgment. *Child Development* 45:291–298.

Walker, L. 1984. Sex differences in the development of moral reasoning: a critical review. *Child Development* 55:677–691.

13   ADOLESCENTS OVER TIME:
A LONGITUDINAL STUDY OF
PERSONALITY DEVELOPMENT

HARVEY GOLOMBEK AND PETER MARTON

Preface

This work grew out of the interest of one of us (Harvey Golombek) in adolescent personality development and the sharing of that interest with the coauthor (Peter Marton) and other collaborators (Bob Stein and Marshall Korenblum). The literature, in the early to mid-1970s, at the inception of the Toronto Adolescent Longitudinal Study, offered two rival hypotheses regarding the nature of adolescent personality development. The turmoil hypothesis was based on the work and observations of a number of influential psychoanalytic thinkers (Blos

To be successful, such an undertaking as the one reported on here requires the effort of a dedicated research team and the support of a broad range of individuals and institutions. The individuals and contributors have been too numerous for us to be able to mention everyone. The Ontario Ministry of Community and Social Services provided funding for this research through their prevention research program, which was administered by the Ontario Mental Health Foundation. The Laidlaw Foundation provided support for Harvey Golombek to spend a research year in England, where consultation could take place with colleagues at the Maudsley Hospital, the Tavistock Clinic, and the Brent Consultation Centre. Angus Hood, then director of the C. M. Hincks Treatment Centre, provided the support and facilities for the research project. We are very grateful to the Etobicoke Board of Education and the teenagers and their families who participated in the longitudinal study. Bob Stein and Marshall Korenblum have been active collaborators throughout the study. Over the years, a number of individuals assisted with the collection of data: Sally Allon, Dawn Redmond, Russell Westkirk, Cathy Leanord, and Maria Churchard. Computer assistance was provided throughout by Cathy Spegg. Secretarial support was provided by Carol Kehm, Rozaleen Heller, and Luciana Dolabaille. Audiovisual assistance was provided by Barry Thompson.

1962; Freud 1958) and reflected their experience with their adolescent patients. On the other hand, Daniel Offer (1969), through empirical study of a select group of middle-class high school students, posited that adolescent personality development was a continuous, largely uneventful process. Our knowledge at the time was further advanced by the epidemiological work of Michael Rutter and his colleagues (Rutter, Graham, Chadwick, and Yule 1976) on the Isle of Wight. This groundbreaking research provided additional ideas and evidence regarding adolescent turmoil.

Our understanding of adolescent personality development and the extent of adolescent turmoil was limited to the available data. Each of the previous studies made a contribution to the field but was subject to limitations. The samples were either clinic patients, healthy middle-class students, or rural adolescents. The time spans examined were relatively short. In order to describe the personality development of a broad range of adolescents throughout their teenage years, the Toronto Adolescent Longitudinal Study was conceived. This study was guided by the previous work just mentioned. The collaborative group contributed a variety of theoretical perspectives. The research strategy was to use multiple measures, to contact a variety of key informants in the adolescent's life, and to use different methodologies: interviews, psychological and academic testing, behavior checklists, physical examinations, and reviews of existing school records. Each adolescent and his or her family joined our research team for a full day each year from age ten through age eighteen.

A study of this magnitude took several years to plan, eight years to execute, and some time to analyze, digest, and write up. A number of articles have appeared to date on some aspects of the study, but this is the first major exposition of the work. Such a lengthy project provides a detailed continuous view of the personality development of our teenage subjects. It is, like all longitudinal studies, limited by the measures that were selected at the inception and that we were thereafter required to continue. Although we inquired into many areas, there are of course questions and measures that could have been, should have been, but nevertheless were not asked or used. The material that follows presents a detailed account of the changes and continuities in personality functioning of a broad range of youngsters in early, middle, and late adolescence. It examines the extent and vicissitudes of turmoil throughout the adolescent years. Furthermore, it describes the relationships of affects, attitudes, behavior problems, and self-image with the personality functioning status of the developing adolescent.

1. *Introduction: Adolescent Personality and the Toronto Adolescent Longitudinal Study*

Adolescence represents a distinct phase in the human life cycle. It commences at the height of physiological pubescence and ends with entry to adulthood. The beginning of adulthood is defined as the point where the young person assumes responsibilities for the self in relation to physical, psychological, social, and economic needs. In the industrialized world, adolescence commonly spans eight years of life between ages twelve and nineteen, a period that can be lengthened or shortened according to socioeconomic and cultural influences.

This rapid phase of growth and change in body and in functional capacity is accompanied by both temporary and enduring changes in the psychology and personality of the adolescent. Although there is much theory and opinion, there is little empirical evidence available as to how maturation influences personality development and mental health.

This work describes the development of personality during adolescence. Findings are presented from a longitudinal research study of a group of nonclinical children. The primary aim of this report is to describe the continuity and discontinuity of personality characteristics and the occurrence of turmoil. In the final section, we discuss the clinical relevance of the research findings and consider the question of how an understanding of personality functioning status aids the clinician in diagnosis and treatment.

"Personality" describes preferred ways of relating and coping with the world during both stressful and quiet times. At its core, the concept "personality" refers to personal characteristics that have some endurance over time. Various investigators have approached the study of personality from different perspectives, including a focus on traits (Allport 1937; Eyseck and Eyseck 1980; Tyrer and Alexander 1979), a focus on specific underlying conflicts, anxieties, and defenses (Blos 1962; Freud 1946), a focus on external environmental determinants (Mischel 1969), and a focus on the internal world with its working model (Bowlby 1988).

THEORY OF ATTACHMENT

Attachment theory, as proposed by John Bowlby and his followers (e.g., Bretherton and Waters 1985), suggests the buildup of an "internal working model" as the core of personality organization. This core develops and changes throughout the life cycle and is composed of representational models of the self and of attachment figures that are progressively internalized. It is proposed that this internal mental representation is essential to the development and maintenance of relationships and therefore to the manifestations of personality traits. This theoretical position assumes both the existence of an internal developing structure within personality and the continuous effect of new external environmental experiences (i.e., an ongoing interaction takes place between environmental experiences and preexisting internal structure). This interaction constantly promotes further development of the internal working model.

DURABILITY OF PERSONALITY CHARACTERISTICS

Continuity and stability of personality characteristics over time have been variously examined. In their study of the self-concept during adolescence, Dusek and Flaherty (1981) report that the self-concept develops in a basically continuous and stable fashion. They concluded that the adolescent's self-concept does not evidence dramatic change as it develops and that any change that occurs is gradual. They note both continuity and stability in personality characteristics over time. In a report on the findings of the longitudinal studies of the Berkeley Institute of Development, Block (1971) similarly indicated that it has been shown that correlational continuity, as judged by the number of personality variables reaching the threshold of statistical significance, is impressive. For boys and girls, respectively, 96 and 89 percent of the junior to senior high school Q-sort item correlations were significant beyond the .05 level.

Clinical experience has demonstrated that psychiatric illness observed during adolescence tends to persist and is not a phase-related, transient phenomenon. In a five year follow-up of a clinical group of adolescents, Masterson (1967) demonstrated that functional impairments tend to persist from childhood to adulthood, as do psychiatric diagnoses. Rutter et al. (1976) reported that about 8 percent of early adolescents studied in the Isle of Wight were found to present with diagnosable psychiatric disorder. About half these cases seemed to have developed problems for the first time during adolescence, while the other half represented disorders originating in childhood.

ADOLESCENT TURMOIL

Personality development during adolescence is influenced by phase-specific changes—biological, psychological, and social. A proportion of adolescents are reported to present with significant personality dysfunctioning at particular points in development, and this is frequently described as turmoil.

Moriarty and Toussieng (1975) have reported that their adolescent subjects experienced rebellious feelings and excessive mood swings only during the junior high school years (i.e., ages twelve to fourteen). They indicate that this brief rebellious period was usually over by age fifteen and that, subsequently, a much more emotionally serene period began, marked by the adolescent turning toward the wider world while avoiding alienation from parents. In a study of fourteen- to fifteen-year-olds, Rutter et al. (1976) indicated that 20–40 percent of their study population reported feelings of misery, self-depreciation, and ideas of reference as manifestations of turmoil (depending on the symptom). Offer (1969) also found that about 20 percent of a normal group of adolescents experienced turmoil. In a study of relationships in adolescence, Coleman (1974) described early adolescence (ages thirteen and fourteen) as a transitional phase that has issues and themes that are different from other ages. During this phase, parents and authority figures are valued, while solitude and heterosexual relationships are areas of conflict.

Historically, psychoanalytic theory (Freud 1958) has asserted that tumultuous change in personality functioning (turmoil) is normal and to be expected during adolescence (i.e., internal personality disorganization and external behavioral disruption are normative). Recent empirical research data, derived from the study of nonclinical adolescents, have challenged this position. Offer (1969) has reported that about two-thirds of a nonclinical population show no significant symptomatology during adolescence, while Rutter et al. (1976) similarly have reported that half to two-thirds of their research population demonstrated no significant disturbance.

217

THE INTERNAL WORKING MODEL

John Bowlby (1973) has presented a conceptual model that allows for the beginnings of an integrated approach to the issues presented. He has asserted that all individuals are internally motivated to seek attachment relationships. The theory of attachment emanates from observations of the behavior of children in defined situations (separation and reunion). Individuals are perceived as motivated to attain or maintain proximity to some other clearly identified individual, one who is conceived as better able to cope with the world. The availability of a significant other (attachment figure) provides a strong and pervasive feeling of security and so encourages the person to value the relationship and continue it. The attributed biological function is protection. As a result of continuing experiences with important others, the individual gradually internalizes a representational model of the other as well as of the self. As these internalizations coalesce, there develops an internal working model that dramatically influences all existing and future relationships.

The concept of the internal working model is an appealing one in that it presents a bridge between the various theoretical schools of personality development. It asserts constitutional characteristics (traits) and needs (i.e., the need for attachment); it emphasizes the role of experience (i.e., relationships with significant others); it places importance on the psychodynamics of internalization, which allows for internal structuring and durability of representational models and core conflicts; and, most important, it emphasizes the ongoing interaction among all these variables. Attachment theory can thus further our understanding of issues related to durability and turmoil.

The internal working model is a theoretical construct that cannot be directly observed or rated. Consequently, it is necessary to propose specific personality functions that reflect the nature, organization, and consolidation of the internal representational world. This study proposes that key personality functions, which reflect the integrity and competence of the internal working model, can be identified, defined, operationalized, and reliably rated. These functions include identity crystallization, maintenance of identity, verbal communication, self-esteem, role assumption, relatedness, and reality testing. These seven characteristics have been defined as follows.

1. "Identity crystallization" refers to the structure and coherence

218

of mental representations. Competence implies that a sufficient degree of internalization has taken place with development such that the individual presents as neither internally empty or excessively rigid and overly complex. The internalizations demonstrate a degree of patterning that allows for feelings and thoughts about the self and others to appear as organized and interwoven.

2. "Identity maintenance" refers to the ability of an individual to maintain an organized and independent inner world of internalizations in varied relationships and circumstances. Competence allows for consistency in the perception of self and others.

3. "Self-esteem" refers to the feelings about the self with regard to adequacy, worth, self-acceptance, and self-confidence. These feelings are clearly rooted in self-representations that are developed in response to experiences with significant others.

4. "Relatedness" refers to the ability of an individual to develop some satisfying emotional involvement with others. Competence in relatedness implies a capacity for empathy and sensitivity to interpersonal cues. This function depends extensively on the quality of the internal working model. Internalized object representations need to be somewhat benign, loving, and understanding for the individual to be able to engage in interpersonal relationships characterized by a sufficient degree of trust and intimacy.

5. "Verbal communication" refers to the ability to communicate about one's self and others with some coherence, precision, and discrimination. Internal self- and object representations need sufficient crystallization to allow for the adequate clarity of personal characteristics as well as those of others. Disturbed communication appears as sparse, inefficient, confused, garbled, illogical, or alternatively as somewhat pedantic, overly precise, or repetitive.

6. "Reality testing" (regarding self and others) refers to competence in being aware of the feelings and thoughts of self and others. Most important is the ability to differentiate one's own thoughts and feelings from those of important others: this reflects the quality and sophistication of the internal mental representations of self and object. A person with disturbed reality testing demonstrates distortion regarding the thoughts and feelings of others and/or difficulty with the accurate awareness of his or her internal world of feelings, impulses, and fantasies.

7. "Role assumption" refers to an ability and a willingness to assume

age-appropriate roles (i.e., student, child, employee, friend) with an average degree of flexibility. Role aspirations are judged according to their realistic nature, capabilities, and social context. Competence in this area reflects the internalization of multiple self- and object representations that are age appropriate, satisfying, differentiated, flexible, and sufficiently integrated.

The specific personality pattern of an individual becomes clear in the context of relatedness to other individuals and requires an understanding of how a person feels, behaves, communicates, and adapts with others. For the study reported here, it was necessary to develop a specific assessment procedure, the Relationships Interview, which would make it possible to rate the seven personality functions defined above and thereby allow for an assessment of the internal working model (see p. 227).

THE TORONTO ADOLESCENT LONGITUDINAL STUDY

The Toronto Adolescent Longitudinal Study was launched in 1977 to examine personality development in a nonclinical sample of children from age ten through age nineteen. Fifty-nine boys and girls, selected to represent the general population, participated throughout the study until its completion in 1985. Each year, the students and at least one of the parents attended our center for a full-day evaluation. A comprehensive battery of measures was used over the eight years of the study to assess their psychosocial characteristics. As part of this battery, the research group developed a procedure that could reliably, validly, and economically assess personality functioning.

Adolescents are not easy to interview, are usually reluctant to discuss personal matters with adults, and are resistant to and often scornful of probing psychological questionnaires. They are, however, usually willing to share concerns about and success in social relationships, an area about which they have considerable interest. Keeping this in mind, a forty-five minute semistructured Relationships Interview was designed by the investigators to allow for systematic inquiry into important and significant relationships. It was our view that interviews focused on interpersonal relationships would reveal the nature of the adolescent's personality organization and reflect the internal working model.

Our sample was interviewed at ages thirteen, sixteen, and eighteen.

Based on this interview material, clinical ratings of the seven complex personality functions previously described were made. Associated affects, behaviors, attitudes, and self-concept areas were simultaneously rated using measures to be described in the sections that follow.

The results derived from the interviews, and the battery of measures made it possible to develop new perspectives in four areas of adolescent personality development: (i) the subphases of adolescence (early, middle, and late); (ii) the routes of passage through which adolescents proceed (stable clear, fluctuating, and stable disturbed); (iii) adolescent turmoil (affects, attitudes, and behavior); and (iv) self-image development. These perspectives will be described in sections 3, 4, 5, and 6, respectively.

2. Overview of Methods

This section presents a description of our study population and sampling strategy and an overview of our procedures. In subsequent sections, we will present more detail about the procedure for specific measures.

STUDY POPULATION AND SAMPLING STRATEGY

In 1977, all children ($N = 669$) attending regular classes in grade 5 in one region of an urban school district were screened using the Conners Teacher Rating Scale (Conners 1969). Since there was Board of Education approval, it was possible to obtain 100 percent teacher compliance. In addition, every student took home a Parent Behavior Checklist (Arnold and Smeltzer 1974). This was completed by 81 percent of the families. This "cooperative sample" screened with both parent and teacher scales numbered 534 and was almost equally divided between boys and girls. No significant difference was found on the Teacher Rating Scale scores between the children whose parents returned checklists ($N = 534$) and those whose parents did not ($N = 129$). Thus, the screening procedure did not introduce a significant bias in terms of behavior observable in the school (see table 1).

The cooperative sample was stratified as follows: the total scores obtained for each of the two behavior rating scales (teacher and parent) were separately rank ordered and separately categorized as high (highest 10 percent), middle (middle 80 percent), and low (lowest 10 per-

TABLE 1

COMPARISON OF COOPERATIVE AND NONCOOPERATIVE GROUPS

	Conners Teacher Scores	
	Mean	(S.D.)
Total population screened ($N = 669$)	19.6	(16.1)
Noncooperative: parent checklist not completed ($N = 129$)	22.8	(16.4)
Cooperative: parent checklist completed ($N = 534$)	18.8	(16.0)

NOTE.—Cooperative sample screened vs. noncooperative population is not significant.

cent). The children themselves were classified by combining the ratings of both teachers' and parents' scores in the following manner: high (high by at least one rater), middle (middle by both raters), and low (low by at least one rater). (For a breakdown of the distribution of children in each group, see fig. 1.)

Having classified the cooperative sample, we selected the study subjects by sampling randomly from each of the three groups. In order to increase the likelihood of selecting children who would demonstrate disturbance during adolescence as well as to guard against the possibility of greater attrition by more disturbing children, we sampled disproportionately from the cooperative population, incrementing each group stepwise by about 25 percent. Thus, we selected eighteen children from the low-, twenty-three children from the middle-, and twenty-

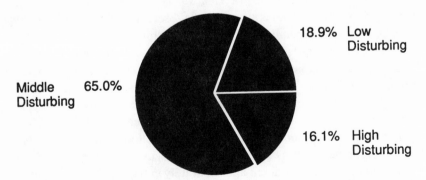

FIG. 1.—Distribution of subjects by category of behavioral disturbance

TABLE 2
DISTRIBUTION OF SUBJECTS BY CATEGORY OF BEHAVIOR DISTURBANCE

Cooperative Sample	N	Study Sample	N
Low disturbing	101	Low disturbing	18
Medium disturbing	347	Medium disturbing	23
High disturbing	86	High disturbing	29
Total	534	Total	70

TABLE 3
CONNERS TEACHER SCALE TOTAL SCORE

	Cooperative Sample			Study Sample	
	Mean	(S.D.)		Mean	(S.D.)
Low ($N = 101$)	7.2	(8.8)	Low ($N = 18$)	12.2	(9.5)
Medium ($N = 347$)	16.7	(9.5)	Medium ($N = 23$)	18.9	(12.5)
High ($N = 86$)	40.6	(21.6)	High ($N = 29$)	38.7	(19.7)

NOTE.—Cooperative sample vs. study sample is not significant. Comparison of groups (low, medium, and high), $F(2,529) = 178.38$, $p < .0001$.

TABLE 4
PARENT BEHAVIOR CHECKLIST TOTAL SCORE

	Cooperative Sample			Study Sample	
	Mean	(S.D.)		Mean	(S.D.)
Low ($N = 101$)	12.4	(11.5)	Low ($N = 18$)	7.3	(9.2)
Medium ($N = 347$)	28.2	(13.1)	Medium ($N = 23$)	27.8	(14.0)
High ($N = 86$)	60.6	(26.4)	High ($N = 29$)	64.8	(23.6)

NOTE.—Cooperative sample vs. study sample is not significant. Comparison of groups (low, medium, and high), $F(2,529) = 165.12$, $p < .0001$.

nine children from the high-disturbing group in order to form our initial study sample of seventy children (see table 2). As expected, the groups were significantly different from each other on the teacher, $F(2,529) = 178.38$, $p < .0001$, and parent, $F(2,529) = 165.12$, $p < .0001$, scale scores (see tables 3 and 4).

It is important to note that the group in the study sample did not differ on the basis of behavioral ratings from the groups in the cooperative sample from which it was selected. The study subjects were thus judged to be representative of the whole range of behavioral presentations from very quiet, nondisturbing to very boisterous and troublesome. The study sample was also balanced for gender. The socioeconomic status, assessed using the Blishen Scale (Blishen 1967), was found to be predominantly middle and lower class. Over the course of eight years, fifty-nine of the original seventy youths, together with their families, continued to participate in the study. This represents an adherence rate of 82 percent; therefore, the validity of our results is not compromised by significant attrition. The data presented in this chapter are from the fifty-nine adolescents repeatedly assessed over the entire course of the study (see table 5).

PROCEDURE

The study was conducted over a period of eight years. Each year, the students and at least one of the parents attended a children's mental health center for a full-day evaluation. A comprehensive battery of measures was used to assess psychosocial characteristics. Each adolescent underwent structured and semistructured interviews and completed self-ratings to evaluate personality characteristics, self-concept, identity status, relationships with family and peers, affects, and the presence of psychiatric disorder. The subjects were administered a

TABLE 5

AGE, SEX, AND SOCIOECONOMIC STATUS OF CHILDREN IN THE STUDY SAMPLE IN 1977, 1979, 1982, AND 1984

	1977	1979	1982	1984
Sample size (N)	70	63	61	59
Sex:				
Male (N)	36	32	31	30
Female (N)	34	31	30	29
Age (years):				
Mean	10.6	13.0	16.5	18.7
S.D.	.6	.4	.4	.4
SES (Blishen Scale):				
Upper third (%)	8.3	9.5	9.8	10.2
Middle third (%)	33.3	30.2	29.5	30.5
Lower third (%)	58.4	60.3	60.7	59.3

psychometric battery to assess cognitive abilities, style, and perceptual-motor coordination. They were examined by a pediatrician to establish their level of physical maturation and to note medical or physical abnormalities. A parent, usually the mother, was interviewed, and rating scales were completed that provided family information about demographic characteristics, family functioning, psychosocial functioning of individual family members, and developmental and behavioral characteristics of the adolescent. The school provided teacher ratings of behavior. Information about academic achievement, attendance, and special services was provided by the Board of Education.

In this report, we present data on a subset of these measures in order to describe the developmental course of personality functioning at three points: early, middle, and late adolescence (sec. 3). In addition, we describe changes over time in affects and attitudes (sec. 4), behavior (sec. 5), and self-image (sec. 6). The specific measures utilized are described in the individual sections.

DATA ANALYSIS

Each set of variables was analyzed using a consistent plan of data analysis. First, overall comparisons of a group of measures were made differentiating personality functioning, gender of the teenagers, and the age at which performance was examined using a multivariate analysis of variance with repeated measures (group × sex × age). If significant differences were found on the multivariate analysis, they were followed with univariate analyses of variance to examine differences in personality functioning on individual measures.

The data in each of the following sections are presented in the following order. First, comparisons are made examining changes associated with development from early to middle to late adolescence. These are followed by a determination of the continuity of individuals over time using Pearson product-moment correlation coefficients. Next, differences associated with personality functioning are explored. Finally, there is an investigation of differences associated with gender.

In order to present data in as clear a manner as possible, we have attempted to illustrate the results with figures. In most cases, the actual numeric data with means and standard deviations are also presented in the Appendix.

3. *Personality Functioning in Early, Middle, and Late Adolescence*

Students of child development have attempted to define subphases of personality growth. For prepubescent childhood, they have attempted to describe and differentiate the infant, toddler, preschool, and middle childhood subphases. There is also considerable interest in understanding how transitions are accomplished from one subphase to another and whether certain characteristics remain stable while others are more prone to change. Study has focused on psychological, social, and biological areas. It is evident that information derived from developmental studies can inform responsible caretakers as to how to plan for the needs of children effectively. Armed with developmental information, it becomes possible to structure the home, institutional environments, and community programs in ways that make these places more appropriate for children at different developmental levels. This kind of informed planning is recognized as essential by parents, educators, social and health care providers, and recreational leaders.

Over the last twenty years, similar attention has been directed toward adolescent development. Those who work with teenagers and youths readily recognize that pubescent youngsters differ considerably from middle teenagers, who in turn differ substantially from the preadult youth.

Adolescence is ushered in by the physical changes associated with puberty, and a clear transition is evident in biopsychosocial functioning. Personality changes as the youngster attaches meaning and feeling to his or her changed physical appearance, intensified sexual and aggressive impulses, and altered perceptions and expectations of the social environment. We proposed that the quality and quantity of these changes would be best revealed through an examination of interpersonal relationships. It is through interaction with others and the degree to which attachment needs can be satisfied that youngsters learn about their identity, their ability to relate, their self-esteem, their communication skills, and their ability to assume a variety of roles necessary for adaptation in varying circumstances. Developmentally heightened affects and attitudes are recognized and distinguished as core relationship wishes are either satisfied or frustrated. "Early adolescence" describes the period from twelve to fourteen, while "middle adolescence" refers to the period from fifteen to sixteen. A period of "late adolescence" has been described for young people seventeen to nineteen. As will become clear from the data to be reported in this section, early teenagers differ considerably from middle and late teenagers and require separate planning and different caretaking by adults.

PROCEDURES

At ages thirteen, sixteen, and eighteen, all the study adolescents were seen by one of two psychiatrists for the purpose of conducting a "Relationships Interview." Each interview lasted forty-five minutes and was administered in a semistructured format. The interview was videotaped, and, following each interview, both the interviewer and another psychiatrist rated the material using a personality functions rating scale. In addition, affects and attitudes were rated on two additional scales. All ratings were conducted independently and blindly by the two raters.

THE RELATIONSHIPS INTERVIEW

The Relationships Interview systematically inquired into the adolescent's perception of his or her relationships with significant others. During each interview, a list of persons important to the adolescent was made, consisting of individuals living in the home, extended family members, close friends, and any additional important persons such as teachers, religious leaders, athletic instructors, employers, or fellow employees. For each person listed, details were sought concerning age, vocation, and health status. The subject was asked to describe each person in detail in response to such open-ended questions as, "What kind of person is . . . ?" Inquiry was made into perceived closeness by asking about the intensity of the relationship and aspects that contribute to feelings of closeness or its absence. Subjects were asked if they felt free to discuss personal problems with each of the individuals listed and, if so, to give examples. Areas of agreement and disagreement were solicited, and the subject was asked how differences were resolved. Finally, he or she was asked about the extent of shared activities and the amount of time spent with each person in a week. Typically, adolescents identified between eight to ten persons with whom they felt close. From this information, clinical ratings of personality functions, affects, and attitudes were made.

The Personality Functions Rating Scale was modified from a scale developed by Giovacchini and Borowitz (1974). The seven areas of personality functioning defined in section 1 (see pp. 218–220) were individually rated using specific criteria. For each area, a clinical judgment was made as to whether the adolescent's functioning was disturbed or clear of disturbance. The seven areas and the criteria employed for the ratings were as follows.

1. *Identity crystallization.* A clear rating indicated that feelings and thoughts about self and others were coherent. Disturbance indicated that thoughts and feeling of the internal representational world were somewhat incoherent. If there was too little structure, the adolescent presented as unstable, empty, or amorphous; if there was too much structure, the adolescent presented as excessively defended and rigid.

2. *Maintenance of internal sense of identity.* The adolescent was considered to be clear if he or she can usually retain an accurate perception of self and others across varied relationships and settings. Disturbance was rated if there was significant fluctuation in mental representations of self and others across relationships and settings.

3. *Self-esteem.* A clear rating indicated feelings of adequacy, self-worth, self-acceptance and self-confidence usually sustained in most relationships. Disturbance indicated significant feelings of one or more of the following: inadequacy, self-doubt, self-depreciation, worthlessness, or a moderate to marked overestimation of self in most relationships.

4. *Relatedness.* This scale was rated clear if there was some satisfying emotional involvement with others and if the adolescent demonstrated the capacity for empathy and some sensitivity to others while retaining self differentiation. Disturbance was rated if there was significant inability to establish or maintain satisfying emotional involvement with others and if there was an inability to be sensitive to others without losing self differentiation (e.g., a tendency to withdraw from others or to become chameleon-like or to merge with the needs or demands of others).

5. *Verbal communication.* A clear rating was made if the adolescent was able to communicate about self and others with some coherence, precision, and discrimination. Disturbance was rated if there was

significant difficulty with communication about self and others (e.g., inefficient, confused, garbled, illogical, or pedantic communication or overly precise, insistent, or repetitive communication).

6. *Reality testing regarding self and others.* This scale assesses awareness of feelings and thoughts of self and others. Adolescents were rated as clear if they were usually able to differentiate thoughts and feelings of self from thoughts and feelings of others. Disturbance was rated if there was significant distortion of thoughts and feeling of others or an inaccurate awareness of the subject's own feelings, impulses, or fantasies.

7. *Role assumption.* No disturbance indicated an average degree of flexibility and willingness to assume a variety of age-appropriate roles. The adolescent's role aspirations were assessed as realistic for his or her age, capabilities, and social context. Disturbance indicated significant difficulty with role flexibility. There was an unwillingness to assume age-appropriate roles and to acquire and maintain realistic role aspirations.

RELIABILITY

The interrater reliability of ratings on all seven of these items was derived using the kappa statistic (Cohen 1960). All items yielded a kappa at a level indicating that agreements were significantly greater than chance, with an average kappa of .63. The seven items were found to constitute an internally consistent scale (Cronbach's alpha = .93). All children were rated by both psychiatrists, and the ultimate rating used was their average score.

CLASSIFICATION INTO PERSONALITY FUNCTIONING GROUPS

The presence of disturbance in personality functioning was determined on the basis of ratings on the Personality Functions Scale. For each youngster, the number of functions rated as disturbed was determined. Subsequently, those with disturbance on no more than one function were classified as clear of personality function disturbance. Those with disturbance on two or more functions were classified as showing personality function disturbance.

RESULTS

DEVELOPMENTAL CHANGE IN PERSONALITY FUNCTIONING
COMPETENCE FROM EARLY TO LATE ADOLESCENCE

There was an increase in personality functioning competence from early to middle adolescence, and this gain was maintained into late adolescence. There was a significant increase in the total score on the seven items of the Personality Functions Scale over time, $F(2,114) = 5.56, p < .005$. (A subsequent post hoc analysis using T-tests indicated that there was a significant increase in competence from age thirteen to age sixteen, $T[60] = 3.08, p < .003$, and from age thirteen to age eighteen, $T[58] = 2.16, p < .035$, but that there was no difference between competence at age sixteen and age eighteen.) These results are presented in figure 2.

Having found a change in level of competence in personality functioning primarily from early to middle adolescence, we examined the continuity of personality functioning in individual adolescents over time. The intercorrelations of scores among early, middle, and late adolescents on the personality functions scale are presented in table 6.

Considerable continuity in the relative standing of individuals over

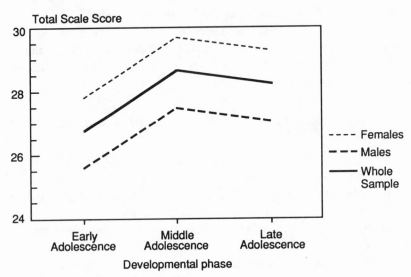

FIG. 2.—Development of personality functioning

TABLE 6
Continuity in Personality Functioning[a]

Variable	Age Spans		
	Early to Middle Adolescence	Middle to Late Adolescence	Early to Late Adolescence
Maintenance of identity	.40***	.69***	.33**
Reality testing	.53***	.48***	.39***
Relatedness	.54***	.50***	.40***
Verbal communication	.44***	.61***	.45***
Self-esteem	.39***	.48***	.41***
Identity crystallization	.37***	.54***	.42***
Role assumption	.33**	.38**	.39***
total scale score	.60***	.70***	.56***

[a] Pearson product-moment correlations.
** $p < .01$.
*** $p < .0001$.

time was found. The intercorrelations on all the measures were significantly greater than zero and ranged from relatively large correlations
on the total score (from the mid-.50s to .70) to more modest correlations on the individual items (from .33 to .69).

PREVALENCE OF PERSONALITY DISTURBANCE AT EARLY,
MIDDLE, AND LATE ADOLESCENCE

Our data indicated that the majority of adolescents (54–67 percent)
presented at any one point in time with little discernible difficulty in
personality functioning. Fifty-four percent of the sample were found
to be clear of personality disturbance at early adolescence, 67 percent
at middle adolescence, and 56 percent at late adolescence. Nevertheless, a substantial portion of adolescents at all three subphases had
personality functioning disturbance. These results are presented in
figure 3.

PATTERNS IN PERSONALITY FUNCTIONING BETWEEN AGES
THIRTEEN AND EIGHTEEN

In addition to examining personality functioning in cross section at
each of the specific ages, we studied patterns of personality functioning

231

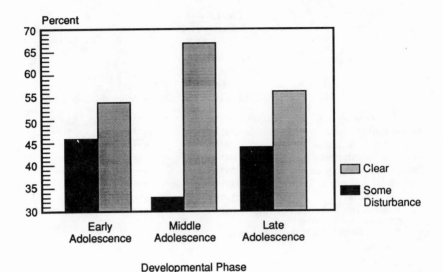

Fig. 3.—Prevalence of personality functioning disturbance

that reflected the course of the adolescent throughout the three sub-phases of adolescence—early, middle, and late. Adolescents who were consistently clear of disturbance were differentiated from adolescents who showed some degree of disturbance at each of the three assessments. Those adolescents who showed clear functioning at one assessment and disturbed functioning at another were classified as a fluctuating group. The distribution of the sample according to the stability over time of their personality functioning is presented in figure 4.

Examination of this table reveals that twenty-one subjects (35.6 percent) remained consistently clear of disturbance from early to late adolescence (consistently clear group), fourteen (23.7 percent) remained consistently disturbed from early to late adolescence (consistantly disturbed group), and twenty-five (40.7 percent) changed their level of functioning (fluctuating group).

SEX DIFFERENCES

The girls demonstrated greater competence in personality functioning than the boys across all three ages. A significant sex difference was found, $F(1,57) = 3.95$, $p < .05$. These results are presented in

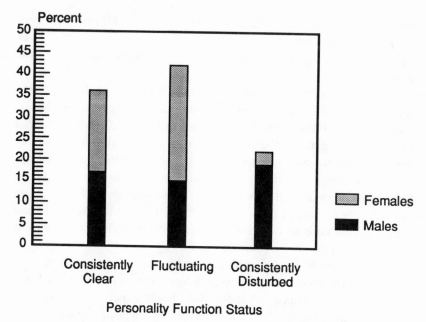

FIG. 4.—Personality functioning in longitudinal perspective

figure 2 above. Comparison of the sex distribution of the three stability groups indicated that there was a significant association between gender and stability of personality functioning status, $\chi^2 = 6.10, p < .047$. Girls were overrepresented in the fluctuating group, while boys made up the majority of the consistantly disturbed group. These results are presented in figure 4.

DISCUSSION

These results indicate that, when studied in cross section, the majority of adolescents (54–67 percent) appear clear of personality disturbance at each developmental subphase: early, middle, and late. Conversely, however, if studied longitudinally, a sizable number (42 percent) experience some personality difficulties at particular points in development. These data, therefore, lend support to the position that adolescent turmoil is a significant phenomenon but is not universal (Rutter et al. 1976). There is evidence for an increase in personality

233

functioning competence after age thirteen. In addition, the sample as a whole showed considerable continuity in functioning over time. At all ages, girls were found to be somewhat more competent than boys.

Most striking was the finding that early adolescents demonstrated poorer personality functioning than did adolescents at later phases. This accentuation of difficulties may result from the accumulation of stresses accompanying the transition from childhood to adolescence, which affects personality organization in the vulnerable child. For our population, potential stresses include the onset of puberty, the change from elementary to high school with the accompanying introduction of a rotating system of classes and new friendships and teachers and the often sudden confrontation with significantly different adolescent role expectations.

Of further interest is the finding that 36 percent of the subjects retained over the entire study period remained clear of personality function disturbance throughout their entire adolescence. To the best of our knowledge, these adolescents never experienced significant turmoil, had a good sense of relatedness to others, had good role differentiation, and were secure in their established identity. This group seemed untroubled by adolescence. Two alternative explanations for this untroubled course of development come to mind. These youngsters may represent a competent group whose internal working models and adaptive skills render them capable of progressing with smooth personality development despite challenging environmental and family influences. Alternatively, this group may have been privileged to experience a growth-enhancing environment, relatively free from disturbing life events. An analysis of family data and life circumstances could help clarify this issue and will be the subject of a future report.

Girls were overrepresented among the group that fluctuated between clear and disturbed status, while the boys were overrepresented among the consistently disturbed group. Perhaps such a difference is due to differences in types of disturbance associated with the two sexes. The difference may reflect the emergence of affective disturbance among females as they mature, while boys are more likely to manifest more consistent conduct problems. Another possibility may be that girls experience a delay of two or three years before manifesting conduct disorder that is similar to the boys' (Offord, Boyle, Szatmari, et al. 1987).

SUMMARY OF MAJOR FINDINGS

PERSONALITY FUNCTIONING IN EARLY, MIDDLE, AND LATE ADOLESCENCE

1. Overall competence in personality functioning increases from early to middle adolescence and remains stable until age eighteen (fig. 2).

2. Personality functioning for individuals demonstrates considerable continuity across all age spans (table 6).

3. At all ages, between 54 and 67 percent of subjects were rated as clear of personality functioning disturbance in cross section (fig. 3 and Appendix table A2).

4. Longitudinally studied from early to late adolescence, 34 percent of the sample remained consistently clear, 24 percent remained consistantly disturbed, and 42 percent fluctuated (fig. 4 and Appendix table A3).

5. Girls demonstrated some modest superiority in overall personality functioning at all ages (fig. 2).

6. For subjects who demonstrate some disturbance during adolescence, boys tend toward consistent disturbance, while girls demonstrate considerable change between disturbed and clear functioning. Similar numbers of boys and girls were found to be consistently clear (fig. 4).

4. Affects and Attitudes

Affects give color to existence and serve as guides to recognizing conflicts and determining future action. It is widely held that affects change both in quality and in quantity during progressive developmental stages. For example, during childhood, infants characteristically show heightened separation anxiety between eighteen and twenty-four months of age. During the "terrible twos," toddlers frequently demonstrate anger in response to frustration and parental control. During the pre-school period, many children show sadness in response to a loss, disappointment, or perceived injustice.

As part of the current study, the investigators were interested in studying how affect changes as youngsters progressed through their adolescent development. Five affects were rated during the course of the study (tables 7 and 8).

TABLE 7
DEFINITIONS OF AFFECTS

1. *Anxiety.* A state of apparent distress, discomfort, tenseness, or panic, as a manifestation of a feeling of fearsome threat, without the child's being able to specify what he or she thinks the threat to be.

2. *Depression.* The emotional state or mood of deep and prolonged sadness. This may be consciously expressed by the child, or it may be inferred from observed inaccessibility to stimulation, a lack of curiosity, or decreased spontaneity or lowered initiative, often accompanied by a prevalence of gloomy or morbid thoughts.

3. *Anger.* An affect characterized by a wish to injure or destroy a person or person-like object.

4. *Pleasure.* The manifestation of a child's present or remembered enjoyment or blissful feelings of people, places, things, or laughter, relaxed and expansive gestures, increased verbalization, etc.

5. *Affection (or tenderness).* A positive emotion toward another creature, which may exhibit no sexual feelings at all or in which sexual and sensual feelings are minor or secondary.

TABLE 8
AFFECTS RATING SCALE

Anxiety	1, Not manifest
	2, Slightly tense
	3, Moderately tense
	4, Much tenseness
	5, Severe anxiety, panic
Depression	1, Not evident
	2, Slight, moody
	3, Moderate
	4, Much obvious sadness
	5, Severely depressed
Anger	1, Not evident
	2, Slight anger
	3, Moderate anger, unkindness
	4, Much anger
	5, Severe anger, sadism
Pleasure	1, Not manifest
	2, Occasional, slight
	3, Moderate
	4, Much pleasure in many areas
	5, Blissful
Affection	1, Not manifest
	2, Slight, limited
	3, Moderate
	4, Much affection
	5, Extremely affectionate

AFFECTS

Anxiety and depression are considered to be the primary affects as they appear to be most common and universally experienced. These two affects are viewed as signals of psychological distress related to changes in the biopsychosocial equilibrium of an individual. It was felt that an understanding of the vicissitudes of these affects would promote a better appreciation of which subphases of adolescence are particularly stressful and which are more tranquil. Anger, pleasure, and affection are regarded as feelings that reflect the capacity of an individual to engage in meaningful relationships with others (either of a positive or of a negative valence). It was anticipated that these feelings would change with substage development and would also reflect overall personality disturbance or healthy functioning.

ATTITUDES

Attitudes are psychological positions that express underlying feelings and thoughts and are constructed out of life experiences that are progressively internalized. They are rooted in constitutional predispositions, self-representations, and object representations as well as in personality deficits and psychological needs. Fantasies created in association with the satisfaction and/or frustration of drives or in association with the satisfaction and/or frustration of needs (attachment, security, mirroring, and idealizing) are often important components of a particular attitude. Attitudes held or expressed at any moment of time clearly represent an interaction of established values, ideals, and beliefs with social expectation and demands.

As part of the current study, we assessed six attitudes—cooperativeness, curiosity, dominance, approval, optimism, and introspectiveness—that could be defined (table 9) and reliably rated (table 10) during early, middle and late adolescence. It was anticipated that attitudes would change with normal maturation but would also reflect personality functioning disturbance or health.

PROCEDURES

THE RELATIONSHIPS INTERVIEW

A semistructured interview was administered to each adolescent in order to provide information regarding the adolescent's perception of

TABLE 9
DEFINITION OF ATTITUDES

1. *Cooperativeness.* Demonstration of willingness to work with another person toward a common goal. May be inferred from the child's willingness not to appear to be deliberately withholding.

2. *Curiosity.* A readiness in the child to discover and absorb information about other people and things. Manifested in such a way as to suggest that an object (human or inanimate) or an event makes a difference or is of concern to the child. Interest may be evident in spontaneous questions or speculations and/or in a willingness to explore imaginatively or physically etc.

3. *Dominance.* The tendency of the child to anticipate an ability to influence other people, particularly those normally in positions of authority in relation to him or her.

4. *Approval.* The opposite of disapproval. An accepting, agreeable, admiring attitude toward a person or behavior, which implies the wish to be like the person or to perform the behavior.

5. *Optimism.* The tendency (amounting to a character trait) for the child to anticipate favorable outcomes or to underestimate obstacles.

6. *Introspectiveness.* The tendency of the child to examine, contemplate, and/or interpret his or her own emotional and psychological state. May be accompanied by speculation as to its origin and consequences. The introspective child demonstrates a readiness to assess his or her feelings and motivations, although he or she may not be willing to articulate them in the interview.

relationships with significant people in his or her life. On the basis of the responses obtained during this interview, ratings were made of affects and attitudes.

At early, middle, and late adolescence, all the subjects were seen by one of two psychiatrists for the Relationships Interview. Each interview lasted forty-five minutes and was administered in a semistructured format. The interviewer asked the adolescent to list persons important in his or her life, and, for each person listed, details were sought concerning age, vocation, and health status. Typically, adolescents identified eight to ten persons with whom they felt close. Once the list was prepared, the interviewer inquired systematically into the nature of each individual relationship.

AFFECT AND ATTITUDES SCALE

Each interview was videotaped. Following each interview, both the interviewer and another psychiatrist rated the material independently

TABLE 10
ATTITUDES RATING SCALE

Cooperativeness	1, Completely uncooperative
	2, Slightly cooperative
	3, Moderately cooperative
	4, Very cooperative, accepting
	5, Exceptionally cooperative
Curiosity	1, No interest
	2, Minimal interest, bland
	3, Some interest manifested
	4, Very interested and curious
	5, Extremely involved
Dominance	1, None evident
	2, Occasionally domineering
	3, Moderately dominating
	4, Very domineering
	5, Extremely dominating, controlling
Approval	1, None manifest
	2, Occasional, with reservations
	3, Moderate, usually accepting
	4, Very approving, generally agreeable
	5, Extremely approving, complete acceptance
Optimism	1, Not evident
	2, Occasionally cheerful
	3, Fairly hopeful
	4, Very optimistic, usually cheerful
	5, Pervasive optimism and ebullience
Introspectiveness	1, Not evident
	2, Minimal self-awareness
	3, Moderate self-awareness
	4, Preoccupied with self
	5, Extreme preoccupation with self

and blindly on an affect and attitudes scale, modified from a scale developed by Giovacchini and Borowitz (1974). Each item was rated on a five-point scale, with 1 indicating relative absence of the variable and 5 indicating a high degree of frequency of the variable. The average of the two ratings by the two clinicians was used as the ultimate score. The interrater reliability of ratings on these items was derived using the kappa statistic (Cohen 1960). These reliabilities are presented in table 11.

The reliabilities were found to be acceptable with an average kappa for affects of .76 (range .66–.87) at age thirteen, .69 (range .58–.75) at age sixteen, and .64 (range .60–.68) at age eighteen. For attitudes, the

TABLE 11
RELIABILITY RATINGS OF AFFECT AND ATTITUDES[a]

Variable	Early Adolescence	Middle Adolescence	Late Adolescence
Affects:			
Anxiety	.66	.58	.60
Depression	.72	.73	.64
Anger	.75	.71	.64
Pleasure	.81	.75	.62
Affection	.87	.69	.68
Mean	.76	.69	.64
Attitudes:			
Cooperativeness	.72	.74	.59
Curiosity	.71	.70	.65
Dominance	.79	.77	.66
Approval	.64	.68	.70
Optimism	.71	.68	.67
Introspectiveness	.72	.66	.61
Mean	.72	.71	.65

[a] Kappa statistic.

average kappa was .72 (range .64–.79) at age thirteen, .71 (range .66–.77) at age sixteen, and .65 (range .59–.70) at age eighteen.

RESULTS

DEVELOPMENTAL CHANGES IN AFFECT AND ATTITUDES FROM EARLY TO LATE ADOLESCENCE

Youngsters experienced more anxiety and depression in early adolescence and in late adolescence than they did in middle adolescence—multivariate $F(2,200) = 5.39$, $p < .00001$; univariate comparisons, anxiety, $F(2,106) = 10.53$, $p < .0001$, and depression, $F(2,106) = 12.04$. During the early adolescent phase, teenagers demonstrated less capacity to feel affection (or tenderness) toward others than at later ages. The ability to experience and acknowledge this emotion increased with age—univariate comparisons, $F(2,106) = 12.3$, $p < .0001$. These results are presented in figure 5.

Early adolescents demonstrated less optimism and introspectiveness than did teenagers during middle or late adolescence. The attitude of

240

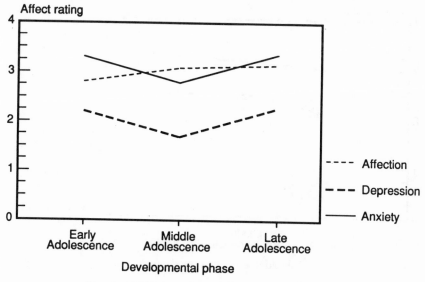

FIG. 5.—Affect in early, middle, and late adolescence

dominance remained unchanged during early and middle adolescence but increased in late adolescence—univariate comparisons, optimism, $F(2,106) = 6.76$, $p < .002$, introspectiveness, $F(2,106) = 22.52$, $p < .00001$ and dominance, $F(2,106) = 4.53$, p .01. These results are presented in figure 6.

The continuity over time of affect and attitudes in individuals is presented in table 12. With the exception of anxiety, there was considerable continuity in affect and attitudes as individuals progressed from one developmental stage to another ($R[59]$ ranging from .44 to .68).

AFFECTS AND ATTITUDES IN RELATION TO PERSONALITY FUNCTIONING STATUS

The three groups classified according to personality functioning status differed in their affective expression—multivariate $F(2,94) = 6.52$, $p < .00001$. The consistently disturbed group was the most anxious and depressed and experienced the most anger, the least pleasure, and the least affectionate feelings. The consistently clear group was most positive in their affects, while the fluctuating group was intermediate. These results are presented in figure 7. (The univariate F-values with

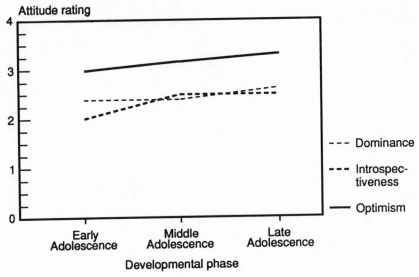

FIG. 6.—Attitudes in early, middle, and late adolescence

TABLE 12
CONTINUITY IN AFFECTS AND ATTITUDES

	Early to Middle Adolescence		Middle to Late Adolescence	
	Pearson Product-Moment Correlation	p	Pearson Product-Moment Correlation	p
Affects:				
Anxiety	.17	N.S.	.28	.02
Depression	.37	.002	.45	.0001
Anger	.32	.006	.50	.0001
Pleasure	.38	.001	.52	.0001
Affection	.38	.002	.52	.0001
Mean affects rating	.32		.45	
Attitudes:				
Optimism	.50	.0001	.69	.0001
Introspectiveness	.44	.0001	.43	.0001
Curiosity	.52	.0001	.44	.0001
Dominance	.25	.03	.44	.0001
Mean attitudes rating	.43		.50	

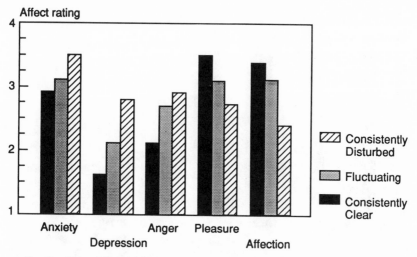

FIG. 7.—The relation between personality functioning and affective expression

2,53 degrees of freedom are the following: anxiety, 7.12, $p < .002$; depression, 26.56, $p < .0001$; hate, 10.28, $p < .0001$; pleasure, 22.93, $p < .0001$; and affection, 23.7, $p < .0001$.)

The three groups showed significant differences in their attitudes—multivariate $F(2,86) = 3.02$, $p < .0001$. Differences were found in cooperativeness, $F(2,53) = 21.34$, $p < .0001$, curiosity, $F(2,53) = 17.4$, $p < .0001$, approval, $F(2,53) = 19.09$, $p < .0001$, optimism, $F(2,53) = 32.67$, $p < .00001$, and introspectiveness, $F(2,53) = 15.65$, $p < .0001$. The consistently disturbed group displayed attitudes that were the most negative; that is, they presented as the least cooperative, the least curious, and the least approving and demonstrated little optimism and little interest in introspection. The consistently clear group were the most positive in all these attitudes, while the fluctuating group fell in between. These results are presented in figure 8.

SEX DIFFERENCES

Girls demonstrated a greater capacity to be affectionate than did boys during middle and late adolescence. During early adolescence, there was no difference in affection between boys and girls—multivariate $F(1,192) = 1.50$, $p < .077$; univariate $F(2,106) = 5.86$, $p < .004$. These results are presented in figure 9.

243

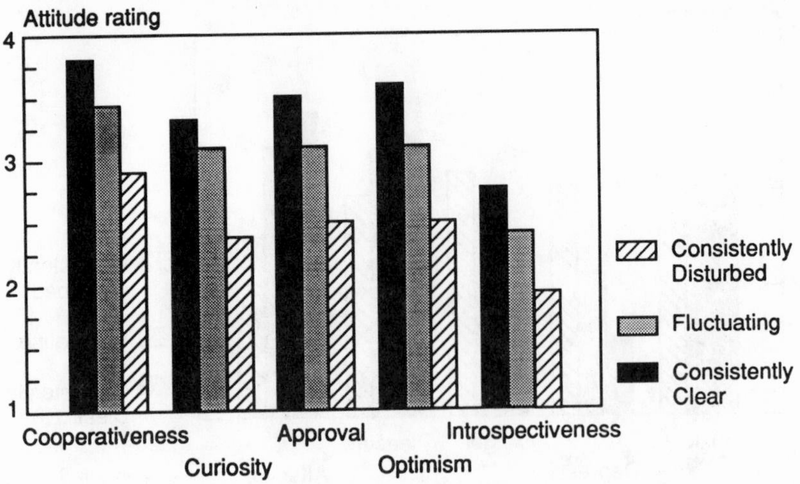

FIG. 8.—The relation between personality functioning and attitudes

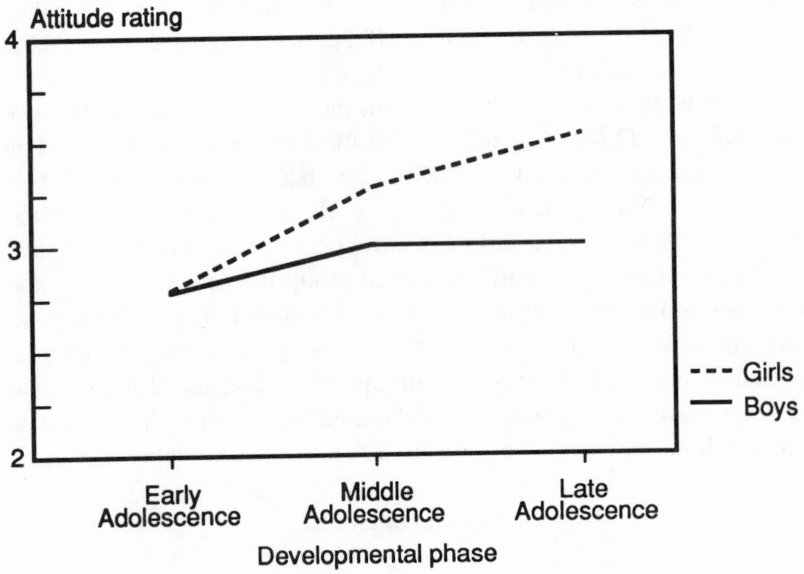

FIG. 9.—Gender differences in the expression of affection

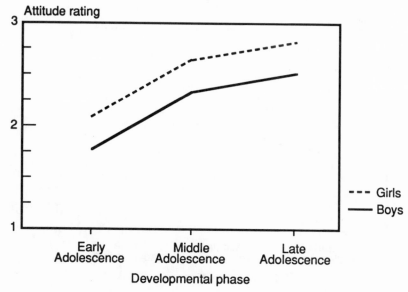

FIG. 10.—Gender differences in the expression of introspectiveness

Girls and boys did not differ in their expression of anxiety or depression during any developmental subphase of adolescence. There were, however, differences in attitudes, with girls demonstrating a greater ability for introspection at all subphases, $F(1,192) = 4.87, p < .009$. These results are presented in figure 10.

In early adolescence, boys demonstrated more curiosity than girls, while, in late adolescence, this was reversed, $F(1,192) = 3.14, p < .047$. These results are presented in figure 11.

DISCUSSION

In early adolescence, teenagers present with higher levels of anxiety and depression than they do in middle adolescence. Compared to later stages, they also appear as the least capable of affectionate feelings and the most troubled by tenderness. In attitudes, they are the least optimistic and seem to have the least interest in introspection. Early adolescent girls feel unsure of their ability to be dominant in the presence of others, and this does not change until they reach their late teenage years. Overall, feelings that are experienced during early adolescence are less consistently sustained into middle adolescence than

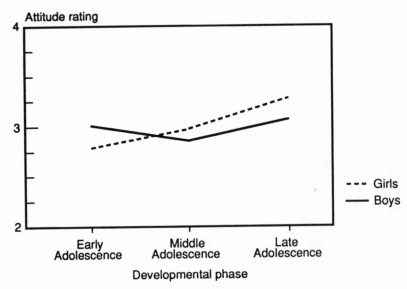

Fig. 11.—Gender differences in the expression of curiosity

is the case during the later transition from the middle to the late teens. It would thus seem that early adolescence is a period of disrupted affect as well as a period that accentuates personality disturbance.

In the previous section, we were able to delineate three separate groups of teenagers who progressed through adolescence demonstrating different patterns of personality functioning. Thirty-six percent of the subjects remained clear of personality function disturbance throughout their teenage development. When this group was assessed with regard to feelings and attitudes, they were readily distinguished from their peers. The consistently clear group presented as the most competent in self-expression and the least anxious, depressed, and angry and gave evidence of experiencing the most pleasure in living.

By contrast, as reported in the previous section, 24 percent of our subjects presented as consistently disturbed in personality functioning at all developmental substages. Compared to the healthy group, these youngsters consistently presented as more anxious, depressed, and angry. They seemed far less able to experience pleasurable feelings, and they presented with the most negative attitudes. They were the least cooperative, the least curious, and the least optimistic. They had the most difficulty demonstrating an accepting, agreeable, and admiring attitude toward others. They were also the most resistant to introspection.

A third group of subjects (40 percent) also described in the previous section was classified as the fluctuating group. These youngsters appeared with personality disturbance at one subphase but clear of disturbance at another. As might be expected, these teenagers presented with feelings and attitudes that were intermediate between their consistently disturbed and consistently clear peers.

In summary, the findings reported in this section further elaborate on those reported in section 3. It is apparent that teenagers traverse adolescence with varying degrees of personality strengths and weaknesses. With the aid of longitudinal assessment, it is possible to distinguish three separate developmental groups.

1. There can be identified a group of youngsters who demonstrate competence in personality functioning from early adolescence into late adolescence. These youngsters consistently demonstrate positive attitudes and are not troubled with persisting painful feelings. They give little evidence of much internal conflict. This group can be considered as demonstrating healthy personality organization.

2. There can be identified a group of teenagers who demonstrate consistent disturbance in personality functioning during all subphases. These youngsters present with painful, distressing, and disorganizing affects throughout their development and give evidence for the most chronically negative of attitudes. It is our hypothesis that the individuals who compose this group have developed personalities characterized by a deficit in the formation of their internal working model. In other words, they are lacking in personality structure resulting from the inadequate internalization of self- and other representations. This group can be considered as demonstrating disturbed personality organization.

3. It has also been possible to identify a group of teenagers who, during their adolescent development, sometimes show healthy functioning and sometimes appear disturbed. They characteristically present as changeable over time. They experience feelings that are inconsistent and intermittently painful. Their attitudes are conflicted and therefore are rated as intermediate between the ratings given to the clear and the disturbed groups. It is our impression that these teenagers represent a group with conflicted internal relationship patterns. We

247

speculate that self- and object representations have been internalized into the formation of an internal working model but that these internalizations are conflicted and distorted. The internal working model of these youngsters is adequate to meet ordinary environmental demands. In reaction to threat, conflicted internal relationship patterns give rise to distorted perceptions of the self and others, which create dysphoria and difficulties in adaptation.

SUMMARY OF MAJOR FINDINGS

AFFECTS AND ATTITUDES

1. Middle adolescents demonstrate the lowest level of anxious or depressed affect when compared to early and late adolescents (fig. 5 and Appendix table A4).

2. Early adolescents are the least affectionate (fig. 5 and Appendix table A4).

3. Early adolescents are the least optimistic (fig. 6 and Appendix table A4).

4. Early adolescents are the least introspective (fig. 6 and Appendix table A4).

5. Late adolescents are the most willing to attempt to exercise influence (dominance) on their environment (fig. 6 and Appendix table A4).

6. Adolescents develop more positive attitudes as they mature (fig. 6 and Appendix table A4).

7. Attitudes and affects demonstrate moderate continuity throughout all the stages of adolescence. There was no significant consistency in anxiety (table 12).

8. The three groups of adolescents (i.e., consistently clear, consistantly disturbed, and fluctuating) were found to differ in the expected direction with regard to their affects and attitudes (figs. 7 and 8 and Appendix table A5).

9. Girls were more introspective than boys at all adolescent subphases (fig. 10 and Appendix table A4). In middle and late adolescence, girls demonstrated more affectionate feelings (fig. 9 and Appendix table A4) and curiosity (fig. 11) than did boys.

5. *Behavior Problems*

Behavioral problems can be classified as falling into one of two categories (i.e., internalizing and externalizing problems; Achenbach 1966). The internalizing group comprises problems within the self, while the externalizing group comprises problems of conflict with the outside world. Behaviors that can be described as reflecting hyperactive, aggressive, or delinquent characteristics are associated with the externalizing group. Alternatively, behaviors that can be described as demonstrating schizoid, depressed, uncommunicative, obsessive-compulsive, anxious, somatic, or social withdrawal characteristics are associated with the internalizing group. Adolescents with behavioral disturbance often present with both externalizing and internalizing problems but usually show a preponderance of one type of difficulties.

Several epidemiological studies have documented that the transition to adolescence is associated with an increase in the presence of behavior problems (Rutter et al. 1976). The effect of maturation on personality functioning has not been examined prospectively in order to determine how this process may give rise to behavior problems.

In the current study, we were interested in documenting the relation between the stages of adolescence and the prevalence and nature of behavior problems. Do behavior problems increase or decrease with age, and do they change in appearance? In addition, do they show continuity over time and across settings? We had already discovered that teenagers traverse their adolescence according to three different patterns of personality functioning, and we wondered what the relation of behavior problems would be to these separate groups.

PROCEDURES

The dependent measures employed were the Teacher's Behavior Rating Scale (Conners 1969) and the Child Behavior Checklist (Achenbach and Edelbrock 1981). The Teacher Rating Scale consists of thirty-nine items rated on a four-point scale by the subject's teacher. Teachers who knew the adolescent well filled out the scale. The Child Behavior Checklist (CBCL) comprises 118 behavior problem items and is designed to be filled out by parents. The Teachers Rating Scale was completed when the subjects were ages thirteen and sixteen but was discontinued at age eighteen, when the items were no longer appropriate. The parent checklist was completed at all three study time periods.

RESULTS

CHANGES IN BEHAVIOR PROBLEMS ASSOCIATED WITH SUBSTAGE PROGRESSION

At school. Teachers reported that the total number of behavior problems tended to decline from early to middle adolescence. The decline was primarily in the area of conduct problems and hyperactivity. (Trends toward significance were found on the univariate tests—total scale score, $F[1,44] = 3.12, p < .084$, conduct problems, $F[1,44] = 3.43, p < .071$, and hyperactivity, $F[1,44] = 3.17, p < .082$.) These results are presented in figure 12.

There was little continuity of behavior problems in school from early to middle adolescence. These correlation coefficients are presented in table 13.

At home. Parents reported a significant decline in behavior problems observed at home with age, $F(2,134) = 2.93, p < .001$. Both

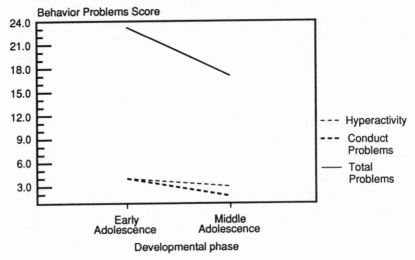

FIG. 12.—Behavior problems at school

TABLE 13
CONTINUITY OF TEACHER BEHAVIOR RATING SCORES FROM
EARLY TO MIDDLE TEENAGE YEARS

Variable	Pearson Product-Moment Correlation	p
Total score	.22	.05
Factor 1: conduct problems	.01	N.S.
Factor 2: inattentive-passive	.33	.007
Factor 3: tension-anxiety	.27	.03
Factor 4: hyperactivity	.27	.03

NOTE.—The comparison is age thirteen with age sixteen.

internalizing problems, $F(2,72) = 9.59$, $p < .0001$, and externalizing problems, $F(2,72) = 11.15$, $p < .0001$, diminished over time. These results are presented in figure 13.

Parents reported that behavior problems that declined were different in boys than in girls. With age, boys improved in the following areas: somatic complaints, $F(2,26) = 5.58$, $p < .01$; uncommunicative, $F(2,26) = 4.96$, $p < .015$; immature, $F(2,26) = 4.69$, $p < .018$; obsessive-compulsive, $F(2,26) = 4.14$, $p < .27$; hostile-withdrawn, $F(2,26) = 3.35$, $p < .051$; aggressive, $F(2,26) = 6.19$, $p < .006$; and

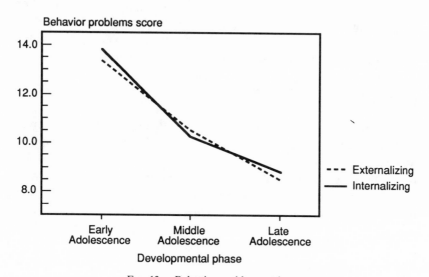

FIG. 13.—Behavior problems at home

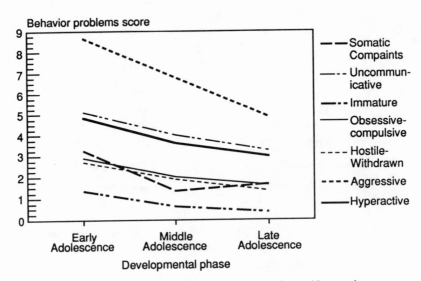

Fig. 14.—Developmental changes in boys' behavior problems at home

hyperactivity, $F(2,26) = 3.23$, $p < .056$. The girls by comparison improved over time only in the immature-hyperactivity factor, $F(2,26) = 4.77$, $p < .017$. These results are presented in figures 14 and 15.

Continuity in behavior problems of boys and girls was evident over time. As expected, externalizing problems were more consistent than internalizing ones. Nevertheless, internalizing problems were also quite consistent. These results are presented in table 14.

BEHAVIOR PROBLEMS AND PERSONALITY FUNCTIONING STATUS

At school. Teachers reported significant differences in the presence of behavior problems among the three differentiated groups of adolescents during the early and middle subphases, $F(2,80) = 4.92$; $p < .008$. The consistently disturbed adolescents displayed the most and the consistently clear adolescents the least problems, while the fluctuating group fell in between. This pattern of results was found on the total scale score, $F(2,44) = 7.00$, $p < .002$, as well as on three of the four factors—conduct problems, $F(2,44) = 4.48$, $p < .017$, inattentive-passive problems, $F(2,44) = 7.60$, $p < .001$, and tension-anxiety, $F(2,44) = 5.53$, $p < .007$. The three groups of adolescents

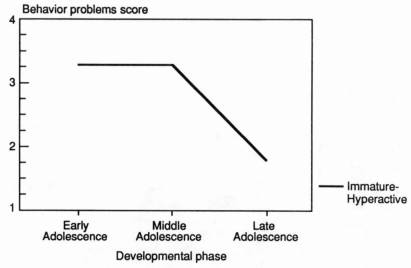

FIG. 15.—Developmental changes in girls' behavior problems at home

were not differentiated by the teachers according to behaviors associated with hyperactivity. These results are presented in figure 16.

At home. The three personality functioning groups differed in the level of externalizing problems, $F(2,36) = 3.90$, $p < .029$, and tended to differ in the level of internalizing problems, $F(2,36) = 2.76$, $p < .077$, presented at home. These results are presented in figure 17.

The girls in the consistently disturbed group showed the most prob-

TABLE 14

Continuity of Internalizing and Externalizing Problems from Early to Middle to Late Adolescence (Parent Ratings)

Variable and Age	Pearson Product-Moment Correlation	p
Internalizing:		
Early to middle	.71	.0001
Middle to late	.67	.0001
Early to late	.62	.0001
Externalizing:		
Early to middle	.81	.0001
Middle to late	.75	.0001
Early to late	.76	.0001

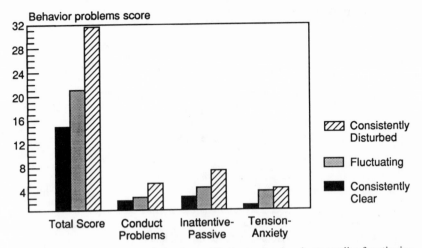

Fig. 16.—Relation between behavior problems at school and personality functioning status.

lems in the area of immature-hyperactivity. The consistently clear girls showed the least problems, and the fluctuating girls fell between— multivariate $F(2,12) = 3.84$, $p < .012$, univariate $F(2,13) = 3.54$, $p < .059$. These results are presented in figure 18.

DISCUSSION

Our results indicate that, as adolescents mature, they demonstrate fewer behavior problems. This process encompasses both externaliz- ing problems (conflict with the outside world) and internalizing prob- lems (conflict within the self) and reflects the continuation of a gradual maturational pattern that begins in childhood (Achenbach and Edel- brock 1981). Parents indicate that their teenagers show considerable consistency in behavior problems over time. These ratings support theories of adolescent development that describe gradual continuous growth throughout the teenage years rather than a discontinuous, un- predictable process (Offer 1969). Other authors (Robins 1966; Rutter et al. 1976) have also reported that conduct problems (externalizing) are persistent over time, as are neurotic (internalizing) problems (Eysenk and Eysenk 1980). In our study, greater consistency was ob- served in the home than in the school. This may be due to the greater

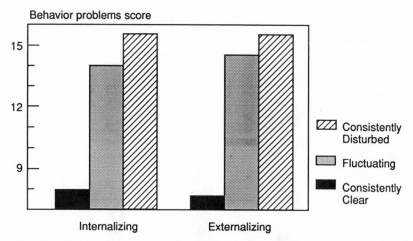

FIG. 17.—Relation between behavior problems at home and personality functioning status.

consistency of ratings when made by the same rater (the parent) rather than different raters (teachers), or it may reflect greater consistency in the home environment than in the classroom. (Perhaps over the years there is more consistency in the home environment than in the classroom.) Differences in ratings between parents and teachers are in keeping with previous reports that suggest that teachers and parents frequently disagree when identifying children whose behavior is disruptive (Offord et al. 1987; Rutter et al. 1976).

Our results show that the behavior of adolescents is related to their personality functions. Those adolescents who differ on the basis of longitudinal personality functioning status also differ in their behavior both at school and at home. These differences are observed at all ages and provide external validation for the clinicians' judgments. Differences were observed in both the internalizing and the externalizing areas. It appears that, when adolescents demonstrate persistent personality functioning disturbance, they also display increased behavior problems of both an externalizing and an internalizing nature. Thus, individuals who demonstrate a persistent pattern of behavior problems throughout their teenage years are the ones most at risk for personality functioning disturbance. Chronic behavior problems can be viewed as characteristic of individuals who have long-standing and pervasive

Immature-hyperactivity score

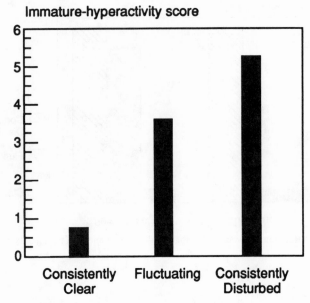

Fɪɢ. 18.—Relation between immature-hyperactivity behavior problems and personality functioning in girls.

difficulties maintaining a positive and realistic sense of themselves and important others. These characteristics result in serious relationship problems that interfere with appropriate family and academic adaptation. Personality dysfunction may manifest in behavior problems of an externalizing or internalizing type, or both. Behavior problems are an outward expression of distortions in the internal working model.

SUMMARY OF MAJOR FINDINGS

BEHAVIOR PROBLEMS

1. Teachers' ratings show a trend toward a decrease in the frequency of behavior problems over time (fig. 12 and Appendix table A6).

2. Little consistency among individuals is reported by teachers between phases (early vs. middle) (table 13).

3. Parents' ratings demonstrate a significant decline in behavior problems between early and middle adolescence in both the externaliz-

ing and the internalizing domains. Internalizing problems declined primarily from early to middle adolescence, while externalizing problems diminished significantly at each subphase, early, middle, and late (fig. 13 and Appendix table A7).

4. Boys and girls demonstrated different patterns of change in behavior problems over time (figs. 14 and 15 and Appendix table A3).

5. Behavior problems at home show continuity between age subphases (table 14).

6. The consistently disturbed group of adolescents displayed the most behavior problems at school and at home (figs. 16 and 17 and Appendix tables A9 and A10).

7. Girls in the consistently disturbed group showed an identifiable pattern (immature-hyperactive) in their behavior problems (fig. 18).

6. *Self-Image*

"Self-image" defines the adolescent's conception of the self in relation to others. It includes thoughts and feelings about the self (self-representations) as well as thoughts and feelings about significant others (object representations). In 1972, Offer and Howard devised the Offer Self-Image Questionnaire (OSIQ) as a self-descriptive test that could be used to measure the adjustment of teenage boys and girls in eleven content areas. These areas were considered to be most important for the assessment of the internal psychological life of the adolescent. Positive responses in each of these areas would predict healthy adaptation and good coping skills. Negative responses in these areas would conversely predict poor adaptation and serious coping difficulties.

In this study, we were interested in determining how self-image changes over time. We intended to determine whether it tends to consolidate and improve with chronological age or to weaken and become disorganized, as might be suggested by the theory of adolescent turmoil. We were also curious to discover whether there would be any differences in the way self-esteem develops in boys and girls. Are there any differences that appear at cross-sectional ages? Does one sex progress in a different manner with regard to self-image development than the other?

As previously described, we were able to distinguish three separate routes of personality development through adolescence. We wondered whether and how adolescents who differed on the basis of longitudinal patterns of personality functioning would differ in self-image. Would there be any significant differences between those following a fluctuating pattern of personality functioning and those who develop with consistent personality functioning? Also of interest was the question of consistency in self-image among individuals over time. Even if developmental changes would become apparent at progressive ages, would individuals show continuity over time in their global self-image?

PROCEDURES

DEPENDENT MEASURES

The dependent measure used was the Offer Self-Image Questionnaire. The OSIQ is a 130-item self-report questionnaire in which the adolescent is asked to rate, on a six-point scale, the degree to which each statement describes himself or herself. Alternatives range from "describes me very well" to "does not describe me at all." The scales assess the following five aspects of the self-image:

1. *Psychological self.*
Impulse control. This scale measures the extent to which the personality is able to contain pressures emanating from either the internal psychological world or the external environment.

Emotional tone. This scale measures the degree of affective harmony within the personality.

Body and self-image. This scale indicates the extent to which the adolescent has adjusted to his or her body.

2. *Social self.*
Social relationships. This scale reflects self- and object representations and friendship patterns.

Morals. This scale assesses the development of conscience.

Vocational/educational goals. This scale measures how well the adolescent is performing as a student and planning for his or her vocational future.

258

3. *Sexual self.*

Sexual attitudes. This scale assesses the adolescent's feelings, attitudes, and behavior toward the opposite sex.

4. *Familial self.*

Family relationships. This scale assesses the quality of the adolescent's relationship with his or her parents.

5. *Coping self.*

Mastery of the external world. This scale assesses adaptation to the immediate environment.

Psychopathology. This scale assesses any overt or severe psychopathology.

Superior adjustment. This scale measures coping ability.

The OSIQ was completed by each adolescent at early, middle, and late adolescence.

RESULTS

CHANGES IN SELF-IMAGE
ASSOCIATED WITH ADOLESCENT DEVELOPMENT

There was a significant improvement with age in the self-image of adolescents, with the most positive self-image found in late adolescence, $F(24,142) = 2.76$, $p < .0001$. This change was found in the following OSIQ scales: impulse control, body image, morals, sexual attitudes, family relationships, mastery of the external world, psychopathology, and superior adjustment. The improvement in capacity for social relationships approached significance. Two scales on which no significant differences were found were emotional tone and vocational/ educational goals. These results are presented in figure 19.

There was a moderate degree of continuity from one substage to another. The average intercorrelation was .55 from early to middle adolescence and .57 from middle to late adolescence. The scales for which there was considerable continuity ($> .40$) over the three age comparisons were impulse control, emotional tone, body and self-image, social relationships, family relationships, psychopathology, and superior adjustment. There was also continuity in the total score. These results are presented in table 15.

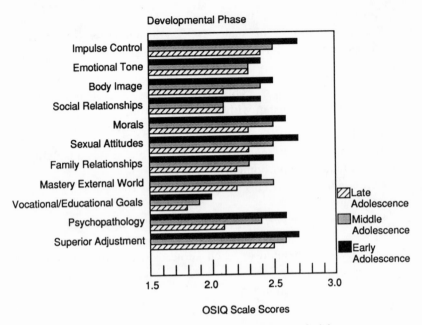

Fɪɢ. 19.—Developmental changes in the self-image of adolescents

THE ASSOCIATION OF SELF-IMAGE WITH PERSONALITY FUNCTIONING

Overall, the consistently clear group demonstrated a more positive self-image than the fluctuating or the consistently disturbed group. There were few significant differences found between these latter two groups. (There was a multivariate main effect for personality functioning groups, $F[24,60] = 1.74, p < .04$.) The differences among the three groups approached significance on the morals scale, but there was no significant difference among the personality functioning groups for sexual attitudes. These results are presented in figure 20.

COMPARISON OF THE SELF-IMAGE OF BOYS AND GIRLS

There were two significant differences found in the self-image of boys and girls at all ages. (There was a significant difference found for the multivariate main effect for gender, $F[24,60] = 1.74, p < .04$.) These differences were found in the body image scale, $F(1,41) = 4.79$, $p < .03$, and in the sexual attitudes scale, $F(1,41) = 14.15, p < .001$.

TABLE 15

CONTINUITY IN SELF-IMAGE FROM EARLY TO MIDDLE TO LATE ADOLESCENCE

Variable and Age	Pearson Product-Moment Correlation	p	Variable and Age	Pearson Product-Moment Correlation	p
Impulse control:			Family relationships:		
Early to middle	.71	.0001	Early to middle	.45	.0001
Middle to late	.69	.0001	Middle to late	.67	.0001
Early to late	.55	.0001	Early to late	.49	.0001
Emotional tone:			Mastery of the external world:		
Early to middle	.65	.0001	Early to middle	.61	.0001
Middle to late	.56	.0001	Middle to late	.53	.0001
Early to late	.52	.0001	Early to late	.25	.04
Body and self-image:			Vocational/educational goals:		
Early to middle	.55	.0001	Early to middle	.32	.01
Middle to late	.64	.0001	Middle to late	.41	.001
Early to late	.46	.0001	Early to late	.21	.07
Social relationships:			Psychopathology:		
Early to middle	.57	.0001	Early to middle	.53	.0001
Middle to late	.54	.0001	Middle to late	.69	.0001
Early to late	.49	.0001	Early to late	.44	.001
Morals:			Superior adjustment:		
Early to middle	.37	.004	Early to middle	.60	.0001
Middle to late	.43	.0001	Middle to late	.53	.0001
Early to late	.26	.03	Early to late	.57	.0001
Sexual attitudes:					
Early to middle	.53	.0001			
Middle to late	.50	.0001			
Early to late	.28	.02			

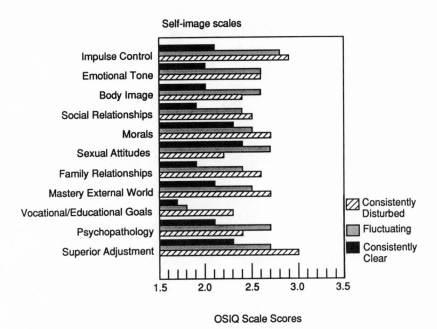

Self-image scales

FIG. 20.—Comparison of self-image among personality functioning groups

The boys demonstrated more positive feelings and attitudes toward their bodies and toward the opposite sex than did the girls. These results are presented in figure 21.

DISCUSSION

The data presented in this section further support the conclusion that the adolescent personality gradually matures during the teenage years. Late adolescents perceive in themselves greater impulse control as well as a more fully developed conscience. They feel increased comfort with their changed bodies and demonstrate more positive feelings and attitudes. They also perceive themselves to have better relationships with members of the opposite sex. Relationships with their families are also perceived to be improved. Late adolescents demonstrate fewer symptoms of psychopathology and appear as the best adjusted.

No significant change takes place in the areas of emotional harmony and vocational/educational goals from early to late adolescence. This

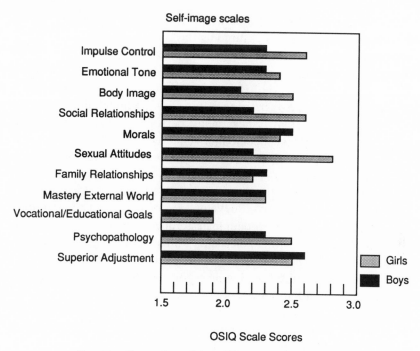

Self-image scales

FIG. 21.—Comparison of the self-image of boys and girls

indicates that older teenagers remain embroiled in some developmental issues. Although considerably more mature than they were at age thirteen, the older teenagers in our study had just entered the late adolescent subphase when vocational and educational problems increase in importance and demand resolution. The continued disharmony of affects noted during late adolescence coincides with the heightened degree of anxious and depressed affect reported in section 4.

These findings support a hypothesis that late adolescence, like early adolescence, is a period of disrupted personality organization. Early adolescents struggle with conflicts surrounding dependence and independence as they mature from childhood. Emotions are aroused as they leave elementary school for the challenges of high school and as they go through the physical and psychological changes associated with puberty. Late adolescents are conflicted as they enter the adult world and are confronted with the tasks of evolving a mature identity in the vocational and educational fields as well as in the area of intimate relationships.

263

A significant degree of continuity over time was noted in seven of the eleven content areas measured by the OSIQ (table 15). This finding is consonant with the findings reported in section 3 that demonstrated considerable continuity of personality functions between all age spans (table 6). This supports a hypothesis that many core characteristics of personality endure over time. Although often affected by substage psychosocial conflictual issues, many personality characteristics do not vary drastically in a specific individual over time. Simply noted, if you know someone well at age thirteen, you will recognize a strong resemblance at age eighteen.

The data reported in this section also clearly demonstrate a difference between teenagers who develop free of personality functioning disturbance and those who demonstrate fluctuating or consistent disturbance. In contrast with adolescents who experience personality disturbance at some points during their development, the adolescents with consistent healthy functioning report significantly better impulse control, emotional harmony, body image, adaptational skills, and adjustment. In addition, they perceive better social relationships and more clearly developed vocational and educational goals; they also report less psychopathology.

It is noteworthy, however, that the nondisturbed adolescents do not differ significantly from their disturbed peers in the areas of conscience development (although a trend is evident) and sexual attitudes. This suggests that adolescence continues as a time of considerable ongoing experimentation, with the areas of morality and sexuality remaining largely conflicted for the whole population (disturbed and nondisturbed).

It seemed surprising to discover that the self-image of the fluctuating group was similar in most areas to the self-image of the consistently disturbed group. Even transient personality functioning disturbance has marked consequences on the self-image of the adolescent. Both groups share a similar level of poor self-image in the areas of impulse control, emotional harmony, body image, social relationships, family relationships, and psychopathology. It can therefore be suggested that the self- and object representations of both groups are similarly disturbed, leading both groups to experience painful and troublesome relationship conflicts. Although the two groups rate themselves as equally disturbed on the OSIQ, it may be the case that more sensitive measures may reveal significant qualitative differences.

More in keeping with prior expectation was the finding that the fluctuating group was differentiated from the consistently disturbed group by more positive attitudes toward vocational and educational goals and by better coping skills. In other words, even though episodically disturbed adolescents and chronically disturbed adolescents are not generally distinguishable in most areas of self-image assessment, they do view themselves as significantly different in their actual social and reality adjustment. Although both groups question themselves similarly with regard to their internal world, the fluctuating group accurately perceives itself as more accomplished and higher functioning in the external world (i.e., in work and in social relationships).

Boys and girls did not differ in their self-image except in two specific areas, sexual attitudes and body image. Here, boys presented as more positive than girls. This finding is supported by clinical experience that suggests that girls are more aware and concerned about their needs for heterosexual intimacy than are boys. Girls also present as more concerned about body shape and weight than do boys at all ages.

SUMMARY OF MAJOR FINDINGS

SELF-IMAGE AND PERSONALITY FUNCTIONING

1. Self-image improves with increasing age during adolescence. This is most evident when early adolescence is compared to late adolescence (fig. 19 and Appendix table A11).

2. Adolescent self-image demonstrates considerable continuity between developmental subphases, particularly in the areas of impulse control, emotional tone (affective harmony), body image, social relationships, family relationships, psychopathology, and coping ability (table 15).

3. The consistently clear group demonstrated the most positive self-image (fig. 20 and Appendix table A12).

4. The self-image of the fluctuating group and that of the consistently disturbed group were similar in most areas (fig. 20 and Appendix table A12).

5. The fluctuating group was differentiated from the consistently disturbed group by more positive attitudes toward vocational and educational goals and by better coping skills; that is, they demonstrated a more positive social and reality adjustment (fig. 20 and Appendix table A12).

6. Boys demonstrate more positive feelings and attitudes toward their bodies than do girls (fig. 21 and Appendix table A13).

7. Boys demonstrate more positive attitudes toward members of the opposite sex than do girls (fig. 21 and Appendix table A13).

7. Conclusions: Adolescents over Time

This study provides a detailed description of some of the psychological changes that accompany pubescence and physical maturation throughout the teenage years. Early adolescence, with its attendant dramatic physical changes, was found to be a time when youngsters experienced more negative affects and attitudes, a poorer self-image, and more disturbance in personality functioning than during the subsequent substages. In addition, parents and teachers reported the early teenagers' behavior to be the most problematic.

With maturation, there was improvement in all these areas as the youngsters progressively adapted to developmental changes and environmental demands. As our study teenagers matured from early to middle adolescence, they appeared happier and less conflicted. Personality functioning and affective regulation improved. Attitudes became more positive and behavior problems decreased at home and at school. Self-image also improved.

This improvement in personality functioning observed in middle adolescence remained stable into late adolescence. Attitudes and self-image continued to develop in a positive direction. However, levels of anxiety and depression rose again in late adolescence in response to new developmental psychosocial challenges. Internalizing behavior problems decreased most from early to middle adolescence and declined more modestly from middle to late adolescence. By contrast, externalizing problems diminished consistently at each subphase. Overall, our results are encouraging in that they indicate that adolescence is a period of progressive psychological growth and adaptation.

INTERNAL WORKING MODELS

Early adolescence is a difficult phase, encompassing the physical changes associated with pubescence and the psychosocial changes related to revised status from childhood. During this time of major transition, adults alter their reactions to and expectations of young people, as do the teenagers themselves. From the perspective of attachment theory, it appears that these stresses challenge the young person's internal working models, which were developed in childhood and which must now serve to mediate novel and more complex demands. The internal working model represents a relatively stable set of relationship patterns that the youngster brings to any interpersonal situation. During adolescence, relationships change, peer networks enlarge, and newly found heterosexual relationships are experienced. As a result, there is a strong need for the revision of the internal working models. Self- and object representations must undergo considerable change in order to allow for more complicated personality functioning.

Youngsters who were fortunate to have developed coherent and flexible internal working models in childhood responded to developmental challenges in adolescence with healthy personality functioning, a satisfactory self-image, and an absence of behavior problems or symptoms of affective distress. Thirty-four percent of our sample fell into this category.

Teenagers who developed rigid and conflicted internal working models in childhood remained adapted during adolescence as long as pressures were modest. With more intense challenges, they developed transient difficulties in personality functioning. Forty-two percent of our youngsters composed this group, which we propose experienced adolescent turmoil.

A smaller number of our study adolescents appeared to have developed internal working models in childhood that were defective or seriously impoverished. These youngsters responded to most stressful situations in adolescence in a dysfunctional manner. They composed 24 percent of our sample, and we expect that they will continue to present character pathology in adult life.

Despite the significant number of adolescents who fit the turmoil and the consistently disturbed groups, there was considerable continuity in functioning for our sample when considered as a whole as they developed from one substage of adolescence to another. For all the variables we examined, there was evidence of both change and continuity. Such a finding is consistent with a transactional theoretical model like that of Bowlby, which asserts both changes and continuities in the progressive development of the internal working models. The research task ahead is to examine in greater detail those factors that promote change and those that account for continuity.

ADOLESCENT TURMOIL

Investigators of adolescent development have puzzled over the concept of adolescent turmoil for many years. In a seminal paper, Rutter et al. (1976) reviewed this subject in the light of findings from the Isle of Wight epidemiological study. Based on data derived from a general population study of fourteen- to fifteen-year-olds, he suggested that the presence of turmoil can be determined by examining the extent to which the adolescent experiences dysphoria and appears estranged from parents. He concluded that alienation from parents was not common in fourteen-year-olds, However, inner experiences of turmoil were common in early adolescence, with 40 percent of his study population reporting some appreciable misery or depression. In our study, we have had the advantage of tracking teenagers over the entire course of their adolescent development. Between one-third and half of our adolescents were found to demonstrate significant personality functioning disturbance at each cross-sectional adolescent subphase, early, middle, or late. However, when studied longitudinally, it was observed that some of the teenagers demonstrated personality disturbance that fluctuated over the course of their adolescence while others demonstrated disturbance that was continuous. It is the group with temporary dysfunction (42 percent), who showed periods of both normal and disturbed functioning in adolescence, that we concluded were presenting with adolescent turmoil.

A consistently positive correlation was observed in our study between personality disturbance and disturbed affects, disturbed attitudes, and disturbed behavior at home and at school. When adolescents presented with personality disturbance, they also appeared as more alienated and internally miserable. Our results are therefore consistent with those of Rutter et al. but refine the concept by suggesting that adolescent turmoil should be used to describe transient difficulties during adolescence and should not include youngsters with chronic dysfunctions that precede adolescence and endure throughout the period. These latter individuals should be differentiated as persons with ongoing personality disturbance.

SEX DIFFERENCES

We examined differences in the development of boys and girls. Gender-related differences were found to be present, but not to the degree that we had expected from the literature. Physical differences in maturation far outstrip differences in psychological development. There are relatively few differences in the development of psychological functioning in boys and girls during adolescence. Girls demonstrate some modest superiority in personality functioning over boys and exhibit more positive attitudes in a few areas. In behavior problems, girls show a different pattern of change. Behavior problems in girls are delayed, demonstrating less change from early to middle adolescence but a greater change from middle to late adolescence. In the area of self-image, boys are more positive about themselves in just a few areas, but overall there were more similarities than differences.

THE LONGITUDINAL PERSPECTIVE

Differentiating adolescents according to longitudinal patterns of development addresses the question of how individuals grow up over time. Our results suggest that some teenagers traverse their adolescence remarkably free of difficulties and do not consistently appear either excessively conflicted or disturbed in personality functioning. A second group shows considerable variation in personality functioning competence over time. At some points, they function at an adequate level and present with little personality disturbance, while, at other points, they function at a lower level and present with various difficulties. We consider that this second group experiences adolescent turmoil. A third group of individuals grows up always appearing disturbed in personality functioning, attitudes, and feelings and presents with significant behavior problems at home and at school over all the years. These teenagers give evidence for ongoing personality functioning problems. Youngsters who follow the adolescent turmoil pathway and those who follow the disturbed personality pathway both experience difficulties during their development as they endeavor to adapt to new demands and challenges. In addition to the temporal course of their difficulties, the turmoil group can be differentiated from the personality disturbed group by more positive attitudes toward vocational and educational goals, by better coping skills, and by better adjustment to social situations and environmental expectations.

SOME CLINICAL CONSIDERATIONS

Our measurement of personality dysfunction represents a reliable and clearly defined assessment of personality functioning during ado-

269

lescence. At this phase of our work, the assessment offers a means of ordering levels of functioning and making broad differentiations. It does not, however, permit us to make diagnoses (DSM-III-R) since thresholds have not been psychometrically determined. Nevertheless, our measurement of personality functioning disturbance correlates well with measures of behavior problems.

A large proportion of youngsters in the consistently disturbed group would be expected to meet diagnostic criteria for some disorders. This report does not answer questions as to the relation of personality dysfunction and the incidence of diagnosed emotional or behavioral disorders. We are, however, able to address the relation between personality functioning competence and adaptation to developmental challenges. In this regard, our concept of adolescent turmoil is not synonymous with clinical disorder but refers to a profile of symptoms that fluctuate with changes in developmental status.

The accurate assessment of clinical problems necessarily requires both a cross-sectional and a longitudinal point of view. Each perspective contributes different but complementary data. A cross-sectional assessment leads toward diagnosis and a determination of a modality of treatment. A longitudinal assessment informs about etiology, severity of disorder, and prognosis. A primary goal in the assessment of a new patient is to understand the presenting difficulties in the light of current and past life events. To this end, during history taking, a detailed cross-sectional account should be made of the presenting problems (affective symptoms, cognitive disturbances, behavioral difficulties, social dysfunctions and biological disorders).

When this compilation is complete, current difficulties should be reviewed longitudinally in the context of developmental change. A life chart tracing biological, social, and psychological development can be composed that includes both healthy, adaptive, and normative characteristics and maladaptive and psychopathological characteristics. Competencies and difficulties should be reviewed in relation to developmental norms. Behaviors incongruous with developmental norms for a particular stage become a cause for clinical concern. Where difficulties originate prior to adolescence and continue through successive adolescent stages, they are likely to signify ingrained personality disturbance. Thus, a longitudinal perspective brought to bear on cross-sectional information helps discern whether problems have become internalized or are part of a fluctuating personality organization. Problems that develop a clearly recognized response pattern and become part of the adolescent's cognitive structure should increase the clinician's concern. Distinguishing between a fluctuating pattern of maladjustment and a persistent pattern of personality functioning disturbance is exceedingly useful for the clinician in determining appropriate treatment and formulating prognosis.

IMPLICATIONS OF ADOLESCENT SUBSTAGES FOR TREATMENT

Adolescent life stages are commonly divided into three periods, that is, ages thirteen and fourteen (early adolescence), fifteen and sixteen (middle adolescence), and seventeen to nineteen (late adolescence). Each stage has been described by psychodynamic theory as having separate characteristics, tasks to be accomplished, specific conflicts that successively become manifest, and particular patterns by which relationships are sought and formed.

In considering the early adolescent phase, psychoanalytic theory has suggested that the typical adolescent undergoes intrapsychic disruption as a result of the physical changes associated with maturation and demonstrates behavior that tends to show a disorganized, erratic quality, with a decreased willingness to accommodate to the expectations of parents and other adults. Mood swings are said to dominate the emotional life.

This description has been somewhat corroborated by our study findings. At age fourteen, as our cohort progressed from childhood into adolescence, the youngsters demonstrated increased anxiety and depression combined with a reduction in their ability to differentiate their thoughts and feelings from those of others. They also showed a decreased ability to communicate clearly about their problems. Although this was the general developmental trend in our sample, our findings indicate that these consequences are less dramatic than those suggested by dominant psychoanalytic writers. Youngsters who demonstrated notable turmoil were in the minority, albeit a sizable one.

Our data suggest, therefore, that, for early adolescent patients who present with difficulties that begin immediately after puberty, the clinician, having first ruled out the presence of a major clinical disorder, is advised to consider such presenting problems as developmental in origin. Extensive or complex intervention is often not required, al-

271

though supportive therapy, parental counseling, and periodic follow-up can be helpful. If the symptomatology is assessed to be particularly severe or markedly painful, then short-term focused intervention should be considered. By contrast, early adolescents presenting with symptomatology that has continued from childhood should be considered differently. Such teenagers are likely to represent a more disturbed group who will usually require more intensive help.

Psychodynamic theory has proposed that the typical presentation of the teenager traversing the middle adolescent phase is marked by exaggerated rebelliousness defending against concerns of regression back to early childhood conflictual issues. Our research does not corroborate this generalization for the middle adolescent. For most teenagers, middle adolescence seems to be a quiet time sandwiched between the disruption that many experience during early adolescence and the anxieties associated with changing status during late adolescence. Our observations conform more closely to a model such as Bowlby's, suggesting that by middle adolescence teenagers have had ample opportunity to adapt internal working models to the demands of the developmental period.

From a clinical perspective, our data suggest that adolescents who show significant disturbance at age sixteen, particularly persisting from age thirteen, must be regarded with considerable concern by the clinician. Symptomatology presenting during middle adolescence is not likely to result from developmental factors but is more likely related to significant personality disturbance or to disabling stress resulting from difficulties in meeting increasing environmental expectations or changes in family or social networks. Prompt and multifocused treatment is often required for these patients.

Regarding late adolescence, psychodynamic theory has proposed that symptoms are related more to an upsurgence of psychological conflict than to problems associated with personality transformation. The late adolescents that we studied corroborated this description. The reemergence of difficulties at age eighteen appears to be associated with the stresses that accompany the transition from adolescence to young adulthood. During late adolescence, there appears to be a developmentally related increase in distress. From a clinical point of view, symptomatology appearing for the first time during late adolescence may again be first considered as developmental, as was the case for early adolescents. Many late teenagers with developmental disturbance can also benefit from brief supportive intervention. (It should be noted, however, that adult forms of mental illness such as schizophrenia and affective disorder frequently appear for the first time during late adolescence; these syndromes, when diagnosed, will require particular and specialized treatment.)

Psychological disturbance appearing in late adolescence that follows difficulties experienced during middle and early adolescence must again be regarded differently and of more serious consequence. In these cases, the patients are more likely to have problems of disturbed personality functions and organization. Treatment of these problems will often require extensive work over a prolonged period and has guarded prognosis.

In summary, our research suggests that adolescent turmoil is common during early and late adolescence and unusual during middle adolescence. Problems that persist from one developmental phase to another are considered to be more resistant to treatment and will often require more intensive interventions. Serious psychopathology becomes evident from longitudinal historical data. Brief, focused, goal-oriented psychotherapy has a useful place in the treatment of developmental problems that are more common in early and late adolescence. With regard to middle adolescence, most difficulties are usually not developmentally related. Problems presenting during this stage are most likely related to persistent personality functioning difficulties or to specific and intense life stresses.

Appendix

TABLE A1

Total Score on the Personality Functioning Scale

	Early Adolescence		Middle Adolescence		Late Adolescence	
	Mean	(S.D.)	Mean	(S.D.)	Mean	(S.D.)
Whole sample	26.7	(5.3)	28.6	(4.7)	28.1	(4.7)
Males	25.7	(5.4)	27.5	(5.0)	27.0	(4.6)
Females	27.8	(5.2)	29.7	(4.2)	29.2	(4.5)

Note.—Scores range from 0 to 35, with a high score indicating competence in personality functioning.

273

TABLE A2
PREVALENCE OF PERSONALITY FUNCTIONING DISTURBANCE DURING
EARLY, MIDDLE, AND LATE ADOLESCENCE

Developmental Phase	Clear (%)	Some Disturbance (%)
Early adolescence	54	46
Middle adolescence	67	33
Late adolescence	56	44

NOTE.—Sample size is fifty-nine.

TABLE A3
PREVALENCE OF PERSONALITY FUNCTIONING DISTURBANCE
THROUGHOUT ADOLESCENCE

	Consistently Clear	Fluctuating	Consistently Disturbed
Subjects (N):			
Male	10	9	11
Female	11	16	2
Total (N)	21	25	13
% of Sample	35.6	40.7	23.7

NOTE.—Sample size is fifty-nine.

TABLE A4
AFFECT AND ATTITUDES IN EARLY, MIDDLE, AND LATE ADOLESCENCE

	Early Adolescence		Middle Adolescence		Late Adolescence		*p*	Post Hoc
	Mean	(S.D.)	Mean	(S.D)	Mean	(S.D.)		
Affects:								
Anxiety:								
Total	3.3	(.7)	2.8	(.9)	3.3	(.6)	.0001	EL vs. M
Males	3.4	(.6)	2.8	(.9)	3.4	(.6)		
Females	3.2	(.7)	2.8	(.9)	3.1	(.7)		
Depression:								
Total	2.2	(1.0)	1.7	(.9)	2.3	(.8)	.0001	EL vs. M
Males	2.2	(.9)	1.8	(1.0)	2.3	(1.0)		
Females	2.1	(1.0)	1.7	(.7)	2.3	(.7)		
Affection:								
Total	2.8	(.8)	3.1	(.7)	3.2	(.6)	.0001	E vs. ML
Males	2.8	(.8)	3.0	(.8)	3.0	(.6)		
Females	2.8	(.8)	3.3	(.5)	3.5	(.6)		
Attitudes:								
Optimism:								
Total	3.0	(.8)	3.2	(.7)	3.3	(.6)	.002	E vs. ML
Males	2.9	(.8)	3.1	(.8)	3.2	(.7)		
Females	3.0	(.7)	3.3	(.5)	3.3	(.5)		
Introspective-ness:								
Total	2.0	(.8)	2.5	(.6)	2.6	(.6)	.0001	E vs. ML
Males	1.8	(.7)	2.4	(.6)	2.5	(.7)		
Females	2.1	(.9)	2.7	(.6)	2.8	(.5)		
Dominance:								
Total	2.4	(.9)	2.4	(.7)	2.7	(.6)	.013	EM vs. L
Males	2.5	(.9)	2.4	(.6)	2.6	(.6)		
Females	2.4	(.8)	2.3	(.8)	2.8	(.6)		

NOTE.—Scores range from 1 to 5, with 1 = little and 5 = much. Univariate *F*-tests with 2,106 degrees of freedom. E = early, M = middle, and L = late adolescence.

TABLE A5

Affects and Attitudes among the Consistently Clear, Consistently Disturbed, and Fluctuating Groups

	Group Mean Ratings							
	Stable Clear		Fluctuating		Stable Disturbed			
	Mean	(S.D.)	Mean	(S.D.)	Mean	(S.D.)	*p*	Post Hoc
Affect:								
Anxiety	2.9	(.5)	3.1	(.4)	3.5	(.4)	.002	CF vs. D
Depression	1.6	(.5)	2.1	(.5)	2.8	(.5)	.0001	C vs. F vs. D
Anger	2.1	(.4)	2.7	(.6)	2.9	(.6)	.0001	C vs. FD
Pleasure	3.5	(.4)	3.1	(.3)	2.7	(.3)	.0001	C vs. F vs. D
Affection	3.4	(.4)	3.1	(.5)	2.4	(.3)	.0001	C vs. F vs. D
Attitudes:								
Cooperativeness	3.8	(.4)	3.4	(.4)	2.9	(.3)	.0001	C vs. F vs. D
Curiosity	3.3	(.4)	3.1	(.4)	2.4	(.4)	.0001	CF vs. D
Approval	3.5	(.4)	3.1	(.5)	2.5	(.4)	.0001	C vs. F vs. D
Optimism	3.6	(.3)	3.1	(.5)	2.5	(.3)	.00001	C vs. F vs. D
Introspectiveness	2.7	(.3)	2.4	(.5)	1.9	(.4)	.0001	CF vs. D

Note.—Scores range from 1 to 5, with 1 = little and 5 = much. C = clear, F = fluctuating, and D = disturbed group.

TABLE A6

Comparison of Behavior Problems in School from Early to Middle Adolescence

	Age				
	Thirteen		Sixteen		
Variable	Mean	(S.D.)	Mean	(S.D.)	*p*
Total score:					
Total	22.9	(21.3)	17.1	(16.2)	.08
Male	29.4	(19.7)	18.8	(16.5)	
Female	13.4	(10.1)	16.8	(8.9)	
Factor 1: conduct problems:					
Total	4.3	(6.7)	2.0	(5.1)	.07
Male	6.1	(6.8)	2.6	(5.5)	
Female	1.8	(3.5)	1.6	(2.0)	
Factor 2: inattentive-passive:					
Total	4.6	(4.8)	3.8	(3.7)	N.S.
Male	6.0	(4.1)	4.5	(4.0)	
Female	2.5	(2.5)	3.4	(1.9)	
Factor 3: tension-anxiety:					
Total	3.4	(3.4)	2.8	(3.2)	N.S.
Male	4.0	(3.0)	2.8	(2.8)	
Female	2.6	(1.9)	2.9	(3.1)	
Factor 4: hyperactivity:					
Total	4.3	(5.3)	2.9	(3.7)	.08
Male	5.9	(5.7)	3.2	(4.0)	
Female	1.9	(2.9)	2.6	(2.4)	

TABLE A7
Comparison of Behavior Problems at Home from Early to Late Adolescence

Variable	Age								
	Early		Middle		Late				
	Mean	(S.D.)	Mean	(S.D.)	Mean	(S.D.)	p	Post Hoc	
Internalizing problems:									
Total	13.8	(10.5)	10.2	(8.8)	8.7	(9.3)	.0001	E vs. ML	
Male	15.4	(9.4)	9.8	(7.7)	8.4	(6.2)			
Female	11.8	(11.7)	10.7	(10.3)	9.0	(12.7)			
Externalizing problems:									
Total	13.4	(11.2)	10.4	(10.0)	8.3	(8.6)	.0001	E vs. M vs. L	
Male	14.6	(10.3)	11.0	(10.0)	9.0	(8.3)			
Female	11.8	(12.5)	9.7	(10.3)	7.3	(9.2)			

NOTE.—E = early, M = middle, and L = late adolescence.

TABLE A8
Comparison of CBCL Narrow Band Factor Scores from Early to Late Adolescence

Variable	Age							
	Early Adolescence		Middle Adolescence		Late Adolescence			
	Mean	(S.D.)	Mean	(S.D.)	Mean	(S.D.)	p	Post Hoc
Boys:								
Somatic complaints	3.2	(3.3)	1.3	(1.6)	1.6	(1.8)	.01	E vs. ML
Uncommunicative	5.1	(2.8)	4.0	(2.9)	3.2	(2.9)	.02	E vs. L
Immature	1.3	(1.6)	.6	(1.0)	.4	(0.5)	.02	E vs. ML
Obsessive-compulsive	2.9	(2.1)	2.0	(2.4)	1.6	(2.7)	.03	E vs. L
Hostile-withdrawn	2.7	(3.1)	1.8	(3.3)	1.3	(1.9)	.05	E vs. L
Aggressive	8.6	(7.0)	6.6	(5.3)	4.8	(5.2)	.01	E vs. M vs. L
Hyperactive	4.8	(3.8)	3.6	(3.8)	2.9	(2.5)	.05	E vs. L
Girls:								
Immature-hyperactive	3.3	(3.8)	3.3	(3.4)	1.8	(2.7)	.02	EM vs. L

NOTE.—E = early, M = middle, and L = late adolescence.

TABLE A9
Comparison of Behavior Problems at School among Personality Functioning Groups

	Group				
	Consistently Clear	Fluctuating	Consistently Disturbed		
Variable	Mean (S.D.)	Mean (S.D.)	Mean (S.D.)	p	Post Hoc
Total score:					
Total	15.0 (10.9)	21.0 (13.5)	31.5 (18.9)	.002	C vs. D
Male	14.5 (11.1)	22.4 (12.4)	31.9 (18.4)		
Female	15.4 (11.2)	20.2 (14.5)	30.0 (25.5)		
Factor 1: conduct problems:					
Total	2.6 (3.8)	3.1 (4.5)	5.4 (5.6)	.02	N.S.
Male	1.8 (2.7)	3.7 (4.8)	5.8 (5.6)		
Female	3.3 (4.6)	2.7 (4.4)	4.0 (6.6)		
Factor 2: inattentive-passive:					
Total	2.8 (2.3)	4.5 (3.3)	7.6 (4.1)	.001	CF vs. D
Male	3.2 (3.0)	4.7 (2.6)	7.2 (3.7)		
Female	2.5 (1.5)	4.3 (3.7)	8.8 (5.8)		
Factor 3: tension-anxiety:					
Total	1.6 (2.5)	3.7 (2.7)	4.4 (2.1)	.01	C vs. FD
Male	2.3 (3.0)	3.3 (2.1)	4.5 (2.0)		
Female	.9 (1.7)	3.9 (3.1)	4.0 (2.6)		
Factor 4: hyperactivity:					
Total	3.5 (3.2)	3.3 (3.7)	4.7 (4.2)	N.S.	
Male	3.1 (2.6)	4.6 (3.9)	5.3 (4.4)		
Female	3.9 (3.8)	2.5 (3.4)	2.7 (3.1)		

Note.—C = clear, F = fluctuating, and D = disturbed group.

TABLE A10
Comparison of Behavior Problems at Home among Personality Functioning Groups

	Group				
	Consistently Clear	Fluctuating	Consistently Disturbed		
Variable	Mean (S.D.)	Mean (S.D.)	Mean (S.D.)	p	Post Hoc
Internalizing:					
Total	8.0 (6.2)	13.8 (10.0)	15.5 (11.2)	.08	N.S.
Male	8.2 (4.9)	11.3 (7.4)	16.0 (12.5)		
Female	7.8 (7.4)	15.3 (11.1)	13.6 (4.8)		
Externalizing:					
Total	7.7 (8.0)	14.3 (10.1)	15.4 (9.2)	.03	N.S.
Male	9.3 (9.7)	14.3 (10.0)	14.9 (9.9)		
Female	6.3 (6.2)	14.3 (10.5)	17.8 (7.5)		

TABLE A11
CHANGES IN SELF-IMAGE FROM EARLY TO LATE ADOLESCENCE

| | Age | | | | | | | |
| | Early Adolescence | | Middle Adolescence | | Late Adolescence | | | |
Scale	Mean	(S.D.)	Mean	(S.D.)	Mean	(S.D.)	p^a	Post Hoc
Impulse control:								
Total	2.7	(.9)	2.5	(.8)	2.4	(.6)	.003	EM vs. L
Male	2.7	(.9)	2.5	(.8)	2.2	(.7)		
Female	2.7	(.8)	2.6	(.8)	2.5	(.6)		
Emotional tone:								
Total	2.4	(.8)	2.3	(.7)	2.3	(.7)	N.S.	
Male	2.4	(.9)	2.2	(.7)	2.1	(.7)		
Female	2.3	(.6)	2.4	(.7)	2.5	(.6)		
Body and self-image:								
Total	2.5	(.8)	2.4	(.8)	2.1	(.7)	.005	EM vs. L
Male	2.4	(.8)	2.2	(.7)	1.9	(.6)		
Female	2.6	(.7)	2.5	(.8)	2.2	(.6)		
Social relationships:								
Total	2.4	(.7)	2.1	(.7)	2.1	(.7)	.08	E vs. ML
Male	2.5	(.8)	2.2	(.6)	2.0	(.8)		
Female	2.2	(.5)	2.2	(.7)	2.2	(.7)		
Morals:								
Total	2.6	(.6)	2.5	(.5)	2.3	(.5)	.08	EM vs. L
Male	2.7	(.7)	2.7	(.6)	2.4	(.6)		
Female	2.6	(.5)	2.3	(.4)	2.2	(.4)		
Sexual attitudes:								
Total	2.7	(.8)	2.5	(.6)	2.3	(.7)	.02	E vs. L
Male	2.3	(.6)	2.1	(.5)	2.1	(.6)		
Female	3.1	(.7)	2.7	(.6)	2.4	(.6)		
Family relationships:								
Total	2.5	(.8)	2.2	(.6)	2.0	(.5)	.0001	E vs. M vs. L
Male	2.6	(.8)	2.2	(.7)	2.0	(.6)		
Female	2.4	(.7)	2.2	(.7)	2.0	(.6)		
Mastery external world:								
Total	2.4	(.7)	2.5	(.6)	2.2	(.6)	.009	EM vs. L
Male	2.4	(.8)	2.4	(.6)	2.2	(.6)		
Female	2.4	(.7)	2.5	(.6)	2.2	(.5)		
Vocational/educational goals:								
Total	2.0	(.6)	1.9	(.5)	1.8	(.5)	N.S.	
Male	2.1	(.6)	1.9	(.5)	1.9	(.6)		
Female	2.0	(.5)	1.9	(.5)	1.8	(.5)		
Psychopathology:								
Total	2.6	(.7)	2.4	(.6)	2.1	(.6)	.0001	EM vs. L
Male	2.5	(.7)	2.4	(.5)	2.0	(.6)		
Female	2.6	(.7)	2.5	(.7)	2.2	(.6)		
Superior adjustment:								
Total	2.7	(.6)	2.6	(.6)	2.5	(.6)	.02	EM vs. L
Male	2.7	(.5)	2.6	(.6)	2.5	(.7)		
Female	2.6	(.6)	2.6	(.6)	2.5	(.5)		

NOTE.—Scores range from 1 to 6, with 1 denoting most positive self-image. E = early, M = middle, L = late adolescence.

[a] Univariate F-tests with 2,41 degrees of freedom.

TABLE A12
Comparison of Self-Image among Personality Functioning Groups

Scale	Consistently Clear Mean	Consistently Clear (S.D.)	Fluctuating Mean	Fluctuating (S.D.)	Consistently Disturbed Mean	Consistently Disturbed (S.D.)	p^a	Post Hoc
Impulse control:								
Total	2.1	(.6)	2.8	(.7)	2.9	(.9)	.002	C vs. FD
Emotional tone:								
Total	2.0	(.5)	2.6	(.7)	2.6	(.8)	.005	C vs. FD
Body and self-image:								
Total	2.0	(.6)	2.6	(.8)	2.4	(.7)	.005	C vs. F
Social relationships:								
Total	1.9	(.5)	2.4	(.8)	2.5	(.6)	.007	C vs. FD
Morals:								
Total	2.3	(.6)	2.5	(.5)	2.7	(.5)	.07	
Sexual attitudes:								
Total	2.4	(.7)	2.7	(.7)	2.2	(.7)	N.S.	
Family relationships:								
Total	1.9	(.5)	2.4	(.7)	2.6	(.7)	.002	C vs. FD
Mastery external world:								
Total	2.1	(.5)	2.5	(.7)	2.7	(.6)	.006	C vs. FD
Vocational/educational goals:								
Total	1.7	(.4)	1.9	(.5)	2.3	(.6)	.001	C vs. F vs. D
Psychopathology:								
Total	2.1	(.6)	2.7	(.7)	2.4	(.7)	.006	C vs. F
Superior adjustment:								
Total	2.3	(.5)	2.7	(.5)	3.0	(.5)	.001	C vs. F vs. D

NOTE.—Scores range from 1 to 6, with 1 denoting most positive self image. C = clear, F = fluctuating, and D = disturbed group.

[a] Univariate F-tests with 2,41 degrees of freedom.

TABLE A13
COMPARISON OF THE SELF-IMAGE OF BOYS AND GIRLS

Scale	Boys		Girls		p^a
	Mean	(S.D.)	Mean	(S.D.)	
Impulse control	2.30	(.84)	2.56	(.53)	N.S.
Emotional tone	2.27	(.74)	2.40	(.65)	N.S.
Body and self-image	2.14	(.71)	2.47	(.76)	.03
Social relationships	2.21	(.70)	2.18	(.67)	N.S.
Morals	2.52	(.60)	2.38	(.44)	N.S.
Sexual attitudes	2.20	(.57)	2.77	(.68)	.001
Family relationships	2.27	(.66)	2.16	(.63)	N.S.
Mastery of external world	2.34	(.41)	2.34	(.40)	N.S.
Vocational/educational goals	1.91	(.55)	1.92	(.52)	N.S.
Psychopathology	2.30	(.61)	2.45	(.69)	N.S.
Superior adjustment	2.61	(.60)	2.53	(.57)	N.S.
Total score	23.00	(5.13)	23.42	(4.60)	

NOTE.—Scores range from 1 to 6, with 1 denoting most positive self-image.
[a] Univariate F-tests with 1,41 degrees of freedom.

REFERENCES

Achenbach, T. 1966. The classification of children's psychiatric symptoms: a factor-analytic study. *Psychological Monographs* 80(no. 7, whole no. 615).

Achenbach, T., and Edelbrock, C. 1981. Behavior problems and competencies reported by parents of normal and disturbed children aged 4 through 16. *Monographs of the Society for Research in Child Development* 46(serial no. 188).

Allport, G. W. 1937. *Personality: A Psychological Interpretation.* New York: Holt, Rinehart & Winston.

Arnold, L., & Smeltzer, M. 1974. Behavior checklist factor analysis for children and adolescents. *Archives of General Psychiatry* 30:799–804.

Blishen, B. A. 1967. A socioeconomic index for occupations in Canada. *Canadian Review of Sociology and Anthropology* 4:41–53.

Block, J. 1971. *Lives through Time.* Berkeley: Bancroft.

Blos, P. 1962. *On Adolescence.* New York: Free Press.

Bowlby, J. 1973. Susceptibility to fear and the availability of attachment figures. In *Attachment and Loss,* vol. 2. London: Hogarth.

Bowlby, J. 1988. Developmental psychiatry comes of age. *American Journal of Psychiatry* 145:1–9.

Bretherton, I., and Waters, E., eds. 1985. Growing points of attachment theory and research. *Monographs of the Society for Research in Child Development* 50(serial no. 209).

Cohen, J. 1960. A coefficient of agreement for nominal scales. *Educational Psychology Measurement* 20:37–46.

Coleman, J. 1974. *Relationships in Adolescence:* London: Routledge & Kegan Paul.

Conners, C. K. 1969. A teacher rating scale for use in drug studies with children. *American Journal of Psychiatry* 126:152–155.

Dusek, J., & Flaherty, J. 1981. The development of self-concept during the adolescent years. *Monograph of the Society for Research in Child Development* 46(serial no. 191).

Eysenck, M. W., & Eysenk, H. J. 1980. Mischel and the concept of personality. *British Journal of Psychology* 71:191–204.

Freud, A. 1946. *The Ego and the Mechanisms of Defense.* New York: International Universities Press.

Freud, A. 1958. Adolescence. *Psychoanalytic Study of the Child* 13:255–278.

Giovacchini, P., & Borowitz, G. 1974. An object relationship scale. *Adolescent Psychiatry* 3:186–212.

Masterson, J. F., Jr. 1967. The symptomatic adolescent five years later: he didn't grow out of it. *American Journal of Psychiatry* 123:1338–1348.

Mischel, W. 1969. Continuity and change in personality. *American Psychologist* 24:1012–1018.

Moriarty, A., & Toussieng, P. 1975. Adolescence in a time of transition. *Bulletin of the Meninger Clinic* 39:391–408.

Offer, D. 1969. *The Psychological World of the Teenager: A Study of Normal Adolescent Boys.* New York: Basic.

Offer, D., & Howard, K. I. 1972. The Offer self-image questionnaire for adolescents. *Archives of General Psychiatry* 6:529–537.

Offord, D.; Boyle, M.; Szatmari, P.; et al. 1987. Ontario Child Health Study II: six-month prevalence of disorder and rates of service utilization. *Archives of General Psychiatry* 44:832–836.

Robins, L. 1966. *Deviant Children Grow Up.* Baltimore: Williams & Wilkins.

Rutter, M.; Graham, P.; Chadwick, O.; and Yule, W. 1976. Adolescent turmoil: fact or fiction? *Journal of Child Psychology, Psychiatry and Allied Disciplines* 17:35–56.

Tyrer, P., & Alexander, J. 1979. Classification of personality disorder. *British Journal of Psychiatry* 135:163–167.

OTHER PUBLICATIONS OF THE TORONTO ADOLESCENT LONGITUDINAL STUDY

Golombek, H., and Kutcher, S. 1990. Feeling states during adolescence. *Psychiatric Clinics of North America* 13(3): 443–454.

Golombek, H., and Marton, P. 1989. Disturbed affect and suicidal behavior during adolescence. *Israel Journal of Psychiatry and Related Science* 26(1–2): 30–36.

Golombek, H.; Marton, P.; Stein, B.; and Korenblum, M. 1986. Personality functioning and behaviour disorder in early adolescence. *Journal of the American Academy of Child Psychiatry* 25(5): 697–703.

Golombek, H.; Marton, P.; Stein, B.; and Korenblum, M. 1986. A study of disturbed and nondisturbed adolescents (the Toronto Adolescent Longitudinal Study). *Canadian Journal of Psychiatry* 31:532–535.

Golombek, H.; Marton, P.; Stein, B.; and Korenblum, M. 1987. Personality functioning status during early and middle adolescence. *Adolescent Psychiatry* 14:365–377.

Golombek, H.; Marton, P.; Stein, B.; and Korenblum, M. 1989. Adolescent personality development: three phases, three courses and varying turmoil: findings from the Toronto Adolescent Longitudinal Study. *Canadian Journal of Psychiatry* 34:500–504.

Korenblum, M.; Golombek, H.; Marton, P.; and Stein, B. 1986. The classification of disturbed personality functioning in early adolescence. *Canadian Journal of Psychiatry* 32:362–367.

Korenblum, M.; Marton, P.; Golombek, H.; and Stein, B. 1987. Disturbed personality functioning: patterns of change from early to middle adolescence. *Adolescent Psychiatry* 14:407–416.

Korenblum, M.; Marton, P.; Golombek, H.; and Stein, B. 1990. Personality status: changes through adolescence. *Psychiatric Clinics of North America* 13(3): 389–399.

Marton, P.; Golombek, H.; Stein, B.; and Korenblum, M. 1987. Behavior disturbance and changes in personality dysfunction from early to middle adolescence. *Adolescent Psychiatry* 14:394–404.

Marton, P.; Golombek, H.; Stein, B.; and Korenblum, M. 1989. The relation of personality functions and adaptive skills to self-esteem in early adolescence. *Journal of Youth and Adolescence* 17(5): 393–401.

Stein, B. A.; Golombek, H.; Marton, P.; and Korenblum, M. 1986. Personality functioning and clinical presentation in early adolescence. *Canadian Journal of Psychiatry* 31:536–541.

Stein, B.; Golombek, H.; Marton, P.; and Korenblum, M. 1987. Personality function and change in clinical presentation from early to middle adolescence. *Adolescent Psychiatry* 14:378–393.

Stein, B.; Marton, P.; Golombek, H.; and Korenblum, M. 1991. Consistency and change in personality characteristics and affect from middle to late adolescence. *Canadian Journal of Psychiatry* 36(1): 16–20.

PART III

PSYCHOPATHOLOGY IN ADOLESCENT EMOTIONAL DISORDERS

EDITOR'S INTRODUCTION

Efforts at clarifying diagnostic consideration during adolescence are most difficult owing to the rapid developmental changes that characterize this period of life. Aggression, which once was comfortably handled during childhood, is now expressed more intensely toward family members, school, community authorities, and friends. Sexual identification is demanded always earlier. On the other hand, the teenager may become passive and withdrawn, gradually eliminating many well-established activities. In this frame of reference, major diagnostic groups must be recognized, clarified, and properly treated. Among those clinical entities to be considered are the mood disorders, anxiety disorders, borderline personality organization, psychotic reactions of adolescence, and the effect on developmental character formation of these psychopathological states.

Michael H. Stone examines suicide in 500 severely disturbed adolescents, a group that shows an increase in self-destructive behavior for the past twenty-five years. Stone sketches, in detail, some of the case histories from among the adolescent suicides. This aids in the discernment of patterns, specifically the events and emotional climates that predispose to suicide in young persons. He describes the concatenation of events in borderline disorders, psychotic disorders, and cluster disorders that may lead to suicide. The study also discusses risk factors and warns that schizoaffective males constitute a group at extreme risk. Stone concludes that adolescents with borderline and psychotic disorders are at high risk for suicide but can be recognized and treated.

Allan M. Josephson and William D. Erickson write how Huntington's Disease dramatically alters the life of the victim, the unaffected spouse, and the psychological development of their children. A turbulent relationship with a violent father, father loss through suicide and institutionalization, and an ensuing hostile dependent relationship with mother significantly altered the development of two male adolescents whose fathers were afflicted with Huntington's Disease. The corresponding changes in family interaction offer insight into the genesis of personality disorders and illustrate critical factors in male adolescent development.

Benjamin Garber, in the Joel Handler Memorial Lecture to the Chicago Society for Adolescent Psychiatry (1990), discusses the learning disabled adolescent. He concludes that the young person may pay a high price emotionally for the effects of early ego interference with growth. Garber describes the personality as demonstrating a prominent narcissistic cast but capable of benefiting from psychoanalytic psychotherapy.

Loretta R. Loeb and Felix F. Loeb, Jr., describe a psychodynamic correlation that they observed in adult manic-depressive patients, which enables them to make an earlier diagnosis in adolescents. They present a review of the literature and case studies to clarify their findings.

14 SUICIDE IN BORDERLINE AND OTHER ADOLESCENTS

MICHAEL H. STONE

Much attention has been focused recently on the mounting suicide rate among adolescents. Solomon and Murphy (1984) have shown, in their cohort studies, the steady increase in this rate over the twenty-five-year span beginning in 1950. The group at greatest risk is white males, in whom the rate, expressed as completed suicides per 100,000 per year, rose from 3.7 to 13.0 in fifteen- to nineteen-year-olds between 1950 and 1975. The increase in white females in this age bracket has been more modest, from 1.9 to 3.1. Rates among nonwhites have been and remain lower, but here too there has been an increase over the last generation in both genders. Diekstra and Moritz (1987) have noted the same phenomenon in Europe during these past several decades and have also drawn attention to some probable underlying factors, including the increasing divorce rate, the declining influence of the church, and, partly as an offshoot of the "baby boom" following World War II, diminished economic opportunities for young people, especially males, entering the work force.

Despite the alarming surge in adolescent suicide deaths that these investigators have documented, suicide remains a comparatively rare event. For this reason, suicide, as a crucial issue in psychiatry, is more accessible to the epidemiologist than to the average clinician. In my follow-up research, I came to occupy a middle position, having identified within the 550 patients I attempted to trace forty-nine suicides, far fewer than would suffice for epidemiological work but many more than a therapist would confront during his or her professional lifetime.

I have already made a number of brief reports on the follow-up study, which, for reasons both of simplicity and of homage to Ming Tsuang's "Iowa-500" (Tsuang and Winokur 1975), I have called the "P.I.-500" (Stone 1987, 1988a, 1989a; Stone, Hurt, and Stone 1987; Stone, Stone, and Hurt 1987). The P.I.-500, 95 percent of whom have now been traced, consisted of 206 patients with borderline personality disorder (BPD) by DSM-III criteria, ninety-three meeting Kernberg's (1967) criteria for borderline personality organization but not for BPD, ninety-nine (DSM-III) schizophrenics, sixty-four schizoaffectives, thirty-nine manic depressives, thirty-six schizophreniform patients, and a small number who did not fit into these major categories. These patients, having been hospitalized at the New York State Psychiatric Institute between 1963 and 1976, have been followed an average of 16.5 years. Of the 520 thus far traced, forty-nine are suicides (i.e., 9.4 percent of the total). To put this figure in perspective, the suicide rate in this group amounts to 673 per 100,000 per year. Most of these patients were in their twenties when they died. This means that their risk of suicide was more than twenty-five times higher than the risk for males in this age bracket during the late 1970s and more than sixty times the risk in white females of comparable age and cohort. The suicide rates within the different diagnostic categories of the P.I.-500 varied little in either direction from 9.5 percent; this was true for both adolescent and adult BPD patients, with the exception of the higher rate noted in the schizoaffectives, 22.5 percent.

As for the adolescent suicides, their number depends on the arbitrary cutoff age one uses in defining the adolescent group. Twenty-one of the suicides occurred in patients who had been twenty or younger when first hospitalized; of these, eleven had been under eighteen. If we restrict our focus to the adolescent suicides, properly speaking (i.e., to those who died at twenty or younger), nine such cases remain.

Of the nine adolescent suicides, five were borderline (all satisfying DSM-III criteria), and four presented with a psychosis—manic depressive in one case, schizoaffective in the other. Life events such as loss of a caretaker or traumatic experiences often figured importantly as precipitants or background characteristics in the lives of eventual suicides. Traumatic events within the family tend to be more pathogenic in this regard than those external to it; those of particular significance include incest (especially transgenerational—father-daughter, uncle-niece, etc.), physical brutality on the part of a parent, or intense

290

TABLE 1
P.I.-500: SUICIDES OCCURRING DURING ADOLESCENCE

Case	Sex	Age at Admission	Age at Death	Life Events			
				Loss	Incest	Parental Brutality	Parental Humiliation
Borderline patients:							
1. .... Female	Female	19	20				
2. .... Female	Female	15	18		+		+
3. .... Male	Male	17	19				+
4. .... Male	Male	16	19	Adoptee	+		
5. .... Female	Female	14	15	Divorce		+	+
Patients with psychotic conditions:							
6. .... Female	Female	16	17				
7. .... Male	Male	17	18			+	+
8. .... Female	Female	18	19				
9. .... Male	Male	17	18	Death/father			

verbal humiliation by close family members (Browne and Finkelhor 1986; Murphy and Brown 1980; Stone 1988b, 1990a; van der Kolk 1989). Table 1 shows the intrafamilial life events experienced by the nine adolescent suicides as well as the ages at index hospitalization and at death.

The small numbers of patients in the two main groups—borderline and other (psychotic)—do not permit statistical comparison, despite the appearance of more "life events" per patient in the borderlines. Actually, in the P.I.-500 as a whole, this distinction could be supported: parental brutality, for example, occurred twice as often in the early years of the borderline than in the psychotic patients (11 percent as against 5½ percent [Stone 1990b], reaching χ^2 significance levels for $p < .05$).

With regard to incest, division of the forty-nine suicides in the series as a whole into those with BPD as their admission diagnosis ($N = 17$) versus those with all other diagnoses ($N = 32$) revealed a higher frequency of this traumatic event among the borderlines (six of the seventeen, compared with two out of thirty-two [$\chi^2 = 6.35$, with Yates' correction, $p < .05$]).

291

In several of the suicides in both the adult and the adolescent groups, the relation between a traumatic episode and death was so close, with respect to the psychological effect of the event and the impulse to suicide, and the timing was so proximate as to suggest a causal linkage. It will be useful in this connection to sketch in detail some of the case histories from among the adolescent suicides. This anecdotal material constitutes the most relevant contribution of this follow-up study to the understanding of adolescent suicide. When the data from this series, for example, are added to similar data from other large-scale follow-up studies, the resulting N would be great enough to aid in the discernment of patterns—specifically, the typical chains of events and emotional climates that predispose young persons to suicide. Brief vignettes of the nine suicides follow.

Clinical Examples

A. THE BORDERLINE PATIENTS

1. A nineteen-year-old woman was admitted to the hospital after a fourth serious suicide attempt with hypnotics in two years. The first of these attempts occurred shortly after leaving home for college. The summer before college she had become depressed, irritable, and bulimic. She had been raised in an affluent family with perfectionistic standards, high expectations of their three children, and much attention to social form and polish. The least attractive or bright of the children, she had come to feel like the failure, the "ugly duckling," and had difficulty making friends at college. Her first suicide attempt followed her first sexual intercourse, which she allowed to prove to herself that she was not homosexual. The overdose that led to admission to our unit occurred after an affair with an orderly at the hospital where she had been taken for the tracheotomy required by her third attempt. While on our unit, she tried to kill herself by injecting cleaning fluid into a vein. She was kept on suicide watch for seven months. Her depression lifted to the point where it seemed safe to let her resume extramural life. She began an affair with an aide on another unit of our hospital. When her therapist made it clear this would have to be revealed to the administration, she obtained a pistol owned by a relative, drove to a secluded area, and shot herself. A few weeks before her death, she reported a dream to her therapist in which she was sent to

the gas chambers to be executed and died. Not having been physically or sexually abused during her upbringing, she more likely succumbed to a combination of predisposition to unipolar depression plus a set of dynamic factors relating to severe narcissistic injury over not "measuring up" to her parents and siblings. She became caught in a "vicious circle," where concern about her appearance led to inappropriate affairs, deepening shame, further lowering of self-image, and greater agitation.

2. A fifteen-year-old girl had been admitted to our unit because of washing rituals, starting after her menarche at twelve, which had begun to consume so much of her day as to preclude going to school. She had become irritable, hostile, and defiant, after having been described, before age twelve, as docile and compliant. On the unit, her defiance expressed itself as a refusal to participate in the usual activities. She was negativistic and openly contemptuous of the staff. At times, especially before her therapist's vacations, she became depressed, making suicide gestures and, eventually, committing acts of self-mutilation. Her facade of toughness mellowed somewhat after two years in residential treatment, but, because she was still not yet ready for extramural life, she was transferred to another hospital. A few months later, she hanged herself. Toward the end of her stay on the unit, she began to divulge the family secret. Her depressed and alcoholic father had sexually molested her from the time she was eleven and a half. Dynamically, this seemed to be the genesis of the ensuing feelings of unworthiness, shame, hostility, and the related obsessional washing symptom.

3. A seventeen-year-old male was transferred to our unit from another hospital, where he had been admitted because of hallucinogen-induced delusions (that he was God and could control traffic with his mind). His illness began at age fourteen, when, at summer camp, he witnessed some boys engaging in homosexual activity. Reacting with panic, he had been brought home by his parents. That fall, his personality changed. He became abrasive and argumentative. He began to abuse LSD, peyote, mescaline, and hashish and to live in the street with a number of other runaways. During his childhood, his mother had been seriously depressed for a year. His father had been verbally, though not physically, abusive. Family life had always been characterized by high "expressed emotion," everyone taking turns criticizing and screaming at each other. He spent eight months on the unit, the first half on suicidal precautions because of several episodes of wrist

cutting when first admitted. He appeared less suicidal when discharged, but he was never really able to reintegrate, return to high school, or make appropriate friends. At seventeen, he killed himself by overdosing. In retrospect, this patient's suicide seemed to have more to do with his antisocial features than with a biologically based depressive illness. As with many antisocial borderlines, suicide is a response to feeling cornered or trapped.

4. A sixteen-year-old male patient was transferred to our unit from another hospital, where he had been admitted because of rapid deterioration in his personality and habits. He had become truant, depressed, drug abusing, and delinquent. The latter involved homosexual prostitution to get money for the at least nine different drugs he was abusing. He lived in the streets as a "hippie." He had been adopted at birth by a wealthy couple whose relationship both with each other and with their son was completely chaotic. The parents argued constantly and threw dinner plates at each other during meals; they finally divorced when the patient was twelve. He then joined a teen gang and began carrying a pistol. At first, he remained with his father, but two years later he moved in with his mother. Both were extremely permissive with him. Shortly before his first hospitalization, his mother, an alcoholic and a flirtatious woman, seduced two of his friends. Later, she seduced him as well. The incestuous relations occurred over a three-week period. He recoiled from them, eventually running away from home and returning to the streets. After four months on the unit, he returned once more to his flagrantly psychotic mother. He continued to abuse drugs and engage in delinquent acts, until, at nineteen, he shot himself.

5. A fourteen-year-old girl was admitted to our unit after being medically cleared from the hospital's emergency room, where she had been treated for a serious aspirin overdose. The suicide attempt followed a rejection by a boyfriend. Her whole life had come to revolve around this boyfriend, owing to the chaotic and destructive conditions within her family. Both her parents were alcoholic and violent. They divorced when she was ten—at about the time of her menarche. She had always been rebellious as a child, the most defiant and irritable of the six children. Her father was especially punitive, hitting her with a stick or a belt for trivial offenses, often until she bled. Once, when she refused to accompany the rest of the family on a picnic, her father ran after her, dragged her to her room, beat her, and then made her stand mo-

tionless in the corner for two hours. After the divorce, she lived for a time with one, then with the other parent. Each threw her out for staying out late, then forced her to live with the other. Shortly before her hospitalization, she stayed out all night with her boyfriend and was told by her mother that she could no longer live at home. She was defiant on the unit as well, brought drugs onto it, was forced to leave, and then jumped to her death.

COMMENT

This patient's life-course exemplifies, in addition to a suicidal denouement to parental rejection, a particular life "script," encountered by Stephens (1987) in a number of female adolescent suicide attempters. Some patients, predominantly depressive and self-effacing, pursue the "humble pie" script, characterized by docility, passivity, and emotional submergence. This was the route taken by the schizoaffective adolescent suicides in this series, but the borderline suicides, as in the present example, show the "cheap thrill" script, consisting of defiance, rebelliousness, drug abuse, promiscuity, and acting out.

Another way of understanding the dynamics of this case example is to recognize the parallel between suicide and violence (as the reverse of the coin whose obverse is murder). Whereas we often think of suicide as the endpoint on the continuum of depression and sadness, many borderline patients suicide as a retaliatory act. This is especially true in the present case. The patient's suicide also signified the abandonment of life that, as Hendin (1987) mentions, equates with a rejection of the abandoning parents.

B. PATIENTS PRESENTING WITH A PSYCHOTIC DISORDER

1. A sixteen-year-old girl was hospitalized because of suicidal ideation, sexual confusion, social withdrawal, and a recent twenty-pound weight loss. She had been hospitalized briefly a year earlier after threatening to jump in front of a train. Shy and withdrawn all her life, she became increasingly withdrawn after her menarche at twelve. She began to develop a delusional system, believing herself to have two selves—one female, whom she found disgusting, and a male self that made her do and say "bad things." On the unit, she made no eye contact, dressed in male attire, laughed inappropriately, and showed

blunted affect. She expressed suicidal ideation and spoke of feeling "unreal" for the past three years. Though bright academically, she had begun having trouble concentrating on her schoolwork. She became preoccupied with dirt and germs. To avoid feelings of hopelessness, she tried to sleep as much as possible, yet she felt that her bed was made of quicksand, into which she would sink and die. Diagnosed schizoaffective, she was given neuroleptics and antidepressants but did not respond. A year later, she was transferred to another hospital. Feelings of despondency deepened. A month later, she took a fatal overdose while on a pass.

2. A seventeen-year-old male was hospitalized because of a suicide attempt with a mixture of pills, which he had ingested shortly before he was to have graduated from high school. A "model" student until age fourteen, he became moody, irascible, and grandiose by turns. At home he locked himself in his room, where he watched television or made morbid drawings. Though he had intercourse with a girl at sixteen, he felt insecure about sex. Shortly before his hospitalization, he asked his father—a highly competitive and explosively angry man—to talk to him "man to man" about sex. His father flew into a rage, screaming, "I'll cut you in two!" He then grabbed a framed photo of his son from the mantel, smashed it on the floor, and stomped on the glass fragments. His mother shouted for the father to stop, saying, "I'm witnessing a murder!" The patient's first response was to try to hang himself. It was a few weeks after being rescued from this attempt that the patient took the overdose that led to hospitalization. Because of alternating bouts of depression and grandiosity, he was diagnosed a bipolar manic depressive. He was given neuroleptics (lithium not as yet available) along with psychotherapy but responded little to either. Transferred to another facility, he took a fatal overdose of hypnotics a year later.

3. A college sophomore suffered a psychotic decompensation after an upsetting holiday with her family. She began to feel that the walls were moving in on her. She would stare for hours in her room, feeling that the world was "slowing down and melting" and that she was "dead." She imagined that "one part of me was talking to another part of me." In this setting, she made a suicide attempt with pills and was brought to the hospital. Her parents had both been Holocaust survivors. Her mother was chronically pessimistic but had never sought help for depression. Several aunts and uncles were described

as "depressed," but the data were not very clear. While in the hospital, with psychotherapy and a combination of thiothixene and amitryptiline, she seemed gradually to improve. After eight months she was discharged, with plans to work for a publishing house until she could resume her studies. But, two months after leaving the unit, she became engulfed once more in feelings of despair and committed suicide with an overdose of her prescribed drugs and sleeping pills.

4. A seventeen-year-old male was admitted to our unit because of a progressively deepening depression that had begun at the time of his father's death, two years earlier. At first he complained of feeling "dead," of having no feelings, or that his body could not function. An outstanding student, he was already a sophomore in college, having skipped several grades toward the end of high school. The drawback to this success was that he was much less mature socially than the other students, did not fit in with the others, and felt completely isolated. An expert at bridge, he began to feel that, if he played the cards in a certain sequence, he would die. Throughout the thirteen months he spent on the unit, he was markedly anhedonic, except for a few weeks toward the end of his stay, when he had a brief hypomanic reaction to phenelzine. Diagnosed "schizoaffective," he was considered at first to be nearer the schizophrenic pole, later nearer the affective pole of the continuum. Though he was in better contact when he left the unit and seemed ready to resume his courses, he went downhill rapidly, became despondent about ever being able to fit in socially, and, just beyond his eighteenth birthday, took a fatal overdose of hypnotic and neuroleptic drugs.

5. One additional vignette must be added if we are to understand more completely a phenomenon relevant to the demise of the first four patients. An important facet of their suicides was the "contagion effect," hypothesized by those who have observed outbreaks of suicide among adolescents in various communities (Hawton 1986). The three schizoaffective patients alluded to in this section were among four young persons who committed suicide within three months of the closing of the inpatient unit during the spring of 1977. The fourth patient was scarcely out of adolescence himself, having been only twenty when he was admitted and twenty-one when he died. These patients had known one another for over half a year, sharing the same group activities, the same staff members, and (in the case of the three males) the same dormitory. The closing of the unit was occasioned by a

change in administration and was perceived by the patients as arbitrary. The net effect was to hurry up the discharge plans of the "old-type" patients still on the unit in order to make way for a restructuring and for accommodation of patients with different clinical pictures. The resulting premature loss of support appeared to have a deleterious effect on the most vulnerable patients. The fourth patient who suicided during this transition had the following history.

C. THE FOURTH CLUSTER SUICIDE

A twenty-year-old college student was admitted in a state of acute depression, following the suicide of his mother a few weeks before. Evasive and guarded, he revealed little of himself throughout the nine months he spent on the unit, save that he berated himself for being "stupid," despite a straight A average during his freshman year at a prestigious university. He was felt to have strong narcissistic features, a hidden grandiosity, and an inordinately harsh conscience. Apart from his mother's mild alcoholism and depression, little seemed remarkable about his family. He was discharged during the abrupt change of administration on the unit—still better and self-critical, but less depressed than before. He continued to work with the same therapist, now on an outpatient basis. A month later, he revealed something of which he had never spoken while at the hospital or to any other person. His mother's suicide was no ordinary suicide. The summer before his hospitalization, she had seduced him into an incestuous relationship that included intercourse. She began to feel guilty about this and, at one point, summoned him to go to the pharmacy to fetch what both knew was to be the means of her suicide. Each carried out their mission. The next day she was dead from the deliberate overdose of sleeping pills. After he left the hospital, he concluded that this incestuous relationship had ruined him for any "normal" relationship to which he might aspire. In addition, he felt guilty at his having been a willing accomplice to a death that, however merited (owing to the shattering effects the incest had on her son), he at the same time wished had not happened. He told his therapist he was "going away for the weekend," went to a motel in a different city, and killed himself with the same compound that his mother had used.

Discussion

A number of recent studies have outlined risk factors in suicide (Asgard, Nordström, and Raback 1987; Pallis, Barraclough, Levey, Jenkins, and Sainsbury 1982; Robins 1986; Roy 1982), mentioning the heightened incidence among those who are white, male, in their twenties (or older than forty-five), single, unemployed, depressed, and middle to upper class socioeconomically. The element of hopelessness has been emphasized by Kovacs, Beck, and Weissman (1975). Sociological factors that could affect the general rate of suicide in various age brackets at different points in time have been addressed, in the earlier literature, by Durkheim (1897) and, more recently, by Diekstra and Moritz (1987). Sociological writers have underlined diminished social cohesiveness (as from increased divorce rate) and decrease in societal control (as from the weakening of religious influence). Focusing on adolescents, Hawton (1986) drew attention, in addition to the general factors highlighted by Durkheim and Diekstra and Moritz, to preexisting psychiatric conditions besides depression, namely, antisociality, schizophrenia, emotional instability (of which borderline personality would be an example), and substance abuse (most especially alcoholism). A history of previous attempts is common—at the level of 40 percent in young persons who complete suicide (cf. Shaffer and Fisher 1981). Some adolescent suicides are characterized by an immediate precipitant. Shaffer (1974) estimated that a disciplinary crisis (such as a school authority informing the parents about truancy) preceded suicide in a third of the cases. Others succumbed to rejection by a parent or by a sexual partner. But for many the buildup to suicide had been more gradual, especially where the adolescent was struggling with general feelings of hopelessness rather than with an acute rebuff. Hawton (1986) also mentions as a risk factor having to live with a seriously disturbed parent.

One can generalize that adolescents are particularly sensitive to any serious blow directed at the set of hopes and aspirations peculiar to their position in the life cycle. They still require support and love from their original families; they are beginning to look forward to selecting a mate and to develop the skills necessary to the kind of work that can sustain them both psychologically (in a job or profession of which they can be proud) and economically.

In the histories of the adolescent suicides in the P.I.-500, one life event could sometimes undermine these hopes in more than one way at a time. The borderline girl (A5), whose boyfriend served as both an alternate family (compensating for her own fragmented and destructive family) and (in her hopes, at least) a potential mate, lost both at once when her mother summarily kicked her out of the house for coming home late.

The young psychiatric population represented by the study group exhibited, as would be expected, all the general risk factors outlined. But only one came from a broken home (A5). Five had a definite or suspected family history of depression (A2, A3, B6, B7, B8), and the mother in the case in section C had commited suicide.

In line with Shaffer's observation, many (55 percent) had made at least one previous suicide gesture or attempt. The diagnostic groups with the highest percentages of previous suicidal acts, in the P.I. series, were the BPD females (64 percent), the schizoaffective females (55 percent), and the BPD males (48 percent). Curiously, among the schizoaffective males, a prior suicidal act was rare: only one of the twenty-three such patients (twenty-two of whom have been traced) had made a previous gesture. If this finding were replicated in other follow-up studies, it would suggest that schizoaffective males constitute a group at extreme risk (22 percent suicided in the P.I. series) and of extreme concern (for the clinician) since they give few warning signals to those who treat them.

As for living with a mentally ill parent, that was the lot of all but one of the borderline suicides (five out of six if one includes the borderline patient of the case in sec. C) and of only one of the patients with a psychosis, the explosively irritable father of B2. A trend such as this, if supported by other studies, suggests that the path to suicide is carved more by genetic/constitutional factors in the psychotic adolescents and more by family-inflicted traumata in the borderlines (cf. Stone 1990b; Zanarini, Gunderson, Marino, Schwartz, and Frankenburg 1989). The ten case examples are too few for statistical purposes, but, with respect to incest, comparisons within the P.I.-500 as a whole indicate that incest was often a proximate cause of suicide in the borderlines and rarely so among those with a psychosis.

In the P.I.-500, as in the smaller series presented here, an incest history was a more frequent correlate of eventual suicide than was physical abuse by parents. Incest appears to heighten suicide risk in adolescents to an extent greater than that noted in victims of physical abuse. Incest, especially transgenerational (namely, father/daughter), usually induces shame, poisons future sexual relationships with age-mates (Stone 1989b), and may be accompanied by death threats from the perpetrator, lest the secret be revealed, as in the celebrated case of Cheryl Pierson (Kleiman 1988). In some instances, incest simultaneously destroys an adolescent's sense of continued support within the family, destroys hope for a trusting intimate relationship with potential mates, and develops unbearable guilt toward the nonincest parent (toward the mother, e.g., in cases of father-daughter incest). Physical abuse does not usually have this combined effect, tending to induce, instead, a sense of righteous indignation against the offending parent. In all likelihood, parental cruelty is a more potent factor in the pathogenesis of aggressive than of suicidal outcomes. Murderers, wife beaters, child abusers, and the like have been victims of cruelty more often than of incest. In addition, incest victims are usually female (the two mother-son cases here are truly rarities), and females are less apt to commit violent felonies regardless of their upbringing.

Arising out of the study of adolescent suicides and of the causes that may underlie these acts are a number of treatment implications. Adolescents with a heredofamilial psychosis (as in the cases of sec. B) may be less likely to have suffered severe intrafamilial traumata than have suicidal borderline adolescents. The incest rate in borderline adolescents, for example, was four times that noted in their schizophrenic and manic-depressive counterparts (Stone 1990b). Treatment should concentrate on situating the vulnerable adolescents in relatively stress-free environments, such as long-term residential treatment facilities and especially staffed treatment communities, where the patients can acquire skills, form friendships, and live with dignity, either for the remainder of their lives, if necessary, or until such time as extramural life becomes tolerable. For seriously traumatized adolescents, in contrast, there is a need not only for removal from the destructive family but for long-term therapy (five or ten years or longer). This should be directed at undoing the ill effects of the incest or other abuse and at a literal reprogramming of the patient, in the hope that the adolescent can develop a more realistic set of expectations about whom to trust, and whom not, in the future. Regrettably, therapists must also recognize that some suicide-prone adolescents are too disordered for treatment to succeed and that suicide may be inevitable. The

301

case in section C probably represents such an example. Here, the therapist and, in the case of adolescents in residential treatment, other responsible personnel must at the same time try their utmost to rescue the patient and yet prepare themselves psychologically for the possibility of failure (lest they succumb to undue countertransferential guilt). In working with suicidal adolescents from highly traumatizing backgrounds, this is a difficult, but necessary, tightrope for the clinican to walk.

A final point concerns the cluster suicides and the so-called contagion effect. In a number of such instances, a wave of suicides has occurred in young people following reports in the media of a particularly dramatic or poignant suicide of an adolescent (Hawton 1986). The suicides all tend to take place in the same locale and often involve mutual friends or acquaintances. Phillips (1974) has written of this under the rubric of the "Werther" effect, alluding to the many suicides in Europe just after Goethe published his famous story. The four young people in the P.I.-500 series who all took their lives within a few months of the closing of the unit did not, of course, catch their drive toward suicide from the media. Rather, they knew each other, shared profound feelings of hopelessness, felt similarly cut off from the (as they must have viewed it) last remaining source of support, and killed themselves one after the other. In all likelihood, each knew who had just commited suicide. Likewise, each suicide would create an atmosphere of even greater despondency for those still alive—heightening even further the vulnerability, perhaps even the sense of "obligation" to suicide, in whoever was still alive. We do not know this for certain, and these adolescents are no longer alive to tell their side of the story. But the circumstantial evidence and the clinical intuition derived from it are fairly compelling. Here, too, there are treatment implications. If a residential facility or a hospital that houses a fair number of suicidal adolescents is about to close down or undergo a drastic change of personnel, extraordinary precautions should be taken to conduct those patients to another, safer facility—preferably, one whose staff has a low rate of turnover in addition to the necessary expertise in dealing with particularly fragile, suicidal adolescents.

Conclusions

Adolescent suicides have been on the increase in America within the past two decades. Suicide risk in adolescents with BPD with a major psychosis appears to be about fifty times greater than the already high risk in the general population. My experience derives from the long-term follow-up of 550 hospitalized patients (the P.I.-500), of whom 520 were traced. A fourth of this group were under eighteen when admitted. There were nine who committed suicide when still under twenty. Parental cruelty, father-daughter incest, and intense verbal humiliation by parents all appeared to heighten suicide risk. Three of the adolescent suicides plus another in a man of twenty-one all occurred as a "cluster-suicide" within three months of the closing of the hospital unit in 1977. A few adolescent suicides occur in circumstances so destructive as to render the suicide well nigh unpreventable. But the majority probably can be prevented with scrupulous attention to the need for ongoing supportive persons and institutions, greater alertness to even faint "early warning signs," and greater awareness of the need, in chronically suicidal adolescents, for very long-term therapy and (in many instances) residential care.

REFERENCES

Asgard, U.; Nordström, P.; and Raback, G. 1987. Birth cohort analysis of changing suicide risk by sex and age in Sweden, 1952 to 1981. *Acta Psychiatrica Scandanavia* 76:456–463.

Browne, A., and Finkelhor, D. 1986. Impact of child sexual abuse: a review of the research. *Psychological Bulletin* 99(1): 66–77.

Diekstra, R. F. W., and Moritz, J. M. 1987. Suicidal behavior among adolescents: an overview. In R. F. W. Diekstra and K. Hawton, eds. *Suicide in Adolescence*. Dordrecht: Nijhoff.

Durkheim, E. 1987. *De suicide: Étude de sociologie*. Paris: Alkan.

Hawton, K. 1986. Suicide in adolescents. In A. Roy, ed. *Suicide*. Baltimore: Williams & Wilkins.

Hendin, H. 1987. Youth suicide: a psychosocial perspective. *Suicide and Life Threatening Behavior* 17:151–165.

Kernberg, O. F. 1967. Borderline personality organization. *Journal of the American Psychoanalytic Association* 15:641–685.

Kleiman, D. 1988. *A Deadly Silence: The Ordeal of Cheryl Pierson: A Case of Incest and Murder*. New York: Atlantic Monthly.

Kovacs, M.; Beck, A. T.; and Weissman, A. 1975. Hopelessness: an indicator of suicidal risk. *Suicide* 5:98–103.

Murphy, E., and Brown, G. W. 1980. Life events, psychiatric disturbance and physical illness. *British Journal of Psychiatry* 136:326–338.

Pallis, D. J.; Barraclough, B. M.; Levey, A. B.; Jenkins, J. S.; and Sainsbury, P. 1982. Estimating suicide risk among attempted suicides. I. the development of new clinical scales. *British Journal of Psychiatry* 141:37–44.

Phillips, D. P. 1974. The influence of suggestion on suicide: substantive and theoretical implications of the Werther effect. *American Sociological Review* 39:340–354.

Robins, E. 1986. Completed suicide. In A. Roy, ed. *Suicide*. Baltimore: Williams & Wilkins.

Roy, A. 1982. Risk factors for suicide in psychiatric patients. *Archives of General Psychiatry* 39:1089–1095.

Shaffer, D. 1974. Suicide in childhood and early adolescence. *Journal of Child Psychology and Psychiatry* 15:275–291.

Shaffer, D., and Fisher, P. 1981. The epidemiology of suicide in children and adolescents. *Journal of the American Academy of Child Psychiatry* 20:545–565.

Solomon, M. I., and Murphy, G. E. 1984. Cohort studies of suicide. In H. S. Sudak, A. B. Ford, and N. B. Rushforth, eds. *Suicide in the Young*. Boston: Wright/PSG.

Stephens, B. J. 1987. Cheap thrills and humble pie: the adolescence of female suicide attempters. *Suicide and Life Threatening Behavior* 17:107–118.

Stone, M. H. 1987. Psychotherapy of borderline patients in light of long-term follow-up. *Bulletin of the Menninger Clinic* 51(3): 231–247.

Stone, M. H. 1988a. The borderline domain: the "inner script" and other common psychodynamics. In J. Howells, ed. *Modern Perspectives in Psychiatry*. New York: Brunner/Mazel.

Stone, M. H. 1988b. Incest in borderline patients. In R. Kluft, ed. *Incest, Trauma and Psychopathology*. Washington, D.C.: American Psychiatric Press.

Stone, M. H. 1989a. The course in borderline personality disorder. In J. Gunderson, ed. *American Psychiatric Association Annual Review*. Washington, D.C.: American Psychiatric Press.

Stone, M. H. 1989b. Psychotherapy of incest victims. *Psychiatric Clinics of North America* 12(2): 237–255.

Stone, M. H. 1990a. Abuse and abusiveness in borderline personality disorder. In D. Spiegel, ed. *Progress in Psychiatry*. Washington, D.C.: American Psychiatric Press.

Stone, M. H. 1990b. *The Fate of Borderline Patients*. New York: Guilford.

Stone, M. H.; Hurt, S.; and Stone, D. K. 1987. The P.I.-500: long-term follow-up of borderline in-patients meeting DSM-III criteria. *Journal of Personality Disorders* 1:291–298.

Stone, M. H.; Stone, D. K.; and Hurt, S. 1987. Natural history of borderline patients treated by intensive hospitalization. In E. Marcus, ed. *Psychiatric Clinics of North America* 10(2): 185–206.

Tsuang, M. T., and Winokur, G. 1975. The Iowa 500: field work in a 35-year follow-up of depression, mania and schizophrenia. *Canadian Psychiatric Association Journal* 20:359–365.

van der Kolk, B. A. 1989. The compulsion to repeat the trauma: reenactment, revictimization, and masochism. *Psychiatric Clinics of North America* 12(2): 389–411.

Zanarini, M. C.; Gunderson, J. G.; Marino, M. F.; Schwartz, E. O.; and Frankenburg, F. R. 1989. Childhood experiences of borderline patients. *Comprehensive Psychiatry* 30:18–25.

15   THE EFFECT OF PATERNAL HUNTINGTON'S DISEASE ON MALE ADOLESCENCE

ALLAN M. JOSEPHSON AND WILLIAM D. ERICKSON

Huntington's Disease, or Huntington's Chorea, is a rare, inherited disease transmitted by an autosomal dominant gene. Each child of a parent with Huntington's Disease is at a 50 percent risk of developing the disease. Clinical manifestations are not noted until adult life, the first symptoms usually being involuntary movement. This often insidious beginning is followed by dysarthria, ataxia, muscular rigidity, and mental changes. The mental changes typically take the form of a progressive dementia and attendant personality deterioration. The disorder is progressive and terminates fatally, most commonly ten to fifteen years after onset.

One poignant aspect of the tragedy of Huntington's Disease (HD) is that the awareness one carries the gene for the disease occurs only after reproduction has taken place. With the onset of HD in a parent, the family experiences the challenges of confronting a devastating disease, dealing with changes in family structure and living with the uncertainty of whether a child, or children, will inevitably become ill. Molecular genetic testing of presymptomatic persons at risk for HD is becoming increasingly precise, offering the hope that in the future child bearing will be less uncertain: potential parents will know whether they carry the gene for the disease (Brandt, Quaid, Folstein, Garber, Maestri, Abbott, Slavney, Franz, Kasch, and Kazazian 1989).

The child of a parent with HD is thus at biological and psychological risk. The sparse literature on the psychological effect of HD on the family has acknowledged the need for support and empathy along with genetic counseling (Lynch, Harlem, and Dyhrberg 1972; Stern and Eldridge 1975; Tips and Lynch 1963). The emotional conflicts of the affected (Werner and Folk 1968) and unaffected spouse have been examined (Hans and Koeppen 1980), but the nature of interactions between these parents and their developing children has been relatively neglected. This gap in the literature is noteworthy for several reasons. First, the importance of family interaction in current theories of psychological development is increasingly recognized (Sameroff and Emde 1989; Thomas and Chess 1980). Second, the psychological environments of HD families have distinctive characteristics that influence the growing child. Affected parents are unable to be healthy role models and may actually be abusive. The resources of unaffected parents are tested by caring for the affected spouse and developing children while struggling with their own feelings of guilt, hostility, and social isolation (Folstein, Franz, Jensen, Chase, and Folstein 1983). Third, Folstein and colleagues have described conduct disorders in the offspring of patients with HD that seem related to the developing child's experience of family disorganization (Folstein, Abbott, Chase, Jensen, and Folstein 1983). In their definition of family disorganization, they include the instability of either parent to maintain discipline and family structure.

The following two cases illustrate the nature of family interaction in HD families and its effect on the emotional development of adolescent males.

Case Example 1

A.B., a thirteen-year-old male in the seventh grade, was admitted to the adolescent psychiatric ward because of a suicide threat. A. called his mother at work, telling her that he was going to take his life. She called his school principal, who went to the home with the police. They found him in a closet, wrapped in a blanket, complaining that he was cold.

Mr. and Mrs. B. married when he was forty-nine and she was twenty-seven. A. was their only child. Mr. B. had concealed his family history of HD from his wife. His first symptom, slurred speech, began when his son was one year old. As his speech worsened, his behavior became more aggressive and moods more labile. Diagnosis was confirmed when A. was seven. Father was increasingly physically abusive toward his wife and A. Two weeks after Mrs. B. requested a divorce because of his abuse, Mr. B. shot himself. A. was ten at the time and witnessed the suicide.

A.'s early development was noteworthy for some difficulty with toilet training and frequent temper tantrums. He had no serious medical illnesses. A learning disability was detected quickly after entry into school, and he subsequently received special education assistance. His peer relationships were unremarkable during his first years. After his father's death, A. became increasingly difficult to control, more demanding, and increasingly angry. At the time of his admission to the hospital, the mother described herself as "powerless" to control his behavior.

A.'s physical examination was normal except for several neurological soft signs consistent with minimal brain dysfunction. CAT scan and EEG were normal. Verbal IQ (WISC-R) was ninety-one, performance IQ 104, with a full scale IQ of ninety-six. Neuropsychological assessment indicated superior perceptual organization and planning abilities, with relatively poor verbal skills. His academic achievement was at expected grade level in mathematics and three years behind expected levels in reading recognition and comprehension. Projective tests suggested that he was dysphoric and angry. Regret about his argumentative relationship with his mother was a clear source of unpleasant affect. He was assessed as defensive and on guard against the expression and experience of affect.

On mental status examination at the time of admission, he was uncooperative and cried frequently, blaming his behavior on dissatisfaction with the hospitalization. When he demanded to see his mother and this was refused, he kicked chairs over and cried that he wanted to return home. He showed no evidence of thought disorder or cognitive dysfunction. He denied vegetative signs of depression, although he described his mood as "a bit depressed."

When interviewed together, A. was calm, and Mrs. B. expressed minor concerns about her son's behavior. When mother was interviewed alone, however, she expressed deeper concerns. She believed that A.'s low frustration tolerance was her fault, a result of her inability to discipline him consistently. She felt "sorry for him" because of the 50 percent chance of his developing HD. Tearfully, she described the verbal and physical abuse that she and A. had experienced during her husband's mental deterioration, ending only with his suicide. She expressed anger toward Mr. B. for having concealed information about his family's history of HD prior to their marriage.

A.'s suicidal references disappeared immediately after hospitalization, and he described his suicide threat as an attempt to get his mother's attention. A recommendation was made that A. be placed in a residential treatment program in order to assure adequate schooling as well as promote independence from his mother. School avoidance had been a serious problem, and it seemed unlikely that Mrs. B. would be able to maintain her son's attendance. He was discharged to his mother pending placement.

His discharge diagnoses (DSM-III) were adjustment disorder with depressed mood; conduct disorder, socialized, nonaggressive (Axis I); narcissistic personality traits (Axis II); and minimal brain dysfunction (Axis III). He was not given a personality disorder diagnosis because of his relative youth. However, his sense of entitlement, grandiosity, and significant anger with the setting of limits was seen as similar to the characteristics observed in adults with the diagnosis of narcissistic personality disorder.

Mother, however, ultimately decided against placement out of the home, appearing to have difficulty initiating such a separation. A. was seen in biweekly individual psychotherapy, focusing on issues of individuation, and his mother received simultaneous counseling for the next year. He refused to return to school at the beginning of the eighth grade. His mother offered him gifts as an inducement to return to school. Her gift giving, described as "making up" for his past family experience, was met with increased demands. When his mother could no longer give, financially or emotionally, A. would become hostile and angry. Mrs. B. would protest, "You're just like your father," but would eventually capitulate.

A. became increasingly truant and was finally placed in a residential treatment center, two years after the initial recommendation. Separation from his mother, imposition of social structure, and peer interaction that held him accountable for his behavior led to a period of remarkable stability, characterized by a decrease in demanding and egocentric behavior. After completion of the program, he returned home, only to drop out of school at sixteen, having completed the tenth grade. He worked intermittently and attended night school, but he was plagued by an inability to follow through with any hopes or plans. He moved in with an older friend but continued to visit his mother three times a day. He explained his frequent visits by telling his mother that he came "just to see how you're doing." He continued to demand money from his mother, and, when she refused him, he would threaten violence. Mrs. B. established a relationship with a supportive male friend and slowly learned to set firmer limits on A.

At follow-up, four years after our initial contact, Mrs. B. was still in counseling. A. had talked with his mother about his fear of dying and of his conviction that there was something wrong with his body. Repeated episodes of hyperventilation and chest pain continued to trouble him. Follow-up neurological exam revealed no evidence of Huntington's Disease. Mrs. B. had used a substantial amount of her modest salary during the previous three years to buy him a minibike, two motorcycles, a snowmobile, a truck, and a car. She felt that she could not marry because of A., who "monopolizes so much thinking time, I don't know my own feelings."

Case Example 2

L.M., a fifteen-year-old tenth grade student, was referred to an adolescent inpatient unit because of failure of outpatient therapy to control his aggressive, provocative behavior or improve his peer relationships and school performance. He had a long history of behavior problems, with impulsive behavior and poor peer relationships since kindergarten.

L. was the youngest of three children. Mr. M. had one sibling, a brother, who committed suicide with the onset of HD. Mr. M.'s father and six of his seven siblings had HD. Mr. and Mrs. M. were married when she was eighteen years old and he was nineteen. Mrs. M. did not know of her husband's family history of HD. The early years of their marriage were difficult, primarily the result of Mr. M.'s alcohol abuse, infidelity, and job instability. Mr. M. first developed motor symptoms of HD when L. was seven years old. Approximately three years after onset of physical symptoms, Mr. M. developed a serious psychosis along with a worsening of motor symptoms, necessitating psychiatric hospitalization. The psychosis improved after several months, but his movement disorder continued to be so severe that he could not return home. He had been out of the home for three years at the time L. was admitted to the hospital.

L.'s birth was the result of a planned pregnancy. His preschool development was notable only for the occurrence of breath-holding spells. In repeated psychiatric evaluations from age six to age fifteen, he was described as testing limits and being a "scapegoat" for his peers. His academic performance had begun to deteriorate in the ninth grade. His behavior contrasted dramatically with that of his two older sisters, who were dutiful and good students.

L.'s physical and neurological examinations were normal. EEG was normal. His height and weight were at the third percentile for his age, but bone age was normal. He had a verbal IQ of eighty-three and a performance IQ of ninety-two, with a full scale IQ of eighty-nine. His academic achievement was at grade level in math and in reading but three years behind in spelling. Projective tests suggested that he had low self-esteem. He described his family in positive terms and was concerned about his father's illness but appeared well defended against affective expression. It was suggested that he was not using all the skills available to him and that he tended to take the easy way out of demanding situations.

On admission mental status, L. appeared small for his age. He initially related to the examiner cautiously, with little inflection in his voice. He did not elaborate any responses longer than a few words. His mild oppositionality lessened toward the end of the interview. He did not have a clear understanding of the need for hospitalization other than that he needed "to get along better" with others his age. L. did not report vegetative signs of depression but appeared sullen. He did not show evidence of thought disorder or organic mental disorder.

During the hospitalization, he required firm limits and active behavioral controls. He made one suicidal gesture, tying a sheet around his neck during a conflict with the staff. He later said that he did it because he was "tired of people telling me what to do." His peer relationships were characterized by the provoking of less competent patients and obsequious following of older, more dominant ones.

His discharge diagnoses (DSM-III) were dysthymic disorder; conduct disorder, socialized, nonaggressive (Axis I); and narcissistic personality traits (Axis II). L.'s dysthymic presentation seemed related to his experience of having his grandiosity challenged and his uniqueness unappreciated. When he was apart from his attentive mother, he did not appear to have the social skills necessary to form relationships with peers, adolescents who naturally did not see him as requiring special attention.

311

L.'s outpatient care consisted of weekly individual psychotherapy for him and behavior management counseling for his mother. He was uncommunicative and frequently would discuss only professional sports rather than reality concerns. His mother reported that L. remained marginally compliant during the eighteen-month therapy.

At age seventeen, L. became involved in shoplifting and truancy. He was increasingly provocative, verbally and behaviorally, with his mother and sisters. He locked himself in the only family bathroom for lengthy periods of time each morning, making it difficult for his mother and sisters to begin the day. Mrs. M. feared that L.'s behavior might be due to early symptoms of HD, and this fear lowered her expectation of behavioral responsibility. This furthered L.'s self-centeredness and imperviousness to discipline. While aware of the effect of her seeing L.'s behavior as out of his control, she could not quiet her concern. She knew that she should expect him to be responsible for his behavior, but she saw this as abandoning him—"I just can't walk away from him if he really has the disease." With the support of his older sisters, who saw how L. was "using" his mother without consequence, Mrs. M. placed L. in a foster home.

One year in foster care and a new school placement led to behavioral improvement. L. was attending school, was not in any legal trouble, and had improved peer relationships. The foster family did not see his negativistic behavior as out of his control, nor did they view him as vulnerable. Because of unrelated problems in the foster family and behavioral improvement, he returned home, only to resume previous habits, including truancy and increase in drinking and use of marijuana.

Three years after initial contact, at age eighteen, he was interviewed again. It was quite evident that his gait was abnormal, his face expressionless, and his thought processes retarded. He was rehospitalized, where neurological examination showed muscle stiffness and cogwheel rigidity. Psychological tests indicated a twelve-point drop in full-scale IQ to seventy-seven. Only when these findings were shared with his mother did she reveal the fact that many family members and his school counselor had called her attention to his gait in the previous six months. L. refused to acknowledge any symptoms and would not accept the diagnosis of HD. On the basis of apathy, depressive ideation, family history of frequent suicides, and a minimally abnormal dexamethasone suppression test (five micrograms/100 milliliters seventeen hours after administration of one milligram of dexamethasone),

L. was started on imipramine. Clinical effectiveness was suggested by his returning home without incident, returning to school with regular attendance, and receiving a graduation certificate. Follow-up dexamethasone suppression test was one microgram/100 milliliters.

Mrs. M. felt that L. needed more structure than she could provide. At the age of nineteen, he moved to a residence for physically and emotionally handicapped young adults. There, he adjusted well. One hot summer day, three years after the onset of symptoms and six years after his initial psychiatric hospitalization, L. went swimming with two friends and drowned.

Discussion

The demanding, self-serving behavior of these two youths seemed to have its roots in a family structure so dramatically altered by HD in their fathers. Both mothers seemed emotionally paralyzed by their sons' extravagant demands and sense of entitlement. Their inability to hold their sons accountable for such behavior seemed related to guilt regarding past family life and anxiety about their sons' potential for illness. It was only through geographic separation that they were able to understand their powerlessness in their relationships with their sons.

The difficulties experienced in these two families may be common. Many members of an HD family are significantly affected, whether they have the disease, are married to that person, or are children whose future life is uncertain. In these families, psychopathology occurs equally frequently in affected and unaffected siblings (Dewhurst 1970; Dewhurst, Oliver, and McKnight 1970; Folstein, Franz, et al. 1983; Oliver 1970). Males are more likely to be antisocial (Folstein, Franz, et al. 1983), and females tend to develop anxiety disorders (Dewhurst et al. 1970). Harper and colleagues noted that "for every overt case of the disease there are at high risk numerous relatives whose lives may be seriously affected, even though they may never develop the disorder" (Harper, Smith, Tyler, Jones, Newcombe, and McBroom 1981). Hans and Gilmore have unequivocally stated that "none of the offspring of choreics escapes the disorder. While only some of the children may inherit the disease itself, all experience the impact through primary social deprivation or secondary personality distortion" (Hans and Gilmore 1968). Folstein and colleagues have less extravagantly stated that conduct disorders observed in the off-

313

spring of HD patients appear primarily as a result of developmental experience, not as a direct effect of the HD gene (Folstein, Franz, et al. 1983).

Our subsequent discussion further examines the effects of altered family structure and interactional patterns of these boys' development.

THE FATHER'S INFLUENCE ON MALE ADOLESCENT IDENTITY FORMATION

The father of a young boy is a role model for the child, offering a realistic view of the man's world of work and life outside the family. He is also a renewed source of support for his wife, who is losing her son, and serves as a wedge between the boy and his mother's need to hold on to him. Fathers influence the processes of moral and cognitive development as well as sex role identification (Lamb 1976).

In a stable home, the process of identity formation and the development of autonomous role functions can proceed smoothly, with the teenager slowly growing into an adult resembling his father in important ways. In families marked by stress, disharmony, and loss, the process of identification is less sure. If parents are unequal in attractiveness, the child often seeks a stable alliance with the more attractive parent because of that parent's competence, power within the family, or love, acceptance, and nurturance. However, the most potent influence on identification seems to be gender similarity (Schwarz 1979). Its pull can never be completely ignored, no matter how unattractive the same-sex parent may be in other respects. If both parents are unattractive models, antisocial outcomes are common.

The importance of the same-sex parent in identification processes is illustrated by M. Despite his physical and mental disability, L.'s father remained an ideal figure, an ideal sustained only by substantial denial. His claim that his father was a good cribbage player at a time when his father could not speak or control his movements and his adamant refusal to acknowledge the presence of obvious symptoms in himself indicated the force of L.'s denial. At about the time his own physical symptoms appeared, L. began to find frequent excuses not to visit his father, and, when he did so, he was tense and surly. His father was not only a poor model for him but also a constant reminder of his own possible future. When that future became a reality with the onset of his illness, L. could only deny both his father's devastation and his own. His denial made practical planning and psychological adaptation nearly impossible.

Mr. B.'s sudden suicide terminated an abusive, unpredictable relationship and also A.'s further identification with him. However, early experiences were influential. A.'s demands and frequent physical threats became a predictable mode of relating to his mother. His mother's response—"You're just like your father"—was engendered by vivid recollections of Mr. B.'s irascibility and brutality.

The specific psychological risk in HD families that could be attributed to the sex of the affect parent has not been assessed. It is not clear whether an abusive, affected father is routinely more deleterious an influence on a son's development than a neglectful, affected mother. But when sex-specific influences are taken into consideration (e.g., the importance of the male adolescent's identifying with his father), those children most at risk would appear to be of the same sex as the afflicted parent.

EFFECT OF LOSS OF FATHER

Father loss during latency and early adolescence has frequently been linked with an increase in behavior disorders, criminal offenses, and psychiatric disorders among male children (Seligman, Gleser, Rauh, and Harris 1974). Rutter (1981) found no such increase in psychological disturbance in boys who lost their fathers through physical illness or accidental death. His studies suggest that the behavior disorders associated with father's absence are in fact linked to marital conflict rather than loss. He reported that psychopathology was as prevalent in conflicted families still living together as in those who have divorced.

Similarly, the stress and conflict occasioned by the affected fathers' behavior in these HD homes were more direct influences than was the loss of father. Death and institutionalization of the father opened the door to intense, difficult relationships between the boys and their mothers.

THE RELATIONSHIPS BETWEEN SONS AND UNAFFECTED MOTHERS

A father's permanent absence dramatically alters family structure and role differentiation. A male child may plunge into a regressive

315

dependent relationship with his mother or may assume a pseudo-adult stance in order to deny these needs, responding to this perceived obligation to care for his mother. These relationships often intensify and can impede the usual growth of autonomy. Newman and Schwam (1979) have described the emotional stress of inevitable developmental shifts and comment, "Sooner or later, however, the break [between mother and son] must be made, and it is often made with guilt, indecision and delay."

With the death of Mr. B. and the institutionalization of Mr. M., the role that the mothers played in their relationships with their sons changed, powerfully influencing A.'s and L.'s development. Guilt for placing their sons at genetic risk was enormous for both women. In an effort to "make it up" to their sons, they became indulgent (e.g., Mrs. B. buying her son several vehicles that she could ill afford). But this indulgence did not assuage the mothers' guilt and led to an increase rather than a decrease of the boys' demands.

These mothers perpetuated tightly bound relationships that impeded development because of their perception of their sons as vulnerable, perhaps carrying HD genes, but clearly having been victimized and psychologically damaged by their father's illness. Individuals at risk for HD are often exquisitely sensitive to their own mood changes, wondering whether they are the harbingers of disease (Elash 1977). These mothers wondered about their son's behavior in similar ways. This uncertainty of whether outbursts are emotional or early HD symptoms, and the mothers' inability to act decisively, created a psychological entanglement in which there were few avenues for normal development. A.'s incessant demands for money and L.'s repeated provocative behavior without reasonable consequences are two examples of this entanglement. There was considerable dialogue around physical symptoms. L. had headaches, and A. complained of shortness of breath. These discussions, similar to those seen in psychosomatic families (Minuchin, Baker, Rosman, Liebman, Milman, and Todd 1975), further intensified the maternal overprotectiveness.

Ambivalent feelings toward the affected spouse may be at the heart of a vacillation between indulgence and frustrated anger. These familiar emotions for many single parents become more intense for the remaining spouse of the HD victim when added to feelings associated with the uncertain future of their children. These tightly bound relationships may be more likely to develop in HD families than in other, less burdened, single-parent families.

When the unaffected parent and child are mother and son, sexual issues become important. The biological push of puberty normally requires the male adolescent to disengage from his mother in order to maintain the relationship without being overwhelmed by sexual feelings. The youth who has grown up in an intense and overinvolved relationship with his mother may feel that he is entitled to a continued special relationship that gratifies his demands. On the other hand, a sense of frustration, anger, and embarrassment results when his mother seems too close. Hostile dependent relationships, evident between A. and L. and their mothers, occur in the life histories of many men with sexual behavior problems (McCord, McCord, and Verdan 1986). These experiences, complicated by early dementia, may help explain the fact that sexual behavior problems are common in male HD victims (Dewhurst et al. 1970). When the unaffected parent is the father and the adolescent a girl, the risk to the girl's development may be that of her volunteering for, being pushed into, or resisting in destructive ways the role of housekeeper and psychological spouse.

THE INDIVIDUAL PSYCHOPATHOLOGY

These two boys were typical of adolescents who are diagnosed as having conduct disorders. They manifested a sense of entitlement. Neither A. nor L. knew how to deal with frustration or denial of their wishes. They had difficulty delaying gratification. These maladaptive patterns of behavior, aspects of which were present early in development, had great influence in their later teen years. Normal adolescent tasks requiring responsibility were not completed, their completion stymied by the boys' lack of persistence. Fantasies of power and interpersonal efficacy served the defensive purpose of protecting them from the stark reality of their failures.

Biological components—constitutional, neurochemical, and genetic —were also important to individual psychopathology. A.'s learning disability and L.'s short stature contributed to low self-esteem. The gradual evolution of L.'s HD also deserves note. His motor symptoms were accompanied by the development of affective symptoms. Depressive syndromes can occur during the prodromal period in HD victims, as well as later in the course, and are often unrecognized (Folstein, Abbott, et al. 1983; Folstein, Franz, et al. 1983). L.'s positive dexamethasone suppression test and response to tricyclic antidepressant therapy underscore the potential contribution of neurochemically mediated depression to HD psychopathology (McHugh and Folstein 1975).

Even in cases with dysfunctional family interaction, adolescents can develop biologically based psychiatric symptoms. Early onset cases are three times more likely to be transmitted through the father and usually present with symptoms of muscle stiffness rather than chorea (Byers and Dodge 1967; Jarvis 1983; Markham and Knox 1965). Boys such as L. are in double jeopardy. They are at earlier genetic risk and are more likely to have destructive experiences with their afflicted fathers.

Intervention

Therapeutic interventions should be based on an eclectic diagnostic approach to psychopathology. In the individual case, a careful weighing of contributing factors may lead to a greater emphasis on familial relationships or disease symptoms. The clinical judgment involved may be among the most challenging in clinical adolescent psychiatry. L.'s shifting clinical picture, from a conduct disorder accounted for by family disorganization to an affective syndrome related to an evolving HD, illustrates the need for intervention to be based on frequent reassessment. Subtle cognitive decline (Cain, Hunt, Weingartner, and Ebert 1978; Lyle and Gottesman 1976) and affective disorders (Folstein, Franz, et al. 1983) may be harbingers of HD.

In the absence of verifiable neurological disease, the question of whether to interpret a conduct problem as emotional in origin or early symptoms of HD should usually be resolved in favor of an emotional interpretation. This strategy was helpful in these two cases and is supported by Folstein, Franz, et al. (1983). This choice will stress individual responsibility, a critical factor in adolescent development. This approach eliminates the indecision inherent in treating any problematic behavior as out of the adolescent's control. Such indecision only fuels the adolescent's narcissism and parents' powerlessness. Obviously, careful clinical observation for cognitive, motor, or affective symptoms suggestive of HD is necessary. These reassessments will assist in determining when, and to what degree, the adolescent may be viewed as less accountable for his behavior.

Concomitant with genetic counseling, families should be made aware of the predictable risks of indulgence, lack of discipline, and the intense, hostile dependent relationships illustrated here. When such relationships are already evident, immediate intervention to free parents from overinvolvement and push adolescents toward responsibility must be made. Individual psychotherapy for parent and child, often in combination with a family approach, should be tried. If the intensity of the hostile dependency does not resolve, out-of-home placement may be necessary. In both these cases, stays outside the home were extremely beneficial. Placement of the boys outside their homes, albeit painful and only reluctantly agreed to, allowed both mothers to gain some perspective not possible through psychotherapy alone.

Conclusions

Our report does have the limitations imposed by a case study method. In addition, our conclusions are tempered by the selective study of affected fathers, sons as the identified patients, and adolescence as the time of psychiatric presentation. The effect of afflicted mothers and the effect of HD fathers on their daughters were not addressed in this study.

The dynamic and developmental issues may be similar to those in other families with a father with a mental disorder. However, we believe that the uniform devastation of the disease and the years of living with the uncertainty of whether a parent will develop the disease make this a unique disorder. Its uniqueness offers further understanding of the normal processes of adolescent individuation and impediments to that process.

With these limitations in mind, we suggest that it is important for clinicians to consider the shifts in family structure induced by a parent with HD and the subsequent effects on developing children. Such an awareness equips therapists to alleviate current distress and aid future coping of parent and child.

REFERENCES

Brandt, J.; Quaid, K.; Folstein, S.; Garber, P.; Maestri, N.; Abbott, M.; Slavney, P.; Franz, M.; Kasch, L.; and Kazazian, H. 1989.

Presymptomatic diagnosis of delayed-onset disease with linked DNA markers. *Journal of the American Medical Association* 261:3108–3114.

Byers, R. K., and Dodge, J. A. 1967. Huntington's Chorea in children. *Neurology* 17:587–596.

Cain, E. D.; Hunt, R. D.; Weingartner, H.; and Ebert, M. H. 1978. Huntington's Dementia: clinical and neuropsychological features. *Archives of General Psychiatry* 35:377–384.

Dewhurst, K. 1970. Personality disorder in Huntington's Disease. *Psychiatric Clinics* (Basel) 3:221–229.

Dewhurst, K.; Oliver, J. E.; and McKnight, A. C. 1970. The socio-psychiatric consequences of Huntington's Disease. *British Journal of Psychiatry* 116:255–258.

Elash, D. D. 1977. At risk for Huntington's Disease. *Psychiatric Annals* 7–8:66–79.

Folstein, S. E.; Abbott, M. H.; Chase, G. A.; Jensen, B. A.; and Folstein, M. F. 1983. The association of affective disorder with Huntington's Disease in a case series and in families. *Psychological Medicine* 13:537–542.

Folstein, S. E.; Franz, M. L.; Jensen, B. A.; Chase, G. A.; and Folstein, M. F. 1983. Conduct disorder and affective disorder among the offspring of patients with Huntington's Disease. *Psychological Medicine* 13:45–52.

Hans, M. B., and Gilmore, T. H. 1968. Social aspects of Huntington's Chorea. *British Journal of Psychiatry* 114:93–98.

Hans, M. B., and Koeppen, A. H. 1980. Huntington's Chorea: its impact on the spouse. *Journal of Nervous and Mental Disease* 168:209–214.

Harper, P. S.; Smith, S.; Tyler, A.; Jones, P.; Newcombe, R.; and McBroom, V. 1981. Decline in the predicted incidence of Huntington's Chorea associated with systematic genetic counseling and family support. *Lancet* 11:411–413.

Jarvis, G. A. 1963. Huntington's Chorea in childhood. *Archives of Neurology* 9:50–63.

Lamb, M. E. 1976. The role of father: an overview. In M. E. Lamb, ed. *The Role of the Father in Child Development.* New York: Wiley.

Lyle, O. E., and Gottesman, I. 1976. Premorbid psychometric indicators of the gene for Huntington's Disease. *Journal of Consulting and Clinical Psychology* 44:229–232.

Lynch, H. T.; Harlem, W. L.; and Dyhrberg, J. S. 1972. Subjective perspective of a family with Huntington's Chorea: implications for genetic counseling. *Archives of General Psychiatry* 27:67–72.

McCord, W.; McCord, J.; and Verdan, P. 1986. Family relations and sexual deviance in lower class adolescents. *International Journal of Social Psychiatry* 8:165–179.

McHugh, P. R., and Folstein, M. F. 1975. Psychiatric syndromes of Huntington's Chorea: a clinical and phenomenologic study. In D. Benson and D. Blumer, eds. *Psychiatric Aspects of Neurologic Disease*. New York: Grune & Stratton.

Markham, C. H., and Knox, J. W. 1965. Observations on Huntington's Chorea in childhood. *Journal of Pediatrics* 67:46–57.

Minuchin, S.; Baker, L.; Rosman, B.; Liebman, R.; Milman, L.; and Todd, T. C. 1975. A conceptual model of psychosomatic illness in children. *Archives of General Psychiatry* 32:1031–1038.

Newman, C. J., and Schwam, J. S. 1979. The fatherless child. In J. Noshpitz and I. Berlin, eds. *Basic Handbook of Child Psychiatry*. New York: Basic.

Oliver, J. E. 1970. Huntington's Chorea in Northamptonshire. *British Journal of Psychiatry* 116:241–253.

Rutter, M. 1981. Epidemiological/longitudinal strategies and casual research in child psychiatry. *Journal of the American Academy of Child Psychiatry* 20:513–544.

Sameroff, A., and Emde, R. 1989. *Relationship Disturbances in Childhood: A Developmental Approach*. New York: Basic.

Schwarz, J. C. 1979. Childhood origins of psychopathology. *American Psychologist* 34:855–879.

Seligman, R.; Gleser, G.; Rauh, J.; and Harris, L. 1974. The effect of earlier parental loss in adolescence. *Archives of General Psychiatry* 31:475–479.

Stern, R., and Eldridge, R. 1975. Attitudes of patients and their relatives to Huntington's Disease. *Journal of Medical Genetics* 12:217–223.

Thomas, A., and Chess, S. 1980. *The Dynamics of Psychological Development*. New York: Brunner/Mazel.

Tips, R. H., and Lynch, H. T. 1963. The impact of genetic counseling upon the family milieu. *Journal of the American Medical Association* 184:183–186.

Werner, A., and Folk, J. J. 1968. Manifestation of neurotic conflict in Huntington's Chorea. *Journal of Nervous and Mental Disease* 147:141–147.

321

16 THE LEARNING DISABLED ADOLESCENT: A CLINICAL PERSPECTIVE

BENJAMIN GARBER

To those who deal with the emotional problems of children and adolescents, it has become obvious in the last two decades that learning disabilities have emerged as an issue of all-encompassing proportions (Rutter 1983). Every child who is seen diagnostically for school-related problems is thought to be learning disabled by someone significant in his or her environment. Every child who does not measure up to academic expectations is considered learning disabled. Even adults who were anything but exceptional students see themselves as having undiagnosed learning disabilities.

It is apparent that learning disabilities and the industry that deals with them have become major players in the mental health arena. If one defines learning disabilities in the broad sense as a failure to learn at a normal rate for whatever reason, then, perhaps, the staggering numbers of learning disabled children make sense. However, if one defines learning disabilities in the narrower sense as problems in the acquisition of developmental skills in academic achievement and social adjustment that are the result of perceptual and linguistic processing deficits, then it becomes evident that the learning disabilities label is grossly misused and abused.

I have seen many children who do poorly in school in response to parental divorce, the death of a parent, or an emotionally disturbed parent. However, owing to administrative expediency, economic considerations, parental pressure, or an avoidance of self-examination,

This chapter was presented as the Joel Handler Memorial Lecture to the Chicago Society for Adolescent Psychiatry on November 7, 1990.

such children are often designated as learning disabled. There follows a lengthy process of psychological testing and neurological evaluation in order to pinpoint the etiology and location of the damaged anatomic substrate. Usually, such a search yields very little. Eventually, the child's immaturities and limitations become so intertwined with intra- and interpersonal issues that the original deficits, if they were there, are obscured from the eyes of the most sophisticated observer.

However, in spite of widespread overkill and the emergence of various diagnostic and treatment cults, there are children with demonstrable learning disabilities. These learning limitations may be the result of a developmental lag, hereditary predisposition, or a vague central nervous system insult in concert with environmental factors.

In the last two decades, there has been an emphasis on school readiness assessment and the remediation of learning deficits in elementary school children. Although follow-up data have presented us with a mixed outcome, these efforts have continued with ever greater expenditures of manpower and money (Schonhaut and Satz 1983; Silver and Hagin 1985). While the remedial and research efforts have focused on the preschool and elementary school child, scant attention has been paid to adolescents with learning disabilities (Kline 1972; Schloss 1971). Research on learning disabled adolescents has been slow in establishing itself. Consequently, clinical impressions have often come from anecdotal reports of teachers and parents. Many of these reports lead to a conclusion that the basic neuropsychological problems that plague these individuals as children do not simply disappear but persist into adolescence and adulthood.

In spite of a heightened interest, interdisciplinary comprehensive clinical studies that seek to understand the developmental interrelations between psychological and neuropsychological factors in learning disabled children have been rare, with virtually no investigations of learning disabled adolescents. Consequently, the psychiatric and psychoanalytic literature that addresses these problems of the high school student has been minuscule (Cohen 1985; Palombo 1979). It may well be that the adolescent's learning deficits have been ignored because it was assumed that the key to problem resolution was early identification and remediation.

It is understandable why intervention with the younger learning disabled child would be deemed more productive. The greater dependency of the child, a lack of chronicity, the lack of ossification of secondary emotional problems, and the lesser complexity would make the younger child an ideal candidate for massive therapeutic efforts. Nevertheless, the relative neglect of the learning disabled adolescent is surprising as most of the current principles, definitions, assessment devices, and treatment procedures were developed by early researcher-clinicians from experiences with adolescents and young adults (Cruickshank 1980).

In the early school years, the learning disabled child exhibits two generalized problem areas: difficulty mastering basic academic skills and a pervasive immaturity. In preadolescence, concerns and anxieties about the learning disabled child increase as emotional and behavioral problems multiply. Consequently, the clinical patterns for the latency child and preadolescent have been well established; however, the clinical picture of the learning disabled adolescent is confusing. For the adolescent, the experience of being learning disabled inevitably becomes interwoven with other concerns, conflicts, interests, strengths, weaknesses, and adaptive strategies. Over time, it becomes more difficult to distinguish the neuropsychological from the psychological and the reactive from the characterological.

There have been several studies that show that learning disabled adolescent boys exhibit significantly more problems in social competence and behavior than do normal boys (Cohen 1985; Cruickshank 1980; Silver and Hagin 1985; Silverman and Zigmond 1983). Studies of twelve- to sixteen-year-old boys showed significantly lower participation in activities, fewer social contacts with organizations and friends, and poorer school performance than in normal boys (McConaughy 1986). These results suggest that deficits in social competence appear at early ages among learning disabled boys and increase in adolescence.

Other studies have focused on the poor social perception of the learning disabled adolescent, which may interfere with progress in academics. There may be an inability to generalize from one situation to another, oversensitivity to the reactions of others, inflexibility in acting, difficulty in accurately interpreting moods and communications (verbal and nonverbal), and difficulty in determining the effect of one's actions on others (Bruininks 1978; Bryan 1974; Wiig and Harris 1974). It may well be that the social-emotional problems of the learning disabled adolescent are more of a hindrance to success and adjustment in life than the mastery of academic concepts. While recent clinical studies have focused on the learning disabled adolescent's social difficulties, other reports indicate that there is a maturational improvement that permeates the adolescent's functioning.

Some studies show that self-esteem appears to rise significantly during adolescence for those youngsters with a learning disability (McConaughy 1986; Silver and Hagin 1985). This rise in self-esteem is more than likely related to improved academic performance. It seems that learning disabled adolescents, having discovered and recognized their academic weaknesses and limitations, tend to concentrate on their strengths and develop compensatory skills. For the first time in their academic careers, they may experience a sense of mastery in circumscribed areas of the curriculum. Having discovered new strengths, it is not surprising that some learning disabled adolescents, unlike the vast majority of younger children with learning disabilities, function better.

The hypothesis that learning disabled adolescents engaged in more delinquent behavior than their peers has not been supported by recent research. A comparison of self-reports with delinquency data indicated that learning disabled and nondisabled adolescents participated in the same kinds and amounts of delinquent behavior (Perlmutter 1987). While a causal relation between learning disabilities and juvenile delinquency has not been demonstrated, it appears that juvenile delinquency may serve as an outlet for some learning disabled adolescents. What emerges then is a conflicting and contradictory picture of the learning disabled adolescent. There is little doubt that maturational factors exert an important progressive thrust that may allow the adolescent to compensate for some of his or her cognitive and emotional deficits. Academic problems still persist, but in a more circumscribed and isolated manner.

The learning disabled adolescent shows a jagged profile in achievement level and an inconsistency in performance. He or she has a pervasive difficulty in dealing with symbols and the ability to synthesize parts into wholes quickly remains unmastered. There is a lack of fluency and a marked laboriousness in written expression, and vocabulary skills are low. In a parallel manner, however, there are changes that occur in the learning disabled adolescent that may be considered more positive.

Hyperactivity in neurologically damaged teenagers diminishes or is characterized by subtler actions. Some studies have shown that hyperactive behavior disappears almost completely in adolescence. As students grow older, they are less easily distracted and pay more attention to tasks (Cruickshank 1980; McConaughy 1986; Mendelson, Johnson, and Stewart 1971; Weiss, Hechtoman, Perlman, Hopkins, and Wener 1979).

In most perceptual and motor areas, the learning disabled show improvement with age. However, it is important to remember that the nonhandicapped also demonstrate refinements and improvements with maturation. The question that remains is whether these improvements are sufficient to modify self-perceptions and how others perceive them. Maturation and/or compensation tend to refine and integrate many perceptual and motor functions. Consequently, problems of incoordination, hyperactivity, distractibility, and poor attention may manifest themselves in more subtle and controlled ways. As handicapped students grow older, some of their disabilities may be reduced or become less distinguishable.

From a clinical perspective, one of the major problems in working with learning disabled adolescents is the heterogeneous nature of their psychopathology. Unlike the younger learning disabled child, whose clinical presentation is more homogeneous, that of the adolescent is quite diverse.

Perhaps the best way to conceptualize a workable assessment of the learning disabled adolescent is via a two-tiered structure. One group of learning disabled adolescents, whose psychopathology is more internally directed, is able to compensate for their limitations. This may result from maturation or may be a function of massive remediation. The other group of adolescents is those who develop further interpersonal, academic, and legal difficulties. These adolescents' symptoms are more externally directed as they experience conflicts with their environment.

The adapting group, while continuing to suffer from academic difficulties and lower peer status than their classmates, has begun to overcome its handicapping conditions by compensatory means. These adolescents have developed strategies for accomplishment by calling on specific areas in which they have worked and proved their competence. The more conflicted learning disabled group will continue to experience difficulties as those adolescents may or may not complete high school or achieve vocational stability.

In order to illustrate the heterogeneous clinical pattern of the learning disabled adolescent, two case examples follow.[1]

Case Example 1

Casey was placed in special education at age eight. At that time, he had a number of evaluations that led to a diagnosis of learning disability and attention deficit disorder with hyperactivity. At age seven he was placed on pemoline, at nine he was started in psychotherapy, and in both instances the results were inconclusive.

The first time I saw Casey he was twelve years old. He was a handsome, clean-cut youngster who transmitted a sense of restlessness and drivenness. There was nothing unusual about his appearance except that his left eye was different. He noticed my curiosity and told me that a boy shot him in the eye with a BB gun two years ago. Subsequently, he developed a cataract, had surgery, and now has poor vision. That was the worst thing that ever happened to him, but he had gotten over it. His biggest concern was being in special education and doing poorly in school. He was bothered by the constant teasing about being a "retard," "mental," and "crazy." His biggest wish was to be in regular classes, and he wondered if I could help. He mentioned five friends and two older brothers who beat him up. He has a constant desire to fix things, and he wants to become a carpenter.

A week later he was equally tense and restless as he explored the limits of the office. He volunteered that he gets along better with his father—who is more patient, talks to him, and takes him to movies and to play golf—than his mother. He used to do bad things—kick doors, throw rocks at kids, steal things—but now he gets blamed even if he does not do anything. His grandfather died last year, and he misses him because he was so nice. He thinks that his grandfather watches him and that each time he gets in trouble his grandfather must be ashamed.

From birth there was an uneasiness that something was not right with him, as he did not act like other children. As soon as he started to crawl and walk, "all hell broke loose." He was into everything, breaking and destroying things. His mother suspected something wrong as he did not talk until he was three and he could not play with other children.

He was screened for kindergarten and labeled immature. The die was cast, and Casey's academic career was off to a bad start. His kindergarten teacher was young and inexperienced, and she did not last the year. Before her departure, she told his mother that something was not right with Casey. However, his first-grade teacher was tough and warm, so he had a good year. In the second grade, things began to fall apart. He was described as immature, unable to follow directions, and destructive. In the third grade, he was placed in a special education classroom. Between the third grade and his present placement, Casey has been in four schools and has experienced a dozen teachers. Toward the end of last year, he was in a class with healthier students where he learned and his behavior improved. This year he was assigned to a behavior disorders classroom, and his functioning deteriorated.

Peer relations have been a source of concern for the parents. Casey is eager to make friends; however, the friendships last a day or two, and then something happens. He may do something silly or goofy, or he will strike out at another youngster. After a fight with his older brother, he grabbed a knife and began to stab at a pillow until it was full of holes. The parents decided that something needed to be done, perhaps a psychiatric hospitalization.

Casey's mother is a short, stocky, ruddy-faced woman who is singularly unattractive and radiates a sense of masculinity. She is thirty-nine years old, and she and Casey's father have been married nineteen years. In addition to Casey, there are two older boys, ages seventeen and fifteen. While the middle son has been a good student, athletic, and popular, the older one has been picked up by the police for hot-rodding and drinking.

The mother has a twenty-seven-year-old brother who is the black sheep of the family: he never finished high school, has had a variety of jobs, and never married. Casey reminds her of this brother, and she worries that he will turn out similarly. Although the mother came across as anxious and concerned, there was a detachment about Casey's plight and joking about his difficulties. The mother showed little emotion and had a masklike face, which was a function of her chronic depression.

Casey's father is a tall, handsome, gregarious man who has a warm manner and an ease with people, which is helpful in his work as a successful insurance agent. He is a reformed alcoholic who has been attending AA for the past eight years. His wife is a moderate drinker; however, she refuses to recognize the problem.

The marriage has been unstable because of their drinking, the mother's depression, infrequent sexual encounters, and problems with the boys, especially Casey. Now things are better, they talk easier, but he hinted at an interest in other women.

Although father seemed more responsive and empathic, he viewed Casey as severely disturbed. He saw his son sometimes as a potential alcoholic and other times as schizophrenic. He expressed a concern that his and his wife's drinking may have damaged Casey's brain. While usually gentle and understanding, the father also beats Casey, afterward feeling guilty and remorseful.

Beginning therapy with Casey was uncomfortable, tension laden, and anxiety provoking. He was painfully self-conscious, compliant, and eager to please. He began treatment by confessing his "crimes." His first dream found him on a ledge suspended over a rushing river; it was dark and rainy, and he struggled to get away from the edge. During the first months, it was difficult to move him from the confessional mode. He had done this with a previous therapist, and he assumed that I expected it since his father advised him to tell everything. In addition to confessing, Casey related a string of painful experiences in which he had been attacked, humiliated, and depreciated.

He began to demonstrate a wonderment and pleasure at my ability to discern his emotional state without telling me how he felt. He was awed by my ability to sense his anxiety, boredom, and anger. He needed to see me as powerful and all knowing so that ultimately I would share these powers with him. I realized that the psychological test scores did not do justice to his capabilities as he possessed an extensive fund of general knowledge and he was keenly observant. There was initial improvement in school, but his behavior at home deteriorated. The turmoil was a function of his mother's increased drinking, which was related to Casey's investment in the treatment. In my excited state of discovery, I pointed this out to the mother; however, her cold, stony, and impassive reaction gave me a palpable taste of what this youngster was up against. Although the mother's depression and Casey's parallel, empty, depressed state were crucial elements of the psychopathology, I was impressed by his restlessness, tension, and agitation. I felt that it was important to impose psychological structure on the tension since he was somewhat aware of its content. He described the anxiety as something crawling in his stomach and as sticks or pins moving back and forth in his chest, arms, and legs.

Six months after we began, Casey told me with some embarrassment about a girl. She was safe because she was from another city and did not know his terrible reputation. When she sent him a picture, he became excited and composed a love song. Apparently, his ardor frightened her, as she did not respond to his calls and letters. He became depressed, and the acting out in school intensified. He was transferred to a school for behaviorally disturbed children. This school, which was isolated in the country, seemed like a jail. His two-year stay there was the low point of his academic career.

This setback led to a critical self-examination that was based on the parental history of alcoholism and his failures in school and with friends. In the new school, the students provoked him as a way to test him while he was struggling to turn over a new leaf. He worked hard at changing his appearance, as if that would magically change his predicament. On one occasion, Casey exposed himself to two little girls, who told their parents. It was agreed not to file charges since he was working on his problems. While being in therapy "saved him," this was also the first time Casey's father complained about the expense of treatment and the lack of progress.

Just as things were at their lowest ebb, Casey found a savior, the church. He became religious and obsessed with notions of what constitutes a good Christian and person. This interest gave him temporary peace of mind. However, the church interest unraveled when he sensed my skepticism and his father's disapproval. At this time, we began to explore the need for constant validation of his actions and beliefs from significant individuals in his life.

About a year into the treatment, two related events had a profound effect on Casey's psychological well-being. After years of denial, his mother signed herself into an alcoholism treatment unit. Soon afterward, Casey was arrested for exposing himself, and there was a possibility of being sent to a correctional facility for juveniles.

For the first time, Casey confronted the emptiness and the loneliness that he had experienced all these years, and he began to appreciate the need to elicit a response from those around him in order to feel alive and intact. The little girls' awed expressions on seeing his genitals was something that he craved and something that he felt embarrassed about and ashamed of since it focused on the possibility that he is a "psycho" and a "pervert." Two court appearances resulted in a year's probation, in part determined by his being in therapy. However, the probation officer told father not to waste his money on "shrinks."

The realization that he flirted with going to jail resulted in a sudden spurt of good behavior. Casey expressed a wish to leave treatment since things were going well and his schoolwork had improved. He discovered music as a calming vehicle and started guitar lessons with fantasies of becoming a rock star. When a current girlfriend left, he was hurt and depressed. He told me about an episode in which he approached two little girls. When I pointed out the possible consequences, he became furious and walked out. His anger persisted until I realized that he was testing my confidence in him. When we reconstructed what happened, he was relieved that I understood his disappointment.

At this time, there was another setback as his mother started drinking again. Casey became angry at her and was able to reconstruct his explosiveness when he was younger. He met a girl that he fought with at age seven and was embarrassed when they talked about how he used to act. He remembered trying to tell his mother what he experienced at school and receiving an uncomprehending blank stare. At those times he would explode, yell, and throw things. Mother would call father or one of the brothers to calm him while she continued in her alcoholic haze.

One of the striking elements in his behavior was the extent to which he mimicked and imitated the behaviors of others. Once he attached himself to a particular individual, that person became his model. Unfortunately, the only youngsters who befriended him experienced similar problems.

A blowup with his father led to a discussion of the damaged eye. Father became so angry with Casey for missing school that he slapped him in the face. The eye became swollen, and Casey recalled the neighbor who shot him. He discussed his weird appearance and his need to wear sunglasses as protection and cover-up. As Casey confronted his limitations, he began to examine me in detail. He noted my accent and commented that my hair looked funny. He wondered why I smoked a pipe and at times I looked tired and glanced at the clock. He wondered why I would work with a "hopeless retard" like himself when I could have been a real doctor. Perhaps I was limited and defective just like he was and that is why I understood him.

Casey went on a fishing trip with his father and enjoyed himself. Although he missed me and his mother, he realized that he was happy to be away. He told me that he was calm during the trip; then he worried whether he had hurt my feelings. After a particularly productive session, he hugged me but became scared that I would think he was turning into a "faggot." We wondered whether his excessive interest in girls was related to fears of becoming homosexual. We discussed his fear of AIDS and looking at guys for clues of homosexuality. He fell asleep during a session to test both of us. If he was relaxed enough to fall asleep, it meant that he trusted me and himself.

Casey befriended the smartest boy at school. In order to emulate and compete, Casey progressed rapidly through the various behavioral levels. The good feelings from school spilled over into the home, and for the first time Casey's mother appreciated him and enjoyed his company.

The next months were spent trying to differentiate the excitement about doing well, with its implied possibilities, from the anxiety of not knowing what is expected of him. There was a fearfulness that, the better he does, the more will be expected. What if he has already attained the maximum functional level? The excitement about going to a regular school, having friends, and driving a car made him physically uncomfortable. He described the feeling as one in which his skin is tearing itself away from the bones; unless he holds on to something or somebody, he feels that he will come apart into little pieces and then will be gone.

The termination phase appeared gradually when Casey talked about attending a special education class at a regular high school. He checked out several schools and found one that felt comfortable. He was tested and interviewed; while the testing showed deficits in certain basic skills, he was accepted conditionally. The earnestness of his manner and the genuine wish to return to a normal environment impressed the staff. Concurrently, he took on his first job as a dishwasher. After three years, a palpable sadness had descended on the analysis as we knew that termination was in the air. On a couple of occasions he became tearful, and I, just like the parents, wondered if he could function without me.

When Casey told his parents that we were finishing, they became anxious and called to see if it was true. The reality of the termination terrified them. Casey was furious because he felt that I would cater to their anxiety with my own and make him come forever. He reported dreams in which a group of kids were beating him up and he was exposing himself to little girls. When we decided that these dreams had something to do with a wish to regress and go back to the beginning, he told me of a dream in which he was visiting a new school with me and his father.

As we considered a termination date, a variety of themes emerged. The first signs of excitement appeared when Casey realized that he was leaving his school; he was finally getting out of jail. The jail sentence was punishment for beating up kids, masturbating, and exposing himself. These sins can be atoned for; however, doing poorly in school could not be helped since he may have been a "retard." He shared the parental fantasy that their drinking damaged his brain but that, since he is young and growing, the damaged brain could grow back.

Casey became curious about my personal life. He wanted to know where I lived, what my family was like, and how I spent my time. He became preoccupied with my accent since it sounded German. He was half German, so we must be alike, which would explain how I understood him. He was still awed by my ability to know what was on his mind; however, he concluded that I understand only as much as he permits. He wanted to invite me to his house so that he could remember me after we stopped since he had difficulty recalling what I look like. This was similar to his learning problems in school: his brain simply goes blank. At times it feels like there is a thick wall and nothing passes either way. He would like to use a hammer or chisel to break it down. It feels like a dark pit in which facts, dates, and numbers sink but nothing comes out. He also feels that his brain is a deep dark pool in which things drop to the bottom and do not float up. The only things that he remembers well are maps and songs. He noted that he remembered more than other kids but that when he felt jumpy he could not remember anything because he was searching for something to make the jumpiness go away.

Casey embarked on a period of depreciation of the treatment and his family. For the first time he wondered about his mother's masculine appearance and father's need to look good in the community. His parents did not fit together. He depreciated his mother's appearance and poor housekeeping, and he recognized that I looked old and tired. He wondered what kind of man spends all day listening to people's problems and playing games with children. He wondered how bad I would look if he got in trouble and did not succeed. If he ever met me outside the office, he would not be able to face me. Just like his dead grandparents, I will be watching him.

The last months of the analysis were spent exploring the causes of his anxiety. The aspect of fooling people was crucial since he worried whether people could tell that he was dumb or was saying things that

333

did not make sense. He worried that he was a fraud, so he kept talking to distract others from figuring him out. He could let me figure him out because he realized that I would not embarrass or make fun of him. With strangers, he was not sure, and, until he could figure out what they would do, he had to pace or do something to make the jittery feelings go away. Since he acted peculiarly, it was seldom appreciated when he did well. I was the only person who was not distracted by his goofy behavior.

During this period, Casey was calm, reflective, and introspective; however, he punctuated the calmness by announcing that he was quitting a month before the time we agreed on. When he approached his parents, they said that it was between the two of us. He was relieved that everyone passed the test. This maneuver was an attempt to short-circuit the sadness that coexisted with the excitement. In the last month, Casey expressed anxiety about not seeing me. Who will he talk to if he has a problem with a girl or gets in a fight in school? Since his mother responds sometimes and his father lectures, then he may talk to his brother, who treats him as an equal.

Casey decided to spend several days fixing up his room and putting things in order, just like with me. He still could not believe that I would allow him to leave at the time we agreed on. He thought that his father was nervous about our finishing, but that is his problem; maybe he should come to see me.

Casey was hopeful that in the end I would tell him all the things that I have not told him before. He hoped I would show him my notes so that he would know everything about himself that needs to be known. Then, and only then, would we be equals.

Case Example 2

By the time I saw Robert diagnostically in his sophomore year, he had a lengthy history of psychotherapy and tutoring. He was the most tutored youngster I have ever seen. Beginning in the second grade, he has been helped by one to three tutors every year. In spite of the help, he was in all low-level classes at a highly competitive, college-oriented high school. He saw himself as having a severe learning disability and a pervasive sense that there was something wrong with his mind and brain. His support for such an assertion was based on a history of enuresis, questionable petit mal seizures, an abnormal EEG, and a history of poor grades. He was envious of his older brother, who was an excellent student, and talked glowingly about his brilliant parents, who were college professors. He was puzzled by his poor school performance, occasional good grades, an inability to concentrate, and failure to complete assignments. He was a responsible youngster, having had a variety of jobs, which he handled expertly. He was athletic, and his peer relations were adequate.

In the first grade, there was a suspicion that he was having difficulty adjusting. Teachers reported that he was easily distracted and restless, that he could not stay on task, and that he was socially immature. In the second grade, he was tested, and a learning disability was diagnosed. While he managed to keep pace with the work, it was decided that he needed assistance with basic reading skills. In the third grade, there began a succession of tutors and learning centers. He plodded along in mainstream classes with constant special education resources as a backup. The school suggested special education placement on three occasions; however, the parents refused. In spite of massive therapeutic efforts, Robert reached a low point in the sixth grade; he was failing and became a nuisance in class. This so infuriated his mother that she hit him and then did not speak to him for weeks. He recalled this incident with sadness and bitterness.

As Robert struggled through junior high school, he developed a predictable pattern. In the beginning of the school year, he impressed teachers with his knowledge, industriousness, and competence. By the first report card, he would begin a downward slide that persisted into early spring. Teachers would become confused by the inconsistency and would consider a special education placement. By the end of the year, Robert would improve and complete on an up note. The three things that kept him out of special education were his parents' refusal, constant tutoring, and not being a behavior problem.

His high school performance was erratic; he would start the year well and then gradually fall behind. He would get an A or an A and a B, and the rest of his grades would be Ds. In classes where the teachers made special allowances, he performed poorly; in classes where the expectations were consistent, he did better.

Robert was depressed. In the diagnostic interviews, he teared easily and bemoaned his fate as a failure incapable of competing with the bright youngsters in the suburbs. His depression was so severe that at times he was paralyzed with inactivity. Although there were two previous attempts at psychotherapy at ages eight and ten, neither one had an impact except for an initially stabilizing effect. In each instance, he complied, catering to parental wishes but feeling like he was being dragged to another tutor. This time he requested help, and the parents felt that he was ready to confront his problems.

Robert's parents were hard-driving, accomplished academicians. To have a child who did not appear ambitious in his studies was exceptionally frustrating. His mother was an only child and an excellent student. She established herself as a much-sought-after teacher and consultant in computer science. The mother was a pleasant, chronically depressed woman. She worried about her son because he seemed so immature, a crybaby, emotional and undisciplined. Yet he could surprise with his maturity, self-sufficiency, and kindness. He seemed forgetful, always late, confused, and easy going, yet he talked about becoming a physician because that was his mother's secret ambition. There was more of a kinship between her and Robert's brother, who was settled, serious, studious, and academically successful. She was a serious individual who budgeted her time so that every minute was used for reading and studying. Her son's lack of interest in reading was devastating, and occasionally she bribed him to read books. She was baffled and confused by the contradictory elements in his functioning. Because of the confusion, she alternated between being angry and being withdrawn. She never knew the right way to approach him.

Robert's father was a pleasant, outgoing man, a successful teacher, but overshadowed by an older brother who is a brilliant research biologist. The father described his own erratic school performance and a younger brother who had learning problems and never completed formal education. The brother lives alone and supports himself with an inheritance and odd jobs. The father saw himself as having similar problems: he gets confused easily, has a poor sense of time, and was recently refused a promotion.

Father was more sensitive to Robert because he saw in him a reflection of his troubled youth. He was a hell-raiser and ladies' man who cared little about schoolwork. He was a disappointment to his father, who was an outstanding surgeon. After holding a variety of menial jobs, Robert's father returned to school when his father died. Although he was almost expelled from college, he completed his studies with a flourish. His life was a pattern of failure followed by success.

Although both parents shared a concern that Robert may turn out like his father's younger brother, the father was more optimistic as he appreciated Robert's abilities and strengths. He was concerned about the appropriate expectations. They have always received confusing messages from professionals; either they are expecting too much, or they are not expecting enough.

Robert was a source of serious disagreement between the parents. Father felt that his wife was overly critical, harsh, and demanding, while she thought that her husband was indifferent and presented an undisciplined model.

Robert was eager to commence therapy. He was anxious to confess his shortcomings, problems, deficits, and academic limitations. He idealized me from the beginning and felt comfortable and understood. He reported a warm and close relationship with father, and there was much resentment and tearfulness when he dwelt on mother's disappointment and anger. There was detailed recall of tutors, teachers, and therapists. Some were considered helpful, while others treated him as if he were retarded. Robert was impressed by the initial shift in parental attitude and felt that I could influence the parents to grant him more independence.

Robert dated girls from other schools since they did not know that he was a poor student. Nevertheless, he would come across as a "sickie" by discussing his problems and poor classroom performance. The boys that he was friendly with had multiple problems, emotional and physical.

He had a strong wish to be with me as he expected something magical would "fix him." He hoped to be transformed into an excellent student as his grades improved during the first months of treatment. The underlying fantasy had to do with my removing the defectiveness from his brain. He nurtured the notion that he was damaged even though the evidence was not compelling. He talked mostly about grades, teachers, and plans to attend college and become a physician.

Robert's stance in the treatment was one of extreme passivity and compliance. During the early phase, he never missed a session and felt ashamed and guilty if he was late. He agreed with everything I said. If I said little, it was his fault for being an uncooperative patient. An early dream was stimulated by a visit to a neurologist. He was in the operating room, and several doctors were huddled in a corner. A tall surgeon stepped out as if he was going to operate on Robert's brain, while the other surgeons left the room. He refused an anesthetic as he felt he could tolerate the pain.

As the treatment deepened, it became evident that Robert studied my face to determine my optimism or pessimism about his future in treatment and school. Robert would spin elaborate plans and then observe my face for a response that would telegraph approval or skepticism.

As his mood improved, his functioning reached a higher level. However, the school situation remained the same as he struggled in most of his classes. One of Robert's strengths was a talent for involving teachers and other adults to help and rescue him. There was a beseeching attitude in his style that elicited caretaking responses. Eventually, the adult would become disappointed with Robert's lack of diligence and perseverance. We realized that he tested people to see if they would help make allowances or cater to his limitations. The more he was left on his own, the better he performed. If the help was excessive, he usually failed.

One of the pivotal times in treatment was graduation from high school. He anticipated the ceremony with a palable sense of dread and foreboding. He felt like a fake, a charlatan, and a fraud as he did not learn and did not deserve to graduate. He felt that he was an embarrassment to the school, his family, and himself. He could not comprehend his parents' pleasure since they had not expected him to finish. The summer after graduation was one of the most difficult times in his life. He collected a number of college applications, but he did not complete them.

Robert entered a local junior college since he needed more treatment and he did not think that four-year schools would accept him. He depreciated the junior college as the teachers were inept and the students were losers like himself.

The notion that his brain was damaged was the key theme of the next two years' work. He concluded that, since he weighed ten pounds at birth, his brain was damaged in the process. The parents maintained a similar explanation. He felt that his mother suspected his deficits from the beginning as she kept detailed logs of his growth and development. He conceptualized his brain as a storage battery that becomes short-circuited or depleted. He frantically turned to others to recharge him intellectually and emotionally. When he was forgetful, the battery was dead; when he was depressed, the battery was poorly charged; and when he gave wrong answers, the wires were crossed. He would hit himself in the head in order to reconnect the circuits. Teachers that were overly helpful saw his damaged battery; consequently, he wanted to get away.

Another significant theme of the treatment was his sense of feeling fraudulent: when he received a good grade, his mother accused him of cheating or the teacher of making a mistake. Consequently, every time he got a good grade he felt that he had fooled the teachers. The good grades were not an accurate reflection of his knowledge since nothing stuck in his brain.

In junior college, he became conscientious about his work, yet each time he wrote a paper he felt that he was plagiarizing and cheating. He wrote papers on obscure subjects so that teachers could not verify his sources. He felt that our ideas about him came from me and that he was parroting them. I was implanting concepts in his head, but these did not stick. He also felt fraudulent because he had difficulty maintaining continuity between sessions; consequently, he was only acting as if he had been here before. Robert remembered his parents telling him that he was pretending to study as he sat for hours in front of open books. He nodded that he understood interpretations but actually did not; it was just an act.

As he began to recognize his competence, the depressive elements lifted. One of his best moments occurred before an exam when he announced that for the first time ever he felt prepared.

He surmised that I was a good student, so I could not possibly comprehend what it feels like not to be prepared. Many of the things that he learned just vanished from his brain. It was as if his brain was a sieve and things fell out. He wondered if there were tests to determine whether his brain was smaller or more porous than others.

As Robert's work improved, there were fantasies of how his father would react to his going away to college. He was overly attached to his father, and he worried about how his parents would manage in his absence. There was a dream in which he and his father were walking along a beautiful campus. He was excited about going to school, but in his father's eyes there was sadness. Suddenly, a strong gust of wind pushed him back.

A parallel anxiety emanated from his parents' expectations. Since he was doing better, they expected good grades to prove to former teachers and tutors that he was brilliant like his brother. They wondered whether he was indeed learning disabled and whether the experts were mistaken after all. This enraged Robert because it gave the impression that he did poorly because he was lazy.

The parents' excitement over Robert's academic progress reached discomforting proportions. He dealt with the tension by regressing in school. The parents' anxiety about his regression was compounded by my anxiety about his seemingly self-destructive behavior. As he began to confront his disappointment and anger with me, Robert reported the following dream. He was piloting an airplane over the water, and the plane started to dive. He glanced over his shoulder and noted how frightened and anxious the passengers became. As the plane was swooping lower and lower, he pulled it up from its dive, and at the last moment it flew away. We agreed that the excitement of inappropriately high expectations made him anxious. To diminish his tension, he made others anxious so that they would expect less.

As we started to discuss termination, he tested me to determine my level of confidence in his departure. He knew that I was pleased with his work and progress. He wondered if I would become depressed just like his father. He referred another patient to take his place, and, when that did not work out, he became anxious about my allowing him to leave.

Robert was excited about leaving treatment and home. For the first time in his life he would not need "helpers" or tutors. The chance to do it on his own would be a new experience.

Robert did leave feeling competent and confident that he could function successfully in school. He felt more intact as he considered the possibility of attending graduate school. There were unresolved issues: his competitive feelings with his brother; his need to study constantly; and his shaky sense of himself as a totally separate and independent human being. However, the resolution of these issues will have to wait for another time; in the meantime, there are many possibilities.

Discussion

Inconsistency and unpredictability of behavior frequently accompany the adolescent state. Dynamic and clinical formulations seem to have far more difficulty explaining the adolescent than they do any other age group. With the constant danger of spontaneous regression, character formation is indeed precarious. Consequently, the adolescent presents a fluid and inconsistent clinical picture in his or her response and adaptation to a learning disability (Garber 1985).

In optimal situations, these youngsters are plagued by anxieties and concerns about their limitations and state of differentness. Because of such anxieties and an academic history replete with failure, depreciation, and rejection, learning disabled adolescents become creative avoiders (Cohen 1985).

The learning disabled adolescent, owing to years of school failure, is unable to develop a global and consistent sense of confidence in his competence. Consequently, he avoids academic and social situations that may threaten his precarious stability. Such youngsters will "cut corners" and take shortcuts in academic endeavors. That means doing the minimum amount acceptable; to go beyond that may result in failure, exposure, and ridicule. Much energy is expended in search of loopholes in assignments and teacher's directions. Papers are plagiarized, and potentially stressful classroom situations are avoided by legitimate and illegitimate means. Frequently, such youngsters are labeled not only as avoiders but also as manipulators. In either instance, the negative self-image is reinforced, which may result in the development of a more elaborate and sophisticated defensive superstructure.

Learning disabled adolescents avoid not only academic exposure but also social situations because there looms the possibility of embarrassment and humiliation. The result is a state of friendlessness or an all-encompassing attachment to someone like oneself. The learning disabled adolescent is most comfortable relating to peers with similar difficulties. Heterosexual involvements are limited or confined to individuals from other places. Consequently, the peer relationships that are so essential to further separation-individuation may be absent or short-circuited.

The avoidance of difficulty and newness enhances a sense of sameness and predictability that can become a prominent element in the elaboration of a rigid character structure. Defensive coping strategies may be employed in a rigid fashion. They rely on a limited number of defensive operations that are utilized with minimal regard for the actual situation. Acting rigidly becomes so ego syntonic that these adolescents demonstrate an exaggerated and tense deliberateness of behavior in novel or anxiety-provoking situations. Their purposiveness becomes so intense that it does not allow deviation or spontaneity. This rigidity may not necessarily become a manifestation of an obsessive compulsive character; often it becomes an important aspect of the adolescents' daily functioning (Cohen 1985).

Learning disabled adolescents, even those who have experienced years of assistance, do not understand exactly what their specific cognitive disability was and is or how it affects their social interactions and learning. It is difficult to differentiate the actual effect of the disability from the meaning that they have given to it. As a result, learning disabled adolescents believe that there is something seriously damaged in their heads. This is a pivotal fantasy around which psychopathology crystallizes. The adolescent will use and embellish the fantasy beyond the point that is reasonable and appropriate. The fantasy is crucial in adolescence because it may have an effect on identity formation. For the learning disabled adolescent, the process of identify formation is made more painful and confusing because it involves thinking about oneself as damaged and inadequate. The presence of this fantasy and its interference with normal identity formation may contribute to the learning disabled adolescent's low self-esteem, which may result in a chronic state of depression. This depression may not be limited to castration and oedipal-related issues but may rather have something to do with one's sense of being an imperfect human being (Aleksandrowicz and Aleksandrowicz 1987; Coen 1986).

While the depression may also be seen as mourning for the loss of the perfect self, it has more to do with not being able to measure up to the expectations of oneself and others. It is not surprising then that shame and embarrassment are constant companions of the learning disabled adolescent.

The primary affective configuration, however, is a high propensity to experience anxiety and distress. Any challenge, novel situation, change, social interaction, or demand to perform will elicit a palpable tenseness and a range of anxiety discharge mechanisms. While the shape and form of the anxiety may be modified and elevated to a more sophisticated level, that anxiety does not necessarily diminish with time or maturation.

Such a chronically pervasive tension state is fed from several sources. Competitive issues and performance concerns are integral components. Increased sexual and aggressive impulses also contribute; however, clinical experience indicates that something more basic is contributing to this tension. Owing to real and exaggerated cognitive limitations, the learning disabled adolescent has difficulty assessing his environment accurately. He is unsure of his ability to evaluate how others see him, what they think of him, and what they expect. He is overly concerned with how he presents himself and feels limited in his capacity to judge the responses of others. Since such cognitive demands may become overwhelming, he will withdraw. When he is unable to withdraw, and when he has to confront daily functional situations, he becomes tense and anxious. Not knowing environmental responses yet having to act as if one does contributes to anxiety and a sense of feeling fraudulent. When he knows his milieu and develops an awareness of what can be expected, he is likely to relax. As he arrives at an impression of how others see him, the anxiety will diminish. Until then, he experiences the gnawing tension that envelops a stranger in a strange land.

Owing to limited social graces, with the stigma of being learning disabled, rigid, lacking spontaneity, depressed, and anxious, the learning disabled adolescent is not considered a worthwhile social companion. He is shunned by mainstream peers. If he develops a talent or skill, he may be accepted by the segment of the student body that shares similar interests. However, the students at large will treat him as a nonentity only to be tolerated.

While the reasons for nonacceptance have been mentioned, there is a more basic explanation why such a youngster does not become an integral part of the school fabric. Owing to his cognitive limitations and an absorption with his emotional pulse, such a youngster is deficient in his ability to be empathic. His self-centeredness precludes his being able to empathize with the feelings of others. While he may be hypersensitive to how others treat him, he is cold and callous to the feelings of peers. He seems indifferent and uncaring, and his comments expose a lack of sensitivity to the hurts that he may inflict unknowingly. For the normal adolescent, who is constantly preoccupied with other people's feelings, such callousness is considered a major crime. The learning disabled adolescent may not know exactly what he does wrong; however, he is aware that his comments turn people off. As he does not know what happens and why and is too embarrassed to ask, he does the only sure thing; he becomes anxious and withdraws (Bachara 1976; Bryant 1982; McGlannan 1977).

Since the learning disabled adolescent doubts his cognitive abilities and the accuracy of his perceptions, he is never sure whether he learned what he should or whether he learned anything at all. He deals with the unsureness by avoidance, by asking repetitively meaningless questions, or by becoming overly rigid and arrogant. Such behaviors may rebuff teachers who might otherwise be understanding. Because of these pervasive doubts and their defensive extensions, the learning disabled adolescent harbors a sense of feeling fraudulent. He feels that he is acting as if he learned but that if he were truly tested it would be obvious that his knowledge is superficial. Consequently, such youngsters may seek the deeper meaning of subjects but feel that a deeper understanding eludes them.

Since the learning disabled adolescent is not sure of his own motives, aims, and true feelings, he also lacks knowledge of the true feelings, motives, and expectations of others. Consequently, he has an overriding need to test people in various direct and indirect ways. Learning disabled individuals, who do not have enough confidence in their cognitive equipment to read the environment accurately, develop other means to determine what is going on. To do so, they make outrageous statements, set up "what if" situations, or paint hypothetical scenarios as a means of eliciting responses from significant adults. These responses may then be used to take their own emotional pulse or to determine a course of action. The various maneuvers are means of dealing with an environment that may be ambiguous or confusing. The more intelligent the adolescent, the more complex the testing maneuver (Garber 1988). These testing maneuvers, which try the patience of parents, teachers, and therapists, often obscure the learning disabled adolescent's strengths and capabilities.

Conclusions

In spite of the various pitfalls and limitations, many of the learning disabled middle- and upper-middle-class adolescents that I have observed seem to make it. Owing to a massive input of educational and emotional resources, such youngsters progress through the system, graduate, and may adapt. They may reach these goals slowly, painfully, and indirectly. Nevertheless, they find their niche and compensate for their limitations. They pay a high price for the progression as they may develop personality distortions with a prominent narcissistic caste.

Parents and teachers gradually diminish expectations, while the young adults may become more realistic about goals, ambitions, and aspirations. An equilibrium is established in which the youngster and his environment become relatively comfortable with one another.

As therapists, we assume that learning disabled adolescents who have received massive academic and emotional tutoring have benefited from the experience. In spite of such benefits, and in spite of having negotiated the educational system, many remain lonely, isolated, and solitary individuals. A pervasive vulnerability to slights, chronic tension, a need to keep proving oneself, and a situational sense of defectiveness may continue to plague the individual for life. We now know that a learning disability is not just a school problem but also a life problem.

The learning disabled adolescents that I have worked with impressed me as being lonely, withdrawn, solitary, and isolated creatures. To the outside observer, they may appear comfortable and self-contained, perhaps even independent and content in their loneliness, yet one has to wonder whether this is the adolescents' true state. It may be an adaptive facade, constructed over years of feeling limited, inept, and defective internally, while seeming different and peculiar externally. Many of these adolescents seem to embrace isolation as they turn away from outside companions and activities. They retreat to the home and put on an appearance of contentment in their solitary pursuits.

If in this chapter I have been able to transmit something about the true nature of the learning disabled adolescent, then perhaps in a small sense I have contributed to diminishing his sense of loneliness and isolation.

NOTE

1. A complete version of case example 1 (Casey) will be published in the *Annual of Psychoanalysis*.

REFERENCES

Aleksandrowicz, D., and Aleksandrowicz, M. 1987. Psychodynamic approach to low self-esteem related to developmental deviations: growing-up incompetent. *Journal of the American Academy of Child and Adolescent Psychiatry* 26(4): 583–585.

Bachara, G. 1976. Empathy in learning disabled children. *Perceptual and Motor Skills* 43:541–542.

Bruininks, V. L. 1978. Peer status and personality characteristics of learning disabled and non-disabled students. *Journal of Learning Disabilities* 11:29–34.

Bryan, T. 1974. Peer popularity in learning disabled children. *Journal of Learning Disabilities* 7:621–625.

Bryant, B. 1982. An index of empathy for children and adolescents. *Child Development* 38:413–425.

Coen, S. J. 1986. The sense of defect. *Journal of the American Psychoanalytic Association* 34(1): 47–68.

Cohen, J. 1985. Learning disabilities and adolescence: developmental considerations. *Adolescent Psychiatry* 12:177–196.

Cruickshank, W. M. 1980. Learning disabilities. In *The Struggle from Adolescence toward Adulthood.* Syracuse, N.Y.: Syracuse University Press.

Garber, B. 1985. Mourning in adolescence: normal and pathological. *Adolescent Psychiatry* 12:371–387.

Garber, B. 1988. The emotional implications of learning disabilities: a theoretical integration. *Annual of Psychoanalysis* 16:111–129.

Kline, C. L. 1972. The adolescents with learning problems: how long must they wait? *Journal of Learning Disabilities* 5:127–144.

McConaughy, S. 1986. Social competence and behavioral problems in learning disabled boys aged twelve–sixteen. *Journal of Learning Disabilities* 19:101–107.

McGlannan, G. 1977. Empathy in learning disabled children. *Journal of Learning Disabilities* 10:42–43.

Mendelson, W.; Johnson, N.; and Stewart, M. 1971. Hyperactive children as teenagers: a follow-up study. *Journal of Nervous and Mental Diseases* 153:273–279.

Palombo, J. 1979. Perceptual deficits and self-esteem in adolescence. *Clinical Social Work Journal* 7(1): 34–60.

Perlmutter, B. 1987. Delinquency and learning disabilities: evidence for compensatory behavior and adaptation. *Journal of Youth and Adolescence* 16(2): 89–95.

Rutter, M., ed. 1983. *Developmental Neuropsychiatry.* New York: Guilford.

Schloss, E. 1971. *The Educator's Enigma: The Adolescent with Learning Disabilities.* San Rafael, Calif.: Academic Therapy.

Schonhaut, S., and Satz, P. 1983. Prognosis for children with learning disabilities: a review of follow-up studies. In M. Rutter, ed. *Developmental Neuropsychiatry.* New York: Guilford.

Silver, A., and Hagin, R. 1985. Outcomes of learning disabilities in adolescence. *Adolescent Psychiatry* 12:197–213.

Silverman, R., and Zigmond, N. 1983. Self-concept in learning disabled adolescents. *Journal of Learning Disabilities* 16:8–14.

Weiss, G.; Hechtoman, L.; Perlman, T.; Hopkins, J.; and Wener, A. 1979. Hyperactives as young adults: a controlled prospective ten-year follow-up of seventy-five children. *Archives of General Psychiatry* 36:675–681.

Wiig, E., and Harris, S. 1974. Perception and interpretation of nonverbally expressed emotions by adolescents with learning disabilities. *Perceptual and Motor Skills* 38:239–245.

17 A PSYCHODYNAMIC APPROACH TO THE EARLY DIAGNOSIS OF MANIC-DEPRESSIVE DISORDER IN ADOLESCENCE

LORETTA R. LOEB AND FELIX F. LOEB, JR.

It is often difficult to diagnose manic-depression during adolescence because adolescent manics may not show the classic adult symptoms of mania (Hugens 1974; Landolt 1957; Olsen 1961). As Laroche, Cheifetz, and Lester (1981, p. 987) wrote, "Current diagnostic criteria and research batteries . . . focus too much on phenomenology and pay inadequate attention to the developmental and psychodynamic processes of childhood and adolescence." In early adolescence, manic patients may present only with symptoms of irritability, aggressiveness, hyperactivity, unsocialized behavior, and depression with self-destructive or suicidal behavior. These patients are often misdiagnosed as having antisocial behavior, adjustment reaction, hyperkinetic reaction, attention deficit disorder, school phobia, anorexia nervosa, or depression (Brown, Ingber, and Tross 1983). Later during adolescence, manic patients may, besides these symptoms, also exhibit psychotic symptoms, and they often are misdiagnosed as schizophrenic (Ballenger, Reus, and Post 1982; Lehmann 1967; Rosen, Bahn, Shellow, and Bower 1965; Weiner 1970).

A psychodynamic correlation that we have observed in adult manic-depressive patients (Loeb and Loeb 1987) enables us to make an early diagnosis of manic-depression in adolescents. We had found that, just before our adult manic patients developed overt manic symptoms, they regularly experienced a sudden abnormal increase in their unconscious sexual drives. They usually kept these drives out of their conscious minds with unconscious ego defense mechanisms (Loeb and Loeb 1987). The resultant unconscious conflict manifested in the psychotherapeutic situation first in parapraxes or dreams and shortly after that in typical manic symptoms.

Having observed this pattern in adults, when we found four adolescent patients desperately trying to use defense mechanisms to keep a sudden abnormal increase in their sexual desires out of their conscious minds, we hypothesized that they too might be suffering from an early, or prodromal, stage of manic-depressive illness. We made this hypothesis even though their overt presenting symptoms did not meet the DSM-III-R criteria for a manic episode. Their overt symptoms included unsocialized behavior, irritability, aggressiveness, hyperactivity, depression, and psychosis. One adolescent had occasional difficulty sleeping, and another spoke slightly faster than normal.[1]

We tested our hypothesis by giving these four patients a trial of lithium carbonate and found that it first reduced their overwhelming, unconscious sexual inclinations and then eliminated their overt symptoms. This enabled them to develop a therapeutic alliance, which allowed them to engage in insight-oriented psychotherapy. In psychotherapy, we learned that our patients' overt symptoms were the consequence of an unconscious conflict between their exaggerated sexual desires and their defenses against them.

Review of the Literature

Abraham (1911), Feinstein (1982), Fenichel (1945), Freeman (1971), Jacobson (1971), Kestenbaum (1980, 1982), Krafft-Ebing (1906), Lewin (1950), Shopsin (1979), Van Putten (1975), and Wolpert (1977, 1981) observed the symptom of hypersexual behavior in manic patients. These observers did not, however, report that their patients had had an increase in their unconscious sexual drive just before they went into overt manic attacks.

Fenichel (1945) and Jacobson (1971) felt that biological factors were causative in mania. Other authors (Sheard 1977; Shou 1978; and Van Putten 1975) observed that lithium reduced patients' sexual drive. Sheard felt that lithium was related to, or had an effect on, the systems that regulate gonadal hormones.

Deleon-Jones, Val, and Herts (1982) reported a case of a forty-three-year-old woman who belonged to a subgroup of subjects who suffer from a subsyndromal affective disorder during their premenstruum. During this patient's premenstrual phase, her MHPG[2] levels were considerably higher than they were during her follicular and luteal phases, and this elevation coincided with the severest manifestations of her symptoms. These elevations did not occur during cycles when she was receiving lithium. Kelly, Koch, and Buegel (1976) also described adolescent and adult cases who had an exacerbation of mood swings premenstrually.

CLINICAL EXAMPLE 1

Toby, an attractive, heavily made-up fourteen-year-old-girl, was brought for therapy by her parents when she threatened suicide. At ten, following menarche, Toby's behavior changed: she became unusually modest about nudity, became verbally belligerent toward her mother and younger sister, and turned her attention toward her father and boys. Once she angrily told her mother that she had whipped the covers off her sister and found her "playing with herself." Because she felt dirty, Toby began washing herself, her home, and her family's clothing incessantly. No longer could she sit still, even to play a board game. She began disrupting the school classes by talking, making crude sexual comments, fighting, or tidying up the classroom. She dressed tough, used excessive makeup, made ink tattoos on her arm, and took drugs. She let the air out of tires, broke windows, smart-mouthed her teachers, was truant, and failed courses. She stole money from her parents to buy seductive clothing and makeup, and she began sneaking out of the house late at night. When confronted with her rebellious, delinquent behavior, Toby lied, swore, and angrily broke things.

Toby's birth had been normal after an uneventful pregnancy. No genetic history of manic-depressive illness was available because Toby was adopted. She was a sweet-tempered baby, but very determined and active. She would not stay in her crib and preferred noisy toys that moved. At nineteen months, after Toby had several dry nights, mother began toilet training. Toby hated soiled diapers and caught on quickly. At two, for two months, Toby would get up in the middle of the night and quietly stand close to her mother's bed. When her mother asked why she was there, Toby denied having nightmares and returned to her bed.

Toby continued to be very active. At three, she loved to swing high on swings, climb to the top of monkey bars, and ride her bicycle as fast as she could. At four, Toby was found in a doghouse with a five-year-old boy. Both had their pants off and were smiling. Toby later told her sister that they had "done it."

During latency, Toby kept her clothing and toys in meticulous order and enjoyed cleaning and tidying up the house. This pleased her compulsively neat father, who was never satisfied with Toby's mother's housekeeping. Toby enjoyed caring for and playing with her younger siblings. Although her family was not religious, Toby became upset if she could not go to church. She became very stubborn if she did not get her way. When she was eight, Toby told her mother that a girl had forced her to take off her clothing, get on top of her, and kiss her. She enjoyed school and doing well academically. She loved to run competitively until she began to win all the races, then she lost interest in running. People fascinated Toby, and she got along with everyone.

During her initial visit, Toby smiled and defiantly said that she had nothing to say because she had no mental problems. Later, she complained that her parents were too demanding, but continued to smile and acted bored. Toby's Rorschach responses were either bland or highly stimulated. She tried to curb her active fantasy life by remaining detached from her overwhelming affects.

After several months of psychoanalytically oriented psychotherapy, Toby reluctantly admitted to her therapist that she had had to sneak out of the house at night to have indiscriminate sexual intercourse with many different boys in sordid surroundings. Before confiding this to her therapist, Toby had successfully concealed this behavior from everyone. She had also defended herself from consciously recognizing the inappropriately excessive and dangerous nature of her nighttime sexual activities.

Toby displayed her unconscious, long-hidden hypersexuality and other symptoms, but she did not manifest the characteristic, adult symptoms of mania.[3] However, because our adult manic psychoanalytic patients, just before they developed their manic symptoms, had regularly displayed either a sudden, abnormal increase in their sexual thoughts, feelings, and fantasies or an increase in their defensive operations against such thoughts, feelings, or fantasies (Loeb and Loeb 1987), we suspected that Toby's symptoms of hypersexuality, obsessionality, excessive modesty, rebellious belligerency, excessive makeup, delinquency, and suicidal threats might be due to an underly-

351

ing manic-depressive disorder. Toby was started on lithium carbonate, and, when her blood lithium level was brought up to 1.5 milliequivalents per liter, her incessant need for sexual activity diminished. Soon after that, her other symptoms, which later turned out to be compromises between her intense sexual urges and her defenses against them, subsided. She stopped wearing excessive makeup, became a delightful, cooperative, well-behaved fourteen-year-old girl, and accepted that she had a mental problem. She realized that she had sexual inclinations that she was unable to control. This knowledge provided the basis for a therapeutic alliance, and Toby could then work in psychotherapy on how to accept and manage her hypersexuality and its symptomatic consequences. In therapy, Toby learned that her inordinate religiosity, neatness, and cleanliness had resulted from her attempt to control her unacceptable, unconscious, hypersexual longings with reaction formations. She also learned that her suicidal thoughts had been due to her unconscious guilt over both her unconscious hypersexual inclinations and her nocturnal hypersexual activities.

In spite of Toby's therapist's efforts to help her parents understand their daughter's conflict between her hypersexuality and her rigid superego, they restricted Toby from being with her boyfriend. Toby then refused to take her lithium unless she was allowed to spend time with her boyfriend. Eventually, Toby's parents allowed her to date and then marry her boyfriend. When Toby became pregnant, she stopped going to high school and stopped taking her lithium. Like most manic patients, Toby was a warm devoted wife and an excellent mother—when she was not acutely manic or hypomanic. Periodically, however, while not taking lithium, she became irrationally "crazy" with her husband and would wear flashy jewelry and heavy facial makeup. During these episodes, Toby, without provocation, would strike her husband.

Two years after Toby stopped her psychotherapy, she and her mother were seen briefly to determine if Toby could be diagnosed as an adult manic-depressive according to DSM-III-R. She periodically had had the following new symptoms: unrestrained buying sprees, further exaggerated neatness and cleanliness, and repeated driving of her husband's car without a license.

CLINICAL EXAMPLE 2

Sue, fourteen, was brought to a psychiatrist because she seemed out of control. Sue's parents said that she had been an amenable, well-behaved child but that, at thirteen, shortly after menarche, she suddenly changed and became impulsive, reckless, and rebellious. She shaved the hair off one side of her head, dressed in odd, ill-matched clothing, took psychedelics, and tied sheets together to climb out her second story bedroom window to have sex indiscriminately with boys. After these episodes, Sue would become tearful, guilty, obsessed with cleaning the house, depressed, and suicidal.

Sue's parents recalled that Sue had enjoyed playing with little boys' penises when three to four. When six, she had enjoyed wiping herself for prolonged periods after urinating. They said that during latency Sue admired big penises and was eager to grow up and have big "boobs." Sue's maternal aunt had suffered from manic-depression, and her maternal grandmother had been hospitalized for depression.

Sue related warmly and with appropriate affect to her psychiatrist. She was irritable, anxious, and spoke with slight rapidity. She had no delusions or hallucinations, but her judgment and insight were poor. Sue revealed that she had been very active sexually because she often felt "horny."

When Sue would no longer listen rationally to her parents, her psychiatrist hospitalized her with the following diagnoses: (1) unspecified substance delirium; (2) oppositional disorder; and (3) borderline disorder. In the hospital, Sue paced back and forth, furiously blaming her mother for keeping her from her boyfriend by hospitalizing her. When frustrated, Sue would burst out in anger and fear she would kill someone. She would then blatantly break ward rules. Once placed in security, she calmed down. Sue wore seductive clothing, continually flirted with the boys, and often had to be removed from the boys' ward. Sue had intercourse with her boyfriend during a home visit; then, after she returned to the hospital, she tried to hang herself with a shirt.

During Sue's first eight weeks in the hospital, she showed none of the typical symptoms of mania except hypersexuality, mild hyperactivity, and slightly rapid speech. It did not occur to Sue's hospital psychiatrist that she might be manic-depressive until he learned of the correlation between increased sexual drive and mania from the authors. He then considered bipolar illness to be a possibility and gave Sue a trial of lithium carbonate.

After one week on lithium, Sue's blood lithium level rose to 1.0 milliequivalents per liter. Her seductive behavior lessened, and her sexual interest in every male on the unit was replaced by a more moderate desire for her boyfriend. Her depression and suicidal ideation stopped. Two weeks after she was started on lithium, Sue felt even calmer, and she again began to dream. Instead of acting out her sexual desires, she could now discuss them with her doctor. After three weeks on lithium, Sue began keeping her room neat, and she was able to pay attention in the hospital school. Although Sue was pleased she had changed, she feared she had become "boring."

After three and a half weeks on lithium, Sue was discharged and transferred to one of the authors for psychoanalytically oriented psychotherapy. Her inpatient psychiatrist continued to manage her lithium—keeping her blood lithium level at about 1.2 milliequivalents per liter with a dose of 1,700 milligrams per day.

Over the next four-year period, Sue was maintained on lithium while she was in psychoanalytic psychotherapy. She gradually became a more conservative dresser, learned to drive a car without difficulty, and began working twenty hours a week after school. Occasionally during this period, however, Sue would have diagnosed hypomanic episodes or acute manic attacks. At these times, she again began to wear her black leather skirt, leather bracelets, and heavy makeup; she again joined the "wild, street-running teenagers." Her lithium dosage was then increased, and she would rapidly revert to her warm, fun-loving self. She would spend her free time with her "sweetheart" and be a considerate daughter and cooperative patient. Eventually, her doctor could again lower her lithium dose to her previous maintenance level without the return of the manic symptoms.

Gradually, in psychotherapy, Sue obtained greater insight into her unconscious sexual drive and her guilt over it, and she could then consciously accept her sexual feelings. This psychoanalytic-psychotherapeutic process was slow since, like all teenagers, Sue had great anxiety and guilt about her sexual drives. Once Sue became aware of her unconscious hypersexual feelings, she could discuss them freely with her analyst. Sue could also use the sudden appearance of such feelings as a signal that she was about to go into a manic attack. She could then avoid manifest manic symptoms and hospitalization by increasing her dose of lithium.

Both Toby's and Sue's sexual impulses regularly increased just before their menstrual periods. They learned to avoid acting out these sexual impulses by increasing their lithium dosage at these times.

Discussion

Manic attacks developed in each of our adult patients as follows. Sexual drives—manifesting as conscious or unconscious sexual thoughts, wishes, fantasies, or behaviors—began to increase markedly. As these drives increased, they threatened the integrity of our patients' egos. This led our patients to use their neurotic ego defense mechanisms and, then, progressively more primitive and regressive defense mechanisms (Freud 1900) against these drives.

In adults, the manifest symptoms of this defensive regression tended to occur in the following overlapping stages (see table 1). First, our patients used neurotic ego defense mechanisms—such as repression, isolation, reaction formation, intellectualization, or doubting—to modify their thought processes. This kept their mounting sexual inclinations out of consciousness and usually resulted in an increase in obsessive thinking and compulsive behavior. Next, if their sexual urges became still stronger, our patients' besieged egos used verbal motor actions to disguise and discharge these urges so that they would not become conscious or acted out directly. They exhibited pressure of speech, played with words, and made puns, jokes, neologisms, and word salads (Kraepelin 1921). Then, if their sexual urges further increased, our patients employed nonverbal motor behaviors to discharge and gratify their urges in the real world (Freud 1915b). They engaged in sexually and aggressively hyperactive interpersonal behavior—acting out their sexual impulses without allowing them to become conscious. Finally, if their sexual needs continued to mount, they used psychotic defenses, such as projection and denial, to distort their mental representations of reality (Freud 1924b): they first had delusions, usually of grandeur, and then experienced hallucinations.

Our adolescent manic patients, like many adolescent manic patients described in the literature, did not exhibit the verbal motor symptoms that are pathognomonic for mania. That is, they did not present with pressure of speech, puns, jokes, neologisms, or word salads. Instead, they displayed only the nonpathognomonic symptoms of the other four stages of regression. This is the reason they were often initially misdiagnosed. Early in adolescence, they usually displayed only the neurotic (often obsessional) mental symptoms of stage 1 and the acting out, nonverbal, hyperactive sexual and aggressive motor behaviors of

TABLE 1
STAGES OF DEFENSIVE REGRESSION IN MANIA AS THE PHALLIC SEXUAL DRIVE INCREASES

Stages	Defensive Operations	Manner of Handling Id Impulses	Symptoms
1	*Neurotic defense mechanisms:* repression, isolation, reaction formation, intellectualization, doubting, generalization, etc.	Direct discharge of unconscious impulses toward objects is inhibited; impulses are modified by unconscious thought processes and discharged indirectly in neurotic symptoms	Neurotic symptoms: obsessions, compulsions, etc. (ego dystonic)
2	*Acting out in verbal motor behaviors* (a hypercathexis of word presentations). *Pathognomonic of mania*	Inhibited unconscious impulses modify word presentations and are discharged in verbal motor behaviors that are directed toward real people	Pressure of speech. Word play: jokes, puns, neologisms, word salads, etc. (ego syntonic)
3	*Acting out in nonverbal motor behaviors* (a hypercathexis of real people)	Unconscious impulses are directly discharged in motor behaviors that are directed toward real people	Hyperactive sexual and aggressive interpersonal behaviors: overspending, overgregariousness, hypersexuality, etc. (ego syntonic)
4	*Psychotic defense mechanisms:* denial (a hypercathexis of thing presentations—the self representation)	Inhibited unconscious impulses are modified by unconscious thought processes and discharged as delusional fantasies about the self-representation	Megalomanic delusions: usually of grandeur (ego syntonic)
5	*Psychotic defense mechanisms:* denial and projection (a hypercathexis of thing presentations—the self and object representations)	Inhibited unconscious impulses are modified by unconscious thought processes and discharged as hallucinatory fantasies about self- and object representations	Wish fulfilling hallucinations (ego syntonic)

stage 3, and they were often misdiagnosed as suffering from attention deficit disorder, hyperkinetic reaction, unsocialized conduct disorder, adjustment reaction, school phobia, or anorexia nervosa (Kestenbaum 1980). Later in adolescence, our patients often also developed the megalomanic, delusional symptoms of stage 4 and the hallucinatory symptoms of stage 5, and they were, therefore, often misdiagnosed as schizophrenic. Unlike the schizophrenic, however, who has a primary disturbance of ego functioning with a resultant defect in thinking and reality testing (Arlow and Brenner 1973), the manic's ego does not initially disavow and detach from a piece of reality (Freud 1924a). It first goes through a characteristic phase of hypercathecting the external world—of displaying extravagant object love.

Perhaps adolescent manic patients tend not to exhibit the symptoms of stage 2 because, although they have the ego ability to use abstraction and verbal symbolism, they have not yet developed sufficient ego capacity to prevent their intensified sexual inclinations from being discharged directly in motor behavior. Like most adolescents, they may tend to act out their newly acquired sexual feelings rather than verbalizing them. They may act them out either directly or in substitute activities such as fast driving, dancing, or sports. Later, when they develop further ego capacity, they can divert their intensified sexual urges into the more abstract activity of playing with words.

All our manic patients reported having had unusually intense phallic sexual inclinations when they were between three and five years old. These sexual inclinations exaggerated their oedipal conflicts. They protected themselves from these conflicts by augmenting the defense mechanisms and adaptational character traits that they had successfully used during their oral and anal phases. This regression adequately controlled our patients' sexual inclinations until their drives substantially increased at puberty. Then, more than in the average adolescent, our patients' sexual drives overwhelmed their egos, producing symptoms.

Although Anthony and Scott (1960) and Thompson and Schindler (1976) felt that the symptoms of manic-depressive illness were not seen before puberty, they felt that the disease could exist as a psychodynamic entity in childhood. Brumback and Weinberg (1977) reported that the manic symptoms of six children, four to thirteen years of age, improved when they were put on lithium. Recently, Varanka, Weller, Weller, and Fristad (1988) reported on ten prepubertal children, six to twelve years old, who had a DSM-III diagnosis of manic episode with psychotic features. All the children improved when treated solely with lithium.

Our observations suggest that the oral-anal character traits and symptoms that are characteristic of adult manic-depressive patients are not due to their having had causative, traumatic experiences in their oral and anal phases of development (Abraham 1911; Fenichel 1945). Instead, these symptoms seem to be the result of a traumatic situation[4] that was precipitated by the intense sexual inclinations that our patients experienced during their phallic-oedipal phase of development. This traumatic experience led our patients to regress defensively back to the oral and anal phases. Wolpert (1981) supports this conclusion. Lewin (1950) also observed that, in all his cases except one, the oral triad was used to defend against external stimuli pertaining to the oedipal situation.

Our observations support Wolpert's (1977) contention that manic-depressive psychoses are genetically determined, actual neuroses in Freud's usage of the term (Glenn 1974; Rangell 1968). Freud (1925) said that the symptoms of actual neuroses are "not mentally determined or removable by analysis, but . . . [are] direct toxic consequences of disturbed sexual chemical processes" (p. 584). We surmise that lithium treatment reduces the abnormally high phallic sexual drives of manic-depressive patients by counteracting certain yet unknown "disturbed sexual chemical processes."

Unlike their increased phallic sexual behavior, the increased angry, belligerent, argumentative, and irritable behavior that our manic patients displayed during their manic attacks did not appear to be primarily biologically determined. This aggressive behavior occurred only when they were unable to gratify their sexual impulses immediately (Freeman 1971; McDevitt 1983) and was often a major symptom in our adolescent manic patients.

During the height of our patients' manic attacks, when their egos and superegos were overwhelmed and disorganized, our patients felt no guilt for their excessive sexual and aggressive inclinations. When their mania subsided, however, and their egos and superegos became reorganized, our patients felt guilty for the sexual and aggressive desires they had experienced, or acted out, during their manic attacks. It was this guilt that caused our patients to denigrate themselves and become depressed and suicidal. Thus, a manic patient's endogenous depression is a consequence of the guilt he or she feels for having experienced or acted out unacceptable, internal, biological sexual pressures. Such depression differs from reactive depression, which is a consequence of guilt over anger against external environmental losses (Freud 1915a). For example, in therapy, Toby learned that she was not suicidal because of an environmental loss but because of her guilt over her excessive sexual wishes and her anger that these wishes could not be immediately gratified. Similarly, Sue became suicidal not when she left her boyfriend to come into the hospital but when she had intercourse with him. Fran, another of our adolescent manic patients, developed neither manic nor depressive symptoms when her beloved father died. These observations are consistent with Roy's (1980) retrospective study of 231 manic-depressive children. He found that, although parental loss was high, such losses were not associated with an earlier onset of bipolar illness.

Psychoanalytic psychotherapy did not diminish our manic-depressive patients' intermittent episodes of biologically determined, heightened unconscious sexuality. Therapy did, however, make them consciously aware of these formerly unconscious urges and their ego defenses against them. This new insight enabled them to prevent overt manic symptoms by increasing their lithium dosage when they experienced sudden and inappropriate increases in their sexual desires.

Conclusions

Our findings will help psychoanalysts and psychiatrists diagnose manic-depressive illness in adolescents who do not show the usual symptoms of the disease. When adolescents present with the symptoms of hypersexuality, unsocialized behavior, aggressiveness, depression, hyperactivity, or psychosis, we should diligently probe for the unconscious psychodynamic[5] forces that produced these symptoms. If these symptoms are the result of a compromise between these adolescents' abruptly increased sexual drives and their defenses against them, we should seriously consider that these patients might be suffering from an adolescent form of manic-depressive illness.

Early diagnosis and treatment with lithium carbonate reduce the overwhelming sexual drives of adolescent manic-depressive patients.

This permits them to engage in psychotherapy and gain therapeutic insight into their maladaptive defenses against their intermittently abnormally intense sexual drives (Feinstein and Wolpert 1973).

NOTES

1. Some authors have preferred to consider a syndrome such as this a lithium-responsive illness rather than an early form of manic-depressive illness. For example, the Committee for Biological Aspects of Child Psychiatry of the American Academy of Child and Adolescent Psychiatry, in a position paper on the use of lithium in children, found lithium to be potentially the best therapeutic agent for manic-depression, emotionally unstable character disorder, intractable aggression, and behavior problems in offspring of lithium-responsive parents (Campbell, Perry, and Green 1977). Delong and Aldershof (1987) feel, however, and we agree, that lithium response rather than specific DSM-III criteria may define those children who have familial bipolar affective disorder.

2. 3-methoxy-4-hydroxyphenyl-ethylene glycol, a breakdown product of norepinephrine that is found in the urine (Pickar, Sweeney, Maas, and Heninger 1978).

3. Although she had occasional insomnia, she did not have elevated moods, nor did she pun, joke, use neologisms, or make word salads. She did not manifest euphoria, distractibility, pressure of speech, flight of ideas, delusional grandiosity, or hallucinations.

4. We use the phrase "traumatic situation" as Freud (1926) did: "In relation to the traumatic situation, in which the subject is helpless, external and internal dangers, real dangers and instinctual demands converge. Whether the ego is suffering from a pain which will not stop or experiencing an accumulation of instinctual needs which cannot obtain satisfaction, the economic situation is the same, and the motor helplessness of the ego finds expression in psychical helplessness" (p. 168). Freud went on to say: "In consequence of the infant's misunderstanding of the facts, the situation of missing its mother is not a danger-situation but a traumatic one. Or to put it more correctly, it is a traumatic situation if the infant happens at the time to be feeling a need which its mother should be the one to satisfy" (p. 170).

5. We are using "psychodynamics" to refer to a body of knowledge and a theory of human behavior that attempt to explain the mental

phenomena in normal and pathological conditions as a result of interacting and opposing goal-directed or motivational forces.

REFERENCES

Abraham, K. 1911. Manic-depressive insanity. In *Selected Papers of Karl Abraham*. London: Hogarth, 1949.

Anthony, J., and Scott, P. 1960. Manic-depressive psychoses in child-hood. *Child Psychology and Psychiatry* 1:53–72.

Arlow, J., and Brenner, C. 1973. *Psychoanalytic Concepts and the Structural Theory*. New York: International Universities Press.

Ballenger, J. C.; Reus, V. I.; and Post, R. M. 1982. The atypical clinical picture of adolescent mania. *American Journal of Psychiatry* 139:602–606.

Brown, R. P.; Ingber, P. S.; and Tross, S. 1983. Pemoline and lithium in a patient with attention deficit disorder. *Journal of Clinical Psychiatry* 44:146–148.

Brumback, R. A., and Weinberg, W. A. 1977. Mania in childhood. *American Journal of Diseases of Children* 131:1122–1126.

Campbell, M.; Perry, R.; and Green, W. H. 1977. The current status of lithium therapy in child and adolescent psychiatry: a report of the Committee on Biological Aspects of Child Psychiatry. *Journal of the American Academy of Child and Adolescent Psychiatry* 17:717–780.

Deleon-Jones, F.; Val, E.; and Herts, C. 1982. MHPG excretion and lithium treatment during premenstrual tension syndrome. *American Journal of Psychiatry* 139:950–952.

Delong, R. G., and Aldershof, A. L. 1987. Long-term experience with lithium treatment in childhood: correlation with clinical diagnosis. *Journal of the American Academy of Child and Adolescent Psychiatry* 131:1122–1126.

Feinstein, S. 1982. Manic-depressive disorder in children and adolescents. *Adolescent Psychiatry* 10:256–272.

Feinstein, S., and Wolpert, E. 1973. Juvenile manic depressive illness. *Journal of the American Academy of Child Psychiatry* 12:123–136.

Fenichel, O. 1945. *The Psychoanalytic Theory of Neurosis*. New York: Norton.

Freeman, T. 1971. Observations on mania. *International Journal of Psycho-Analysis* 52:479–486.

Freud, S. 1900. The interpretation of dreams. *Standard Edition*, vols. 4, 5. London: Hogarth, 1955.

Freud, S. 1915a. Mourning and melancholia. *Standard Edition* 14:237–258. London: Hogarth, 1955.

Freud, S. 1915b. The unconscious. *Standard Edition* 14:159–215. London: Hogarth, 1955.

Freud, S. 1924a. The loss of reality in neurosis and psychosis. *Standard Edition* 19:183–187. London: Hogarth, 1955.

Freud, S. 1924b. Neurosis and psychosis. *Standard Edition* 19:149–153. London: Hogarth, 1955.

Freud, S. 1925. An autobiographical study. *Standard Edition* 20:7–70. London: Hogarth, 1955.

Freud, S. 1926. Inhibitions, symptoms and anxiety. *Standard Edition* 20:77–174. London: Hogarth, 1959.

Glenn, J. 1974. The analysis of masturbatory conflicts of an adolescent boy with a note on actual neurosis. In M. Harley, ed. *The Analyst and the Adolescent at Work*. New York: Quadrangle.

Hugens, R. W. 1974. *Psychiatric Disorders in Adolescents*. Baltimore: Williams & Wilkins.

Jacobson, E. 1971. *Depression*. New York: International Universities Press.

Kelly, J.; Koch, M.; and Buegel, D. 1976. Lithium carbonate in juvenile manic-depressive illness. *Journal of Diseases of the Nervous System* 37:90–92.

Kestenbaum, C. J. 1980. Adolescents at risk for manic-depressive illness: introduction and overview. *Adolescent Psychiatry* 8:344–366.

Kestenbaum, C. J. 1982. Children and adolescents at risk for manic-depressive illness: introduction and overview. *Adolescent Psychiatry* 10:245–255.

Kraepelin, E. 1921. *Manic-Depressive Insanity and Paranoia*. Edinburgh: Livingstone.

Krafft-Ebing, R. 1906. *Psychopathia Sexualis*. Chicago: Logan, 1929.

Landolt, A. D. 1957. Follow-up studies on circular manic-depressive reactions occurring in the young. *Bulletin of the New York Academy of Medicine* 33:65–73.

Laroche, C.; Cheifetz, P. N.; and Lester, E. P. 1981. Antecedents of bipolar affective disorders in children. *American Journal of Psychiatry* 138:986–988.

Lehmann, H. E. 1967. Schizophrenia. IV. clinical features. In *Comprehensive Textbook of Psychiatry*. Baltimore: Williams & Wilkins.

Lewin, B. 1950. *The Psychoanalysis of Elation*. New York: Psychoanalytic Quarterly, 1961.

Loeb, F., and Loeb, L. 1987. Psychoanalytic observations on the effect of lithium on manic attacks. *Journal of the American Psychoanalytic Association* 35:877–902.

McDevitt, J. 1983. The emergence of hostile aggression and its defensive and adaptive modifications during the separation individuation process. *Journal of the American Psychoanalytic Association* 31:273–300.

Olsen, T. 1961. Follow-up study of manic-depressive patients whose first attack occurred before the age of 19. *Acta Psychiatrica Scandinavia* 162(suppl.): 45–51.

Pickar, D.; Sweeney, D.; Maas, J.; and Heninger, G. 1978. Primary affective disorder, clinical state change, and MHPG excretions. *Archives of General Psychiatry* 35:1378–1382.

Rangell, L. 1968. A further attempt to resolve the problem of anxiety. *Journal of the American Psychoanalytic Association* 16:371–404.

Rosen, B. M.; Bahn, A. K.; Shellow, R.; and Bower, E. M. 1965. Adolescent patients served in outpatient psychiatric clinics. *American Journal of Public Health* 55:1563–1577.

Roy, A. 1980. Parental loss in childhood and onset of manic-depressive illness. *British Journal of Psychiatry* 136:86–88.

Sheard, M.; Marini, J.; and Giddings, S. 1977. The effect of lithium on luteinizing hormone and testosterone in man. *Diseases of the Nervous System* 38(10): 765–769.

Shou, M. 1978. The range of clinical uses of lithium. In F. Johnson and S. Johnson, eds. *Lithium in Medical Practice*. Baltimore: University Park Press, 21–39.

Shopsin, B. 1979. *Manic Illness*. New York: Raven.

Thompson, R., Jr., and Schindler, F. 1976. Embryonic mania. *Child Psychiatry and Human Development* 6:149–154.

Van Putten, T. 1975. Why do patients with manic-depressive illness stop their lithium? *Comprehensive Psychiatry* 16(2): 179–183.

Varanka, T. M.; Weller, R. A.; Weller, E. B.; and Fristad, M. A. 1988. Lithium treatment of manic episodes with psychotic features in prepubertal children. *American Journal of Psychiatry* 145:1557–1559.

Weiner, I. B. 1970. *Psychological Disturbance in Adolescence.* New
ˋ York: Wiley.

Wolpert, E. 1977. *Manic-Depressive Illness.* New York: International
Universities Press.

Wolpert, E. 1981. On the nature of manic-depressive illness. In G. I.
Greenspan and G. H. Pollock, eds. *The Course of Life,* vol. 3, *Adult-
hood and the Aging Process.* Maryland: National Institute of Mental
Health.

PART IV

PSYCHOTHERAPY
OF ADOLESCENT
EMOTIONAL DISORDERS

EDITOR'S INTRODUCTION

Psychoanalysts have tended to be cautious about analyzing adolescents, and many therapists have introduced parameters into treatment approaches to adolescents that have resulted in the supportive techniques encouraging repression. With our greater understanding of ego development and structural theory, however, the development of a wide range of dyadic techniques from supportive dynamic psychotherapy to intensive psychoanalytic psychotherapy and psychoanalysis are now more comfortably utilized. Gitelson's perspective that the therapeutic task is not only directed to psychic analysis but should rather result in a synthesis of the adolescent's character is helpful in understanding the psychotherapeutic approach to be utilized. Whatever approach is required to engage the adolescent may be used, but only as a means to the end: eventual dyadic engagement. Further, this should be pursued even if the current definitive treatment plan cannot provide a dyadic experience since, very frequently, a brief period of parametric therapy is followed by a search by the adolescent for a more intensive, dyadic psychotherapy.

Richard C. Marohn, in delivering the William A. Schonfeld Distinguished Service Award address, discusses the vicissitudes of becoming an adolescent psychiatrist and psychotherapist. He focuses on the development of the self of the adolescent psychiatrist. He examines the emergence of "unresolved adolescent issues," the continued presence of important developmental tasks, not yet resolved. He believes that understanding adolescent development and psychopathology "deepens the psychotherapist's capacity to recognize how specific character traits, defensive and compensatory solutions, behavior, and symptoms have become integrated into adult functioning." Further growth can be enhanced by an experience with a competent supervisor or mentor; one is helped discover self-potential and skills. Marohn concludes that

367

self-confrontation leads to further psychological growth and structuralization of the psychotherapist's self and lifelong continuous growth.

Donna L. Moreau defines the clinical problems encountered at psychiatric teaching hospitals that treat adolescent patients on adult wards. A particular psychiatric hospital that utilizes an adolescent consultation service will be the focus for examining specific situations from the viewpoints of the various disciplines involved in the treatment of the adolescent patient on an adult ward. The problems and conflicts faced by patients, nursing staff, adult psychiatrists and residents, and adolescent consultant staff are addressed, citing several illustrative clinical examples.

Further examination of developmental issues was pursued in a joint symposium of the Children's Hospital of San Francisco and the Summit Institute of Jerusalem, Israel. The key presentations are included in a special section, edited by Stanley Schneider and Charles P. Fisher. These studies are presented in an edited version.

18 ON BECOMING AN ADOLESCENT PSYCHOTHERAPIST: HOW AM I GOING TO WORK WITH THESE KIDS?

RICHARD C. MAROHN

I walked onto the Chicago State Hospital unit for adolescent boys in 1962, a second-year psychiatric resident. I was greeted by a tall, angry-looking seventeen-year old, the unofficial leader of the peer group, who punched me on the shoulder.

To him I said, "I'm Dr. Marohn."

To myself I said, "How am I going to work with these kids?"

My terror was no less when a few hours later I met in my office with Ken, one of my two designated psychotherapy cases, a mild and meek, neurotic-looking fifteen-year-old suburbanite who was in public care, not private, because of his father's recent death from cancer and the loss of the family's financial support. At first, it seemed that Ken was like me when I was a teenager: studious, kind of "nerdy," bespectacled, not particularly athletic. This made me a bit anxious, but I soon realized that he was different from me. He had begun having temper tantrums, skipped school, and had fired his father's rifle into the wall of his bedroom. I saw Ken in twice-weekly psychotherapy sessions, under supervision, for about eight months as an inpatient and then on an irregular basis as an outpatient. Because he did not keep office appointments regularly, I alternately felt that he was "resistant" or that I was a failure as an adolescent therapist. When he did show up, it seemed that we did not talk about what I was learning was important:

William A. Schonfeld Distinguished Service Award Address, presented to the American Society for Adolescent Psychiatry, New York, May 13, 1990.

psychodynamic or interpersonal issues. Yet, with very helpful supervision, I recognized that, interspersed with talk of photography and books, Ken was dealing with loneliness, deprivation, and worthlessness.

The anxiety I felt was familiar—not at all unlike what I experienced when, as a sophomore medical student, I worked with chronically psychotic patients. This is not the anxiety of playing in a piano recital, or of asking a girl out for a first date, or of speaking before an audience. This is a less acute but more pervasive anxiety, not anxiety that produces dysfunction because of exhibitionistic or other narcissistic risks, but one that heralds the beginnings of a major reworking and restructuring of the personality, its prejudices, values, and other beliefs.

The American Society for Adolescent Psychiatry (ASAP) was founded as a home and place of refuge for those adult and child psychiatrists who had found the "in-between" age group to be their professional focus. It still remains so and continues to gain recognition as such. When Dan Offer first tried to interest me in the organization through the Chicago society in the late 1960s, I was not quite ready, even though I readily became a member. My personal psychoanalysis had not yet freed up the creative energies that being an adolescent psychiatrist requires. One has to be ready to accept what an organization like ASAP has to offer; one has to be ready to accept the challenges to maturation that adolescent patients can offer the psychotherapist; and one has to be ready to benefit from the developmental tasks of adolescence. Many of us do not reap those benefits until our chronological young adulthood.

My own personal and professional growth has occurred concurrently with the development of adolescent psychiatry and this superb organization. For me, ASAP has become a professional home, and, despite excursions into other professional memberships and liaisons, it will always remain so.

In 1969, I attended the ASAP Conference on Training (Offer and Masterson 1971) in Chicago and heard Jim Masterson's (1971) commanding paper "To Teach Is to Learn Twice," in which he pointed out that "this learning process, much like psychotherapy, consists of . . . engagement, involvement and separation" and that "intellectual learning and the solving of emotional growth tasks go hand in hand" (p. 7) for supervisor, trainee, and patient. I was so impressed by Masterson's focus that I asked him to do a reprise at the 1983 Annual Meeting in New York. I also heard Will Hendrickson (1971) describe how the wife of one of his residents complained that, on the adolescent unit, "he went through hell when he was working with those kids, and so did I; but he ended up doing a lot of growing up. You should know that I once hated you and his patients for what you were doing to him, but now, I must confess, I appreciate it" (p. 21). Hendrickson emphasized that "adolescent patients, especially inpatients, have a way of demanding, with their behavior if words do not suffice, the doctor's attention to painful countertransference realities in a way that makes them relatively undeniable" (p. 32).

Dan Offer gave me one more nudge: I was invited to present a plenary paper alongside Ghilly Godenne and Jim Masterson in Dallas in 1972. I well remember how Ghilly charmed us with Bobby's voyage from adolescence into adulthood (Godenne 1974). By then, Jim Masterson had become a legend in adolescent psychiatry with his work on the borderline adolescent. My own paper "Trauma and the Delinquent" (Marohn 1974) was an attempt to understand the violent behavior of our hospitalized juvenile delinquents at the Illinois State Psychiatric Institute, and it foreshadowed the affinity I later developed for the psychology of the self and the work of Heinz Kohut.

Still later, I was asked to revitalize the ASAP Juvenile Delinquency Committee and was able to be more responsive and feel more competent. That chairmanship led me to organizing the 1976 conference on Juvenile Delinquency in Chicago; the ASAP "elders" took note, and I became more and more involved in the organizational and political aspects of adolescent psychiatry.

These different, but related, aspects of adolescent psychiatry— treatment and research, teaching and writing, and political and organizational activity—are the tripod on which our identity rests, and nowhere has it been better supported than in the foundations of this organization. There is no better way to learn adolescent psychiatry than from the people who discuss their work here. The political and organizational tasks of the ASAP continually confront one with the important developmental and therapeutic issues of adolescent psychiatry. Our committee and parliamentary deliberations are frequently spiced with clinical examples and truisms! In ASAP, I and others have found a nurturing, supportive, facilitating, and holding environment.

Be it from learning from what others present, from the questions and challenges that listeners raise, or from the confidence gained from being heard, ASAP has provided a truly empathic atmosphere.

I want to focus here on the development of the self of the adolescent psychiatrist, more specifically, the adolescent psychotherapist. These are preliminary musings, which I hope before too long will be actualized in some sort of a research study.

My confusion about what to do with my first adolescent patient, Ken, can certainly be understood as a manifestation of my personal development. Yet there is something anxiety ridden for all of us in our first encounters with adolescent patients; it is usually called "unresolved adolescent issues." Such "unresolved" issues persist into the young adulthood of most people, not just those long-term students who were previously thought of as "prolonged" adolescents. Many of the important developmental tasks of adolescence are not resolved by the close of chronological adolescence and are continually reworked throughout the life cycle.

A psychiatrist, psychoanalyst, or psychotherapist who works primarily with adults will often fail to recognize the continuing presence of these adolescent issues in his patients' therapy. Often, they are completely ignored, and the material is considered, inappropriately, as remnants of preoedipal or oedipal psychopathology or as primitive narcissistic or object relation fixations or arrests. An understanding of adolescent development and psychopathology deepens the psychotherapist's capacity to recognize how specific character traits, defensive and compensatory solutions, behaviors, and symptoms have become integrated into adult functioning. The psychotherapist's interventions can be more believable and empathically correct when he has the adolescent perspective in his repertoire.

A learning experience with a competent supervisor or mentor greatly enhances the growth of the psychotherapist-trainee. Such growth necessarily involves mastering, resolving, and integrating adolescent issues, such as comfort with one's and another's sexuality, the integration of ideals and goals, self-esteem regulation, the establishment of a secure self and a commitment to a vocational identity, and the transformation of one's ties to parental and other selfobjects. None of us has resolved all these adolescent interests by the time we enter our training, so the supervisor is in a unique position to help. If he or she understands adolescence, our supervision can be particularly helpful, even crucial, for initiating or maintaining the maturation of a psycho-therapeutic self.

Often, our training has been burdened by the dogmatism and strictures of a more classical approach. The ideal supervisory experience enables trainees to find their own way, especially helping them learn how to use themselves as the agents of empathic contact and change. Roy Grinker (1968, personal communication) once told me that supervision does not change anything—residents pretend to conform to the supervisor's wishes but continue to do things their own way. I think that what each of us takes from our supervisor depends on our own inner configurations. The supervisor's value is in helping the novice psychotherapist discover and develop his or her own potential and skills.

Psychotherapists learn from their adolescent patients as well, if internal configurations will permit. I remember an argument I had with a psychoanalyst-supervisor at the time of my first contact with adolescent patients at the state hospital. He felt that it was the supervisor who informs the data he derived from his supervisee, just as the therapist informs the patient's data. He took offense at my brashness and, I guess, adolescent rebellion when I tried to convince him that therapists could learn from their patients and supervisors from their trainees!

Let me tell you how Kerry has helped me reflect on this odyssey. Kerry was fifteen years old when I first met her at a girls' residential facility twenty-four years ago. She is now a recent graduate from a professional school. Two years before I met her, in sixth grade, she had come to the attention of both the public schools and the Juvenile Court because of academic underachievement, runaways, and sexual delinquency. She had been referred to the treatment center and had been living there about a year when I was asked to see her in consultation because she had become depressed and had ingested some nail polish remover. She was apparently distressed over the impending loss of her housemother, who was being transferred elsewhere.

I began seeing Kerry in weekly psychotherapy sessions. She was often silent and said that she was seeing me only because others wanted her to. She told me a little more about herself only when, after several frustrating sessions, I attacked her wall of silence. I suppose that I was correct in addressing her defensive withdrawl, but I was clumsy. I interpreted that she did not want to become attached to me because she feared she would lose me too. In essence, I was interpreting her narcissism as a resistance to object relating. Her reply was, "Are you going to see me for fifty years?" She expressed her fear of my dying, as had her father, and wanted to terminate therapy.

I began to understand that she could not explicitly acknowledge that she wanted to see me in therapy, but, with her impending release from the group home after six months of psychotherapy, we recognized that she continued with the sessions by her choice, and she acknowledged that therapy had helped her. She became more explicit about wanting my attention. For example, what did I think of her new hairstyle? She also became more serious about her boyfriend and planned to "get a ring for Christmas." She alternately called me the "great psychiatrist" who had helped her, but criticized my tie. She described her boyfriend as a good dresser, brought him to meet me, and was radiant. In sessions, we talked about the parallels between the two relationships, and she recognized not only how much she wanted me to approve of her but how she also wanted me to adore her.

After she had left the group home, the office psychotherapy lasted about one year, until her mother and stepfather discontinued it because of the cost and their belief that she was not motivated to change. Kerry called me to tell me this and said that it "didn't matter" to her, but five months later she asked to return to treatment, troubled by intensified sexual activity with her boyfriend. It distressed her that she was angry so often and did not enjoy sex.

She seemed more committed to our sessions than before, asked me many questions about my work, and said that she now liked talking to me. But, before too long, her participation in therapy became sporadic, and she was pregnant. She missed one appointment because she planned a criminal abortion and thought that I would stop her. We arranged for a therapeutic abortion, after which she became depressed and experienced difficulty talking about both the procedure and the loss. She began using marijuana, amphetamines, and LSD more frequently, continued to miss appointments, and ran away from home. I felt powerless—I could only sit and wait. She finally called and said that she wanted to quit therapy because it was a "waste of time and money."

About four years ago, when I learned that her stepfather had died, I sent her a sympathy note. She wrote back, "It seems like an eternity since I last saw you, although I have not forgotten those sessions." She recounted how, in the intervening years, she had married, had a son three years later, was divorced three years after that, started college within a year, and graduated summa cum laude. She was entering her final year at a prestigious professional school. She thanked me for my expression of sympathy and asked to see me to discuss something. When we met, Kerry told me of her doubts about whether her nine-year-old son should visit his father, who was in prison on drug charges. She thought it would be a good idea to have him continue to see his father, her ex-husband, especially because her son's psychotherapist had recently left the city. She also wondered about his starting with another therapist.

I was pleased, though a little surprised, that she recognized the importance of therapy for her son—surprised until she began to reflect on her own experiences. Kerry talked about her problems with separation and reminisced about her own therapy with me, her inability to talk and express herself, and how worthless she had felt. She said she remembered therapy quite well and enjoyed it but used to wonder why I "bothered" with her; after all, she was "just a piece of shit." The fact that I continued to see her and try to help her, especially with the abortion, was very significant to her. She said that she "stored up a lot of this" but could use it only "later." As a result, she said, she would always feel free to contact me in the future if she felt the need. Today, I can more comfortably see how my functions as a selfobject, both mirroring and ideal, helped Kerry find herself.

Daniel, a current patient of mine, thrives on our meetings but always protests about how slowly the session time passes or why he has to see me twice a week. About two years ago, when he was thirteen, his parents contacted me because of Daniel's recent angry and impulsive behavior: drawing an obscenity on the blackboard at school, throwing a book at a teacher, and setting off a smoke bomb in the school auditorium. Both his parents felt that he needed therapy and were very careful and detailed in working out the referral. They first had him tested for educational and learning difficulties, then thoroughly researched and interviewed me.

Although Daniel's school behavior was the presenting complaint, his father's reasons for referral were more sophisticated: he believed that his son had problems in self-esteem regulation, that he did not seem to understand the complexities of interpersonal interactions, and that he seemed to be having difficulty making the transition to a more adult and autonomous adjustment.

Daniel was hardly a preadult. He was cute, boyish, and short, a fact immediately noticeable to us both! He was bright, verbal, and tried to please me by talking as I had asked, although he denied any psychological or emotional problems and insisted that whatever anxiety or depression he might feel were always related to concrete actual events. He said that he engaged in normal mischief and disavowed any delinquent motives. Two years after beginning twice weekly psychotherapy, his grades have improved, and the "mischief" has disappeared. He comes conscientiously to his sessions, on his skateboard when the weather is tolerable, and, though he continues to protest that these sessions are unnecessary, he is usually reluctant to leave.

My experience with Daniel demonstrates the changes in me. Twenty-five years ago I would have had difficulty thinking Daniel needed treatment—he exhibited no horrendous pathology. Twenty-five years ago I would have had to be intrusively interpretative to prove to myself and him that I was doing something. Twenty-five years ago I would not have felt comfortable simply watching the skateboard maneuvers and tricks he demonstrated for me in the office and would have focused on what he was not able to verbalize. Twenty-five years ago I would not have been at ease with myself to let him sit in my chair and reverse roles with me. Twenty-five years ago I would have continually questioned whether I was doing the right thing—as I did with Kerry. I have developed a sense of myself as a psychotherapist. There has been, silently, some sort of structuralization.

I remember how puzzled I was with Ev Dulit's ideas about doing "pieces" of psychotherapeutic work with his adolescent patients, who would contact him from time to time. Now I find myself doing the same and no longer criticizing myself for not having completed the job the first time around or for not having been able to see the transference neurosis unfold in its entirety.

Just as Ken and Kerry used me as a mirroring selfobject and Daniel still does, they also replicate my personal development as an adolescent psychiatrist.

My reflections begin with my own adolescence: the academic and extracurricular accomplishments; the enrichment from new friendships; the frightening "separation" struggles, most noticeably around religious and moral beliefs; and the loneliness, a loneliness that allowed me to pursue thought, music, and fantasy. Sure, I could have profited from psychotherapy then, but that was as foreign to my family and culture as orthodontia!

My sixteen years with the Illinois State Psychiatric Institute (ISPI) Adolescent Program taught me a great deal. I believe that inpatient work, competently supervised, is still the best way to learn adolescent psychiatry. At ISPI, I could recognize and learn how to manage primitive transferences that I now often manage with ease in my office. Because of such experiences, I believe strongly that a competent psychotherapist of adult patients will profit from work with adolescents, and I strongly advocate adolescent psychiatry as part of the core curriculum of the training of the general psychiatrist.

When I got to ASAP, I found many mentors here and have learned from them. I found many twinships here, in colleagues and friends trying to solve similar issues, expanding my horizons, teaching me about things beyond my own narrow, biased, and provincial world.

Doing psychotherapy with adolescent patients is especially important to the growth of every psychotherapist. To immerse oneself in the psychological life of an adolescent who is herself transforming the representations of her important selfobjects is comparable to the very process of psychotherapy supervision. In supervision, the trainee uses the mentor as a selfobject to develop his own psychotherapy functions and not simply to imitate him.

Adolescent psychiatry is different from child psychiatry, as Dulit (1990) has so beautifully described, and that difference lies in who our patients are—people emerging into, experimenting with, and attempting to integrate their sexuality; people playing with and using their verbal skills and newly found, or developing, modes of thinking; people transforming their relationships with their parents, "separating" psychologically, and using newly found selfobjects to enhance their own competence. These are not children, and they are not adults. Adolescent psychiatry has taken its place in the subspecialties.

The adolescent psychotherapist emerges from such a background of uncomfortable encounters with his adolescent patients and himself, to be supported by peers and colleagues, stimulated by idealized others, and enriched by the understandings his patients give him.

As I said at the annual ASAP meeting last year (Marohn 1989), I believe that competent psychotherapists have the capacity to "right" themselves, to alert themselves to some sort of derailment or deviation of their therapeutic activity and to get themselves "back on the track." This capacity relies on and reveals an internal blueprint whereby we organize experience—in this instance, the experience of the therapeutic encounter—and whereby we develop a psychotherapeutic self.

This self-correcting or self-righting mechanism has been described by a number of authors as an attribute of the healthy and mature personality (Fajardo 1990; Kligerman 1989; Lichtenberg 1989; and Tolpin 1986). This ability is also an important attribute of the competent adolescent psychotherapist, and it is one of the most common challenges in the treatment of the adolescent, when we help him or her get "back on the track." Often, it is our patients who show us how to "get it right."

As the psychotherapist matures, ideas, inferences, and modes become "second nature"; that is, they become structuralized and begin to operate as silent, smooth functions. This is why many beginning psychotherapists experience the kind of anxiety I did. They are exposed to new ideas and new ways of operating, which have not yet become internal structure. This is not conflict or fragmentation anxiety but growth and maturation anxiety. As the psychotherapeutic self becomes established and firmed, we find that it is not necessary to introspect so frequently, or to agonize over a countertransference issue, or to worry about "what to do," or to wonder, "How am I going to work with these kids?"

"Initially, we struggle with various schools of thought, divergent ways of understanding and approaching the patient, the ideas and personalities of our supervisors, and problems we never anticipated" (Marohn 1989, p. 12). Gradually, we become comfortable with our interventions and rarely have to think about them. When we do, we do so because we are still developing the psychological structures to deal with the particular situation. This self-confrontation leads to further psychological growth and structuralization of the psychotherapist's self. Thus, one reward of therapeutic work with adolescents is the prospect of lifelong, continuous psychological growth.

For me, that growth began when I first asked myself, "How am I going to work with these kids?" In doing so, I exhibited a self-reflection that is the first step in the introspective process, in learning how to do psychotherapy. Later, I would wonder how my own adolescence was different from Ken's and why Kerry kept coming to sessions when I did not seem to know what I was doing.

Luckily, in this profession, growth can continue, thankfully with a bit less anxiety than twenty-five years ago. Now, as Daniel banters with me about the fee I earn for each of our sessions, I can think about how I can help him make use of the idealizing transference.

Fortunately, "these kids" always save the day for us. Recently, a high school senior handed me his notebook. In it was his latest entry:

Sunday. Blew off my papers. Got very high with Tom. Let him listen to a lot of [Pink] Floyd. He loved it. Wrote Sally a real long letter. She is going to think I am so strange. I love her and miss her so much. I have a doctor appointment tomorrow. I'm considering giving him this journal, not like he would be able to read it or anything, but I can't seem to tell him. I hope I give it to him.

Well, he and many others have "given it" to me—anxiety and challenge, but also learning and growth. And so has ASAP.

I thank you all.

REFERENCES

Dulit, E. 1990. On the uniqueness of adolescent psychiatry. *Newsletter of the American Society for Adolescent Psychiatry* (Spring), pp. 9–10.

Fajardo, B. 1990. Approaches to the empirical study of resilience and self-righting. Paper presented at the Self Psychology Workshop, Institute for Psychoanalysis, Chicago, March 17.

Godenne, G. D. 1974. From childhood to adulthood: a challenging sailing. *Adolescent Psychiatry* 3:118–127.

Hendrickson, W. J. 1971. Training in adolescent psychiatry: the role of experience with inpatients. In D. Offer and J. F. Masterson, eds. *Teaching and Learning Adolescent Psychiatry*. Springfield, Ill.: Thomas.

Kligerman, C. 1989. The search for the self of the future analyst. In A. Goldberg, ed. *Progress in Self Psychology,* vol. 5. Hillsdale, N.J.: Analytic.

Lichtenberg, J. 1989. *Psychoanalysis and Motivation*. Hillsdale, N.J.: Analytic.

Marohn, R. C. 1974. Trauma and the delinquent. *Adolescent Psychiatry* 3:354–361.

Marohn, R. C. 1989. Identity revisited—the perspective of self psychology. Plenary presentation at the annual meeting of the American Society for Adolescent Psychiatry, San Francisco, May 7.

Masterson, J. F. 1971. To teach is to learn twice: teaching and learning the art of psychotherapy with adolescents. In D. Offer and J. F. Masterson, eds. *Teaching and Learning Adolescent Psychiatry.* Springfield, Ill.: Thomas.

Offer, D., and Masterson, J. F., eds. 1971. *Teaching and Learning Adolescent Psychiatry.* Springfield, Ill.: Thomas.

Tolpin, M. 1986. The self and its selfobjects: a different baby. In A. Goldberg, ed. *Progress in Self Psychology,* vol. 2. New York: Guilford.

19 A MODEL ADOLESCENT CONSULTATION SERVICE IN A PSYCHIATRIC TEACHING HOSPITAL

DONNA L. MOREAU

The psychiatric literature on adolescent psychopathology is replete with a multitude of views on what is considered pathological behavior, what is developmentally normal behavior, and how such determinations are culturally defined (Freud 1958; Levenson, Feiner, and Stockhamer 1985; Offer and Masterson 1971). The issue of treatment begs an immediate answer. Who should provide treatment for adolescents? Where are adolescents requiring psychiatric hospitalization best treated?

The increase in the adolescent patient population (American Society for Adolescent Psychiatry 1971; U.S. Bureau of the Census 1973) was initially not paralleled by an increase in the number of experienced clinicians to treat these patients (Arnoff and Kumbar 1973). In a national survey of psychiatrists conducted one to three years after residency training, many practitioners felt that they had been inadequately prepared for the adolescent treatments they were conducting in their private practices (Looney 1980). While it is agreed that adolescent psychiatrists provide an indispensable portion of the core curriculum to a general residency program (Looney, Ellis, Benedek, and Showalter 1985; Maddow and Malone 1972), there are few recent published data on how adolescent specialists can best be integrated into the structure and function of adult inpatient units that treat adolescents (Hartmann, Glasser, and Greenblatt 1968; Hendrickson 1957; Naumburg 1980).

Adolescents are no longer treated on children's wards, but the debate about whether treatment is best conducted on adult wards or all-adolescent wards remains unresolved. Beskind's review (1962) of the literature concludes that, although there are no sound psychiatric principles supporting either side of the argument, sicker adolescents are best treated on adult wards, where even ill adults can provide some ego supports and controls, and higher-functioning adolescents can be treated on either adult or adolescent units, provided that certain guidelines are adhered to. He concludes that adult units can adequately treat patients fifteen years or older if they compose no more than 15 percent of the total patient population and if appropriate schooling, activities, and therapy are provided (Hartmann, Glasser, and Greenblatt 1968; Slaff 1985).

The difficulties of treating adolescents on adult inpatient units may be attenuated but are not obviated by such measures. Staff members who have no adolescent subspecialty training may find it difficult to diagnose and treat adolescents. This chapter supports the clinical necessity of obtaining a child and/or adolescent psychiatric consultation on all adolescents admitted to adult wards not staffed by their own child and adolescent psychiatry specialist. A psychiatric hospital that admits adolescents to adult units and provides an adolescent program and adolescent consultation service will be described. Two clinical cases will be reported.

Adolescent Psychiatry Consultation Service

THE INPATIENT SERVICE

The inpatient service described here is part of a 104-bed psychiatric hospital affiliated with a major medical center. There are three acute care units with twenty-four beds and one intermediate care unit with twenty beds. The adolescent service is part of the child and adolescent psychiatry division, which is closely integrated into the overall department. No more than five adolescents (defined as younger than eighteen and older than twelve years) are admitted to the adult wards at one time. All adolescents are active participants in the Adolescent Program (AP).

Each unit is directed by a board-certified adult psychiatrist. A PGY-IV is the assistant unit chief. The PGY-II and psychology intern are the primary therapists. Each therapist is supervised by a preceptor, usually an adult psychiatrist. A social worker and a primary nurse are assigned to each patient. The director of adolescent psychiatry oversees the AP and supervises a second-year child and adolescent psychiatric fellow on consultation for all hospitalized adolescents.

This system has three inherent problems. (1) The staff on the wards are separate and autonomous from the adolescent psychiatry staff. (2) Final clinical decisions are the responsibility of the unit chief, who, as noted, has no specialized training in the diagnosis, treatment, or management of adolescent patients. (3) The least experienced therapist provides treatment in a highly specialized area of psychiatry without benefit of direct supervision of those most qualified to provide it.

THE ADOLESCENT PROGRAM

Adolescents attend the AP, which consists of therapeutic activities, schooling, and group therapy. A staff member from the AP is assigned to each unit and attends weekly team meetings. Adolescent Program staff members do not, however, attend the daily meetings where treatment plans are reviewed and revised. Despite their knowledge of the patient's functioning with peers and in daily tasks (most accurately reflecting outpatient life), their assessments are not necessarily integrated into the unit team's assessment and management of each patient.

THE CHILD AND ADOLESCENT PSYCHIATRY FELLOW

The child and adolescent psychiatry fellow is an active member of the adolescent team and serves in an educative and supervisory capacity. He or she, under the supervision of the director, is the intermediary among the various caretakers of the adolescent patient but is not a member of the regular inpatient staff and is thus an "outsider." Support for the recommendations of the adolescent consultant depends on the adult unit chief.

THE ADOLESCENT THERAPIST

The therapist faces transference issues with all patients, but, in the treatment of adolescents, particular countertransference problems arise. The therapist has, in most cases, only recently emerged from a prolonged adolescence. The role of student for the therapist has many parallels to the adolescent experience (Shulman 1980). Themes of identity, autonomy and authority, self-esteem and competence, and activity and passivity are similar (McCaughan 1981). Amid the welter of psychosis, acting out, or intense emotions, the new therapist may attempt to control uncertainty about therapeutic actions and reactions in one of two maladaptive ways: a rigid conception of psychopathology and treatment can be adhered to, or psychopathology obvious to the more experienced clinician may be minimized. The new therapist must learn to distinguish punitive from therapeutic actions and become comfortable with decisions based on sound clinical assessment and theoretical principles that may be perceived by the adolescent as punitive, sadistic, or controlling. Since most of the didactic teaching focuses on adults, and since the unit chief, assistant unit chief, and supervisor are in most cases adult psychiatrists without specialized adolescent training, the adolescent consultant can provide a critical understanding of adolescent patients.

Assessment of the Adolescent Inpatient

While it is expected that adolescents normally undergo psychological, behavioral, and cognitive changes, such changes are not expected to result in major disruptions that impede further growth and development. The three substages of adolescence are normally marked by a progressive decrease of behavioral expression in favor of a more verbal, articulated expression of emotions and thought. The adolescent consultant can help the treating staff empathically understand their adolescent patients in the light of this developmental progression. In particular, the adolescent consultant offers expertise in the assessment, diagnosis, treatment, and management of adolescent psychiatric patients.

A thorough assessment of the adolescent's environment and a complete developmental history, family history, and interpersonal functioning and school reports are necessary to make an accurate differential diagnosis and to determine a treatment plan. Once this information is gathered, it must be interpreted. Diagnosis of an adolescent in the early stages of his or her illness is often difficult. Thus, it is not always possible or desirable to make a diagnosis during the initial stages of hospitalization.

An adolescent's symptoms are often misperceived as "behavior problems." Such behavior problems must be understood psychodynamically as well as interpreted diagnostically (Shapiro 1989). The adolescent consultant can give a more sophisticated understanding of these symptoms. While certain adolescent behavioral disturbances may be manifestations of one of the behavioral disorders or character pathology, they may represent symptoms of an underlying psychosis. In adults, this determination is more readily apparent than in adolescents, whose pathology is just beginning to define itself and is based on nebulous historical antecedents.

The staff must not lose sight of the fact that these patients are teenagers and that a certain amount of testing of limits is normal for this age group. Such behavior should not be assumed to be pathological but should be considered to be an expression of normal developmental processes. The hospital staff have in effect assumed the role of parents for its adolescent patients, and the parenting provided must be consistent, empathic, and nonpunitive. Adult units that operate on the premise of expected self-control of such behavior may find it hard to impose the necessary limits and restrictions on an adolescent whose behavior necessitates containment.

A primary treatment and management decision involves the efficacious and judicious use of medications. When a patient requires medication for an affective disorder, a behavioral disorder, a schizophrenic process, or a hyperactive syndrome, the adolescent consultant can be helpful in recommending appropriate medications and dosage.

The following clinical illustrations highlight how the consultant can best serve the patient and the staff in the areas of diagnosis, treatment, and management.

CLINICAL EXAMPLE 1

M was a fourteen-year-old adopted Korean girl transferred to this hospital from a children's ward where she had been hospitalized for six months following an overdose attempt when she felt rejected by her camp counselor. When her therapist went on vacation, M, who was on an open unit, ran away from the hospital. She hitchhiked and was sexually assaulted by a man who picked her up. She was found on the George Washington Bridge, contemplating jumping, by a family who returned her to the hospital. On her return, the staff placed M on unit restriction. However, the ward was not locked, and this unit status required M's voluntary compliance. The adolescent consultant who had seen M on admission reconsulted and firmly recommended that she be put in bedclothes to minimize the risk of elopement while awaiting transfer to a long-term locked unit.

M was on an intermediate care unit that was adept at treating young adults with borderline personality disorder. When possible, the unit tried to institute and maintain a therapeutic-administrative split. In M's case, the unit attempted to adopt its philosophy of self-control, while dynamic understanding was gained through psychotherapy, to a patient whose pathology would lead her to self-destructive and self-abusive behavior before any therapeutic progress could be achieved. The hospital had as its foremost task in this case to protect M and limit exposure to an external environment that would stimulate her beyond her capacity to control her behavior. The consultant helped make the staff aware of the potential for adult abuse of this young, impressionable, dependent, and needy girl. The consultant's recommendation was initially followed, but, as soon as M was permitted daytime clothes, she ran away from the unit and became involved in another sexually abusive incident. The director, who functioned in an advisory role to that particular unit, interceded. After that, transfer to a locked unit was hastened.

CLINICAL EXAMPLE 2

R was a seventeen-year-old, black, eleventh-grade boy admitted psychiatrically for the first time after a violent fight with his older brother, during which, his father felt, R could have killed his brother had not the father interceded. There was no prior psychiatric history and no history of drug abuse. During assessment, it became clear that R was a paranoid, isolated boy who for the past two years had been having intermittent auditory hallucinations and homicidal ideation toward all the people he perceived as rejecting him. A diagnosis of paranoid schizophrenia seemed warranted, and R was started on haloperidol.

On the ward, where he interacted with adult patients and staff, R seemed to improve. In the AP, however, he was perceived as isolated, paranoid, and frightening to the other adolescents, whom he regaled with his intense, vivid, homicidal fantasies. The unit staff perceived a manipulative, controlling quality to his psychotic symptoms, which would reappear when he was pressed into activities and actions he did not like. They insisted that he continue to attend the adolescent activities. The AP staff interpreted R's behavior as a response to the unmanageable stress of interactions with his peers and felt that his aggressive, belligerent facade was a defense against intense anxiety. The treating therapist and the supervisor tried to approach R's behavior through a psychodynamic understanding, postulating unacceptable homosexual feelings and impulses toward his brother displaced onto his peers. The unit staff was planning discharge home, but the consultant, in agreement with the AP staff, recommended placement in either a residential facility or a long-term hospital. A discharge date was set, but, as R began to become more active outside the hospital, he became more seclusive and began talking about a "hit list" to the unit staff. As his condition deteriorated, the debate raged whether R's behavior was consciously manipulative or psychotic with unconscious dynamic roots.

The AP staff, the ward staff, and the treating therapist and supervisor had different approaches to treating R. There was poor communication between the unit-based treatment team and the AP team. The consultant needed to be particularly active in this case by interviewing the patient, attending unit and AP team meetings, and meeting with the primary therapist and supervisor. However, the ward chief, who was also the supervisor, maintained that the initial assessment of R was, in fact, the correct one and continued to support the treatment plan outlined by the primary therapist and unit staff. A conference to which the fellow and the director were invited was planned to discuss continued treatment and management for R. The director was able to prevail, and a plan with which all were comfortable was developed. R's medications were increased, and no immediate discharge was planned until it was learned that the brother was leaving for college. R returned home with a recommendation for family treatment as well as individual treatment.

Discussion

The preceding cases illustrated ways in which the adolescent consultant, as part of the treating team, contributed to the education of the resident and to patient care. The fellow benefited as well from this role. It provided a supervised opportunity to study adolescent disorders in greater depth and provided an opportunity to develop administrative skills. Each consultation was initiated by a phone call or brief meeting between the primary therapist and the fellow. The auxiliary staff were consulted for their assessment of the patient. In these discussions, key issues pertaining to a particular patient were clarified and highlighted so that the consultation had one or several focal points around which it revolved. The written consultation was placed in the chart with a brief list of references relating to the consultant's diagnostic impression and treatment recommendation and was discussed with the unit staff, primary therapist, and AP staff. Follow-up was provided as appropriate for each patient.

The treatment of adolescents on adult wards that utilize an adolescent consultation service is still subject to difficulties. First, the chain of command is such that the least experienced clinician has primary responsibility for the patient, the least experienced adolescent specialist has the initial and most consistent consultation role, and the final authority for the adolescent patient resides in an experienced clinician with no adolescent training. Second, the unit staff can view the AP staff and the child fellow as "outsiders" who do not have to live with the day-to-day problems associated with a particular patient and, consequently, do not know the patient and what is best for the patient as well as they do. This can be discouraging and demoralizing to the AP staff, who have direct patient contact but no authority. Third, the many areas and levels of care provided by the unit staff, AP staff, and consulting service can be confusing to the adolescent patient and the family, who may hear different assessments and different plans from the various caretakers.

The cases that presented problems were reviewed by all participants so that future problems of a similar nature could be averted. We feel that our consultation service is a good model for hospitals that plan to treat adolescents on adult inpatient units, and we hope that our mistakes as well as our successes will be of educational value to other clinicians and hospital staff.

REFERENCES

American Society for Adolescent Psychiatry. 1971. Position statement on training in adolescent psychiatry. *Adolescent Psychiatry* 1:418–421.

Arnoff, F. N., and Kumbar, A. H. 1973. The nation's psychiatrist: 1970 survey. Washington, D.C.: American Psychiatric Association.

Beskind, H. 1962. Psychiatric in-patient treatment of adolescents: a review of clinical experience. *Comprehensive Psychiatry* 3:354–369.

Freud, A. 1958. Adolescence. *Psychoanalytic Study of the Child* 13:255–278.

Hartmann, E.; Glasser, B. A.; and Greenblatt, M. 1968. *Adolescents in a Mental Hospital.* Boston State Hospital Monograph Series, no. 4. New York: Grune & Stratton.

Hendrickson, W. J. 1957. Adolescent service: neuropsychiatric institute. *Bulletin of the Michigan Society for Mental Health* 13:1.

Levenson, E. A.; Feiner, A. H.; and Stockhamer, N. 1985. The politics of adolescent psychiatry. *Adolescent Psychiatry* 12:94–103.

Looney, J. G. 1980. Psychiatrist transition from training to career: stress and mastery. *American Journal of Psychiatry* 137:32–36.

Looney, J. G.; Ellis, W.; Benedek, E.; and Schowalter, J. 1985. Training in adolescent psychiatry for the general psychiatric resident: elements of a model curriculum. *Adolescent Psychiatry* 12:94–103.

Maddow, L., and Malone, C. 1972. *The Integration of Child Psychiatry into the Basic Residency Program.* Hillsdale, N.J.: Town House.

McCaughan, D. L. 1981. Teaching and learning adolescent psychotherapy: adolescents, therapists, and milieu. *Adolescent Psychiatry* 12:414–433.

Naumburg, G. W. 1980. Organizing an inpatient adolescent program within an adult psychiatric service. In D. R. Heacock, ed. *A Psychodynamic Approach to Adolescent Psychiatry: The Mount Sinai Experience.* New York: Dekker.

Offer, D., and Masterson, J. F., eds. 1971. *Teaching and Learning Adolescent Psychiatry.* Springfield, Ill.: Thomas.

Shapiro, T. 1989. The psychodynamic formulation in children and adolescent psychiatry. *Journal of the American Academy of Child Psychiatry* 28(5): 675–681.

Shulman, D. 1980. Training residents in adolescent psychiatry. In D. R. Heacock, ed. *A Psychodynamic Approach to Adolescent Psychiatry: The Mount Sinai Experience.* New York: Dekker.

Slaff, B. 1985. The history of adolescent psychiatry. *Adolescent Psychiatry* 9:7–22.

U.S. Bureau of the Census. 1973. *Characteristics of the Population.* Washington, D.C.: U.S. Government Printing Office.

IDENTITY, IDENTITY CRISIS, AND IDENTITY DIFFUSION IN ADOLESCENTS AND YOUNG ADULTS: INTRODUCTION TO SPECIAL SECTION

STANLEY SCHNEIDER AND CHARLES P. FISHER

Within my earthly temple
    there's a crowd.
There's one of us that's humble;
    one that's proud.
There's one that's broken-hearted
    for his sins,
And one who, unrepentant, sits
    and grins.
There's one who loves his neighbor
    as himself,
And one who cares for naught but
    fame and pelf.
From much corroding care would
    I be free
If once I could determine which
    is Me.

Edward Sanford Martin
(1856–1939)

In April 1990, Psychiatric Services of Children's Hospital of San Francisco and the Summit Institute of Jerusalem held a joint symposium in San Francisco—"The Fate of the Troubled Young Person: Identity, Identity Crisis, and Identity Diffusion in Adolescents and

Young Adults." Some of the major papers of that symposium are re-printed here.

In working with adolescents and young adults, it is always useful to ask what makes it possible for some young people to go through these developmental phases in a relatively successful way while others are involved in emotional turmoil and upheaval resulting in developmental disturbance or arrest. In this symposium, theoretical contributions by Joseph Sandler and Ana-Maria Rizzuto come to grips with basic ways of viewing and understanding psychological structure in relation to a central theme of adolescent experience—the sense of personal identity. The three additional chapters presented here highlight clinical and cultural concerns related to this theme. These three papers, by Fisher, Schneider, and Rizzuto, have in common the fact that all make use of anthropological as well as clinical data in an effort to explore adolescent development and psychopathology in relation to concepts of identity.

Joseph Sandler's chapter reviews the field of the self and its objects. This chapter serves as an important introduction to our understanding of how normality and pathology diverge. Sandler deftly summarizes contributions he had made to the literature over the past thirty years, describing psychic structure in terms of a representational world. His chapter defines the concept of self-representation with particular care and develops the concept of object representation in a parallel fashion. Sandler reviews his idea of the "shape" of a representation, which provides a convenient way of describing important dynamic and developmental changes. Using these building blocks, Sandler differentiates identification, introjection, and incorporation and relates each to the development of psychic structure. Wishes and defenses are clearly defined from a representational point of view. In his conclusion, Sandler addresses the concept of identity, describing it too in representational terms and bringing us his startling but convincing thesis that the self is our oldest object.

The chapter, "I, Me, Myself . . ." by Ana-Maria Rizzuto investigates identity as a subjective experience. While expressing doubt that the concept of identity can be employed as a theoretical or clinical term, she explores its phenomenology as a sense of knowing or perceiving itself. She describes identity as "the cumulative result of the fantasied elaboration of the history of our loves." It is "a relational narrative in the context of others." She views this subjective experience as the starting point for Freud's theorizing when he moved from the "I" of personal narrative to "the I" or *das Ich*—the ego of psychoanalytic theory. Words—in particular the personal pronouns "I," "me," and "myself"—are crucial to Rizzuto's account of the development of self-knowledge. "Whatever Freud learned about his own private world or the inner life of his patients had to pass through the narrow door of [these] three pronouns." Rizzuto sketches an epigenetic theory based on the child's acquisition of these pronouns— typically between twenty-four and thirty months of age—and traces its evolution into adult development. This developmental vantage point can assist us in achieving a finer understanding of identity as a subjective experience. Rizzuto traces for us a historical understanding of the problem with remarkable insight into the linguistic components of the concepts she uses.

Since Psychiatric Services of Children's Hospital and the Summit Institute both deal with adolescent and young adult patient populations, understanding the complexities of identity formation and its potential pitfalls is of paramount importance. Charles Fisher's chapter pays homage to Erik Erikson's use of the term "identity" and explores a number of ways in which Erikson himself looked beyond it. Identity may function as a resistance in psychotherapy or psychoanalysis and may serve as an "inner arrest" in the individual's relation to the community at large. More pointedly, identity as a created narrative of one's development acquires the features of a "personal myth" of the kind described by Ernst Kris. Finally, Erikson related identity to "the sense of 'I' " that is the individual's central awareness of being a sensory and thinking creature endowed with language, who can confront a self (composed, in fact, of a number of selves). This complex structure, consisting of "I" and multiple selves, is at the root of internal experiences of fluidity, variability, and unexpected change. Fisher utilizes cultural/anthropological examples as well as clinical case material to illustrate his ideas regarding a "look beyond identity" and "transcending one's identity."

Stanley Schneider's chapter arises out of his clinical work at the Summit Institute with Israelis and North Americans. He addresses the issue of how cultural factors affect identity formation in adolescents. Erikson writes that the adolescent period is one of a moratorium, and Schneider examines how a time-out period, in another culture, may *reduce* emotional turmoil—even in the more disturbed adolescent and young adult. Since mental health values are culturally determined, one needs to look at how cultural factors impinge on identity formation. Schneider views the various aspects of cultural impingements as important aspects to be contended with in the coalescing of an identity: "The sense of peoplehood and community (in addition to family) is very crucial in the developmental enhancement of the adolescent's self-image, self-esteem, and feelings of belonging."

Another chapter by Ana-Maria Rizzuto ends this section, by examining how fashion and style define the identity of the adolescent via a definition of the *body* of the adolescent. Shopping, clothes, and grooming become a way for adolescents to express transient or lasting commitments to sexual, economic, and social roles. The interplay between parents and peers is also addressed with "dress" behavior being one of the means by which the adolescent learns to form an identity as distinct from both peers and parents—while utilizing both as identificatory models in the process. Rizzuto discusses these developmental issues as "an area that has been neglected in the literature: the use of clothes and fashion in the process of differentiation from internal objects, their looking eyes, voices, and judgments. . . . Clothes and decoration are signifiers of great subtlety, capable of revealing what is taboo to express in spoken words." In terms both humorous and insightful, she traces a variety of meanings of clothing for the normal and the troubled adolescent.

These chapters constitute a look at several aspects of identity formation—its vicissitudes and complexities. Many questions are asked, not too often coupled with answers. However, the importance lies in the quest.

20 COMMENTS ON THE SELF AND ITS OBJECTS

JOSEPH SANDLER

Although the search for close-fitting and unambiguous definitions in our field is a most important and commendable enterprise, it is inevitable that we need to use some terms that carry a variety of different meanings, even though we might feel dissatisfied with the lack of clarity inherent in the concept. In a sense such concepts are pliable and context dependent. Concepts of this sort serve us well, until they become overstretched, at which point an acceptable reorganization of the concept may, and usually does, emerge. The concept of self is par excellence a pliable one, whose exact meaning at any one time will depend on the particular context in which the term is used. Unfortunately, as things are at present, any precise definition of "self" will of necessity exclude certain meanings of the term that we need for communicating with one another. The extent of contemporary discussion about the self indicates an increasing degree of strain within the concept, and major aspects of the meaning of the concept do need to be separated.

It is generally accepted that the term *das Ich* was used by Freud to refer both to the self (in a variety of meanings) and to the ego as a "structure" in the sense of a large-scale psychological organization. Conscious of the problems generated by using the ambiguous term "ego," a concept that had reached the limit of its elasticity, a distinction was made between concepts of the ego and the self in the United States after World War II. Following a suggestion of Hartmann (1950), Edith Jacobson put forward a concept of self-representation that had the same theoretical status in relation to the ego as had object representation (Jacobson 1954). By distinguishing between ego and self, some

Reprinted with permission. Joseph Sandler. 1962. Comments on the self and its objects. In Lax, Bach, and Berland, eds. *Self and Object Constancy*. New York: Guilford.

of the phenomena of narcissism and masochism could be better understood, and love or hate for oneself could be seen more clearly as paralleling love or hate for the object.

The Emergence of the Sense of Self

The psychoanalytic notion of the self—introduced by Hartmann and Jacobson—is essentially a concept of a self-representation. Such a concept of representation links the ideas of self and the older ideas of body image and body schema, although the self is a broader concept than either. From a number of points of view, the self can be regarded as being (among other things) an elaboration or extension of the body schema or of the body image (for a full discussion of this topic, see Sandler 1962). Such a view probably corresponds to one of the meanings of Freud's remark that "the ego is first and foremost a body ego" (1923), provided that for "ego" we now read "self." One could say that the self-representation can be looked at as a self-schema, an extended body schema, about which Henry Head (1926) said many years ago, "The sensory cortex is the storehouse of past impressions. They may arise into consciousness at images, but more often . . . remain outside central consciousness. Here they form organized models of ourselves which may be called schemata. Such schemata modify the impressions produced by incoming sensory impulses in such a way that the final sensations of position or of locality of the body rise into consciousness charged with a relation to something that has gone before."

It should be noted that the concept of self-representation has at least two main facets and that the term as I shall use it here encompasses both. The sense of the first is conveyed by what one might call the self-schema, a structural organization formed in exactly the same way as Head described the development of the body schema. It is an organized psychological structure that exists outside consciousness and, indeed, I would say, outside subjective experience, in the so-called nonexperiential realm of the mind (Sandler and Joffe 1969).

The second major aspect of the meaning of self-representation is the phenomenal or experiential one, in which the self-representation can be considered to be the image and subjective experience of ourselves that we have at any given moment. Thus, if we have a fantasy involving ourselves, the self-representation in that fantasy is, while we are having the fantasy, an experiential representation of ourselves, usually in interaction with others, that is, with object representation that parallels the self-representation. Such a subjective experience may be conscious, but it may equally be unconscious, for the notion of unconscious experience is a central one in psychoanalytic thinking.

Just as we build up and differentiate self-representations during the course of development, so do we construct object representations, that is, organized schemata and images of the object in our world. This has been put as follows (Sandler 1962):

> From the concept of the self-representation . . . it is not a difficult step to make the further extension to representations which correspond to all the non-self components of the child's world. As the child gradually creates a self-representation, so he builds up representations of others, in particular of his important love and hate objects. In the beginning the representations which he constructs are those which are linked with need satisfaction, but he gradually creates schemata of many other things, activities and relationships. He does all of this as a consequence of the successive experiences of his own internal needs and their interaction with his external environment. He gradually learns to distinguish between "inner" and "outer," a distinction which he cannot make in the earliest weeks and months of life, where the main differentiation between experiences must be based on whether they provide pleasure or pain. Incidentally, this is why I have avoided the use of the term "inner" or "internal" world for the representational world, for these terms . . . refer to only a part of the child's representational world—that part which a child learns to localise as being inside himself.

The concept of the representational world has been an extremely useful tool for the more refined conceptualization and clarification of psychoanalytic concepts (Sandler 1962; Sandler and Rosenblatt 1962). It allowed a new approach to the understanding of processes of internalization, to the superego (Sandler 1960), to the ego ideal (Sandler, Holder, and Meers 1963), and to a variety of other clinical as well as theoretical problems such as childhood depression and processes of individuation (Joffe and Sandler 1965; Sandler and Joffe 1965). In the application of what can be called a representational point of view, it is convenient to speak of the particular "shape" of a self- or object representation "to denote the particular form and character assumed by that representation or image in the representational world at any one moment" (Sandler and Rosenblatt 1962). The idea of the "shape" of a representation allows us to use a convenient shorthand in diagrammatic representations to illustrate, for example, the changes that take place in the representational world when different mechanisms of defense are applied to unconscious psychic content:

> The child who feels angry at one moment, and the subject of attack at another, shows a change in the shape of his self-representation—or alternatively his self image (be it conscious or unconscious) has changed. Moreover, the shape of an unconscious self-representation may be differentiated from that shape which is permitted access to consciousness or motility. Thus we can speak of the child who has an unconscious aggressive wish to attack an object as having a particular shape of his self-representation—the unconscious image of himself attacking the object—which is not ego syntonic and which is only permitted to proceed to consciousness or motility once its shape has been changed by means of defensive activity on the part of the ego. . . . The self-representation can assume a wide variety of shapes and forms, depending on the pressures of the id, the requirements of the external world, and the demand and standards of the introjects. Some shapes of the self-representation would . . . evoke conflicts if they were allowed discharge to motility or consciousness, and the defence mechanisms are directed against their emergence. [Sandler and Rosenblatt 1962]

As self-representations can be considered to be sensorimotor in nature, identification can be regarded as a change in the shape of a self-representation based on the model of another. So, if a little child walks like her mother, we can say she changes the shape of her self-representation on the basis of an object representation (or an aspect of that representation), that is, on the basis of an image of her mother walking. (I do not distinguish here between identification and imitation, which can be differentiated by other criteria.) Of course, identifications are never complete but can be, to varying degrees, partial, temporary, or enduring and (after a point relatively early in development) can occur throughout life.

The sort of identification just described has been referred to as secondary identification. In this process the boundaries between the self and the object remain intact. The object is still perceived as an object, but the shape of the self-representation has been changed. Incidentally, the term "self-boundary" is far more appropriate in this context than "ego boundary." So-called primary identification, in which there is a fusion or confusion between self- and object representation, involves the absence or breakdown of functioning self-boundaries. This phenomenon occurs very early in life, before boundaries between self and object have been established, and later as a regressive manifestation in certain psychotic states. It is also possible to find examples of primary identification in normal adult life. We may find ourselves moving slightly from side to side in a rhythmic fashion while watching ice skaters on television. Or we may catch ourselves as if we were about to fall when we see someone slip and fall in the street.

Although the terms "introjection" and "identification" have often been used synonymously, it is possible to differentiate the two in a meaningful way in terms of the representational world. So-called early introjection can be seen as the process of building up the inner world of representations, a product of the "organizing activity of the ego" (see Hartmann 1939; Sandler 1960). Introjection, of the sort that is thought to result in the formation of an organized superego, can be regarded as the process of attributing to certain object representations a special status so that they are felt to have all the authority and power of the real parents. The child then reacts, when his parents are absent, as if they were present. This does not mean that he copies them any more than before, for that would be the process of identification. Of course, identification can (and often does) accompany introjection of the type described, but from a theoretical point of view the two processes should be sharply differentiated. Incorporation refers to the actual taking into the body of substances or things from the outside, but fantasies or thoughts of incorporation (usually referred to simply as "incorporation," which is very confusing) involve the shape of the self-representation being changed so that it now encloses a representation of something that is "nonself." In one sense thoughts or fantasies of incorporation represent displacements from one part of the representational world to another.

The workings of the mechanisms of defense can be illustrated conveniently in terms of changes in the representational world. Thus, the mechanism of projection, from a representational point of view, becomes a transfer of some aspect of the self-representation to an object representation. The unconscious image of oneself attacking an object, for instance, is transformed into a conscious image or thought of the object attacking the self. The "attacking part of the self" is projected (i.e., displaced within the representational world) onto the object representation. The defense mechanism of displacement is reflected simply in a change in the direction of an activity, originally directed toward one object, toward another. So the child who has a wish to attack his mother, whom he also loves, can deal with his conflict of ambivalence by directing his attacking wishes toward a sibling or other convenient person. In reaction formation the shape of the self can be changed (in certain respects) into its opposite so that an unconscious image of a sadistic self becomes a one of a kind, caring self or an unconscious dirty, messy self-representation is changed into one that is neat, clean, and meticulously tidy. All the mechanisms of defense can be viewed with profit in representational terms.

In a 1963 study of the ego ideal, we put forward the view in the Hampstead Index project that the concept of ego ideal had been stretched beyond its useful limits and proposed that we make use of the motion of an ideal self in many of the contexts in which the idea of the ego ideal had been used (Sandler et al. 1963). The ideal self represented a shape of the self that was the most desirable, in either instinctual or narcissistic terms, at any one time. It could change from moment to moment depending on the state of the individual's unconscious impulses and on his sources of narcissistic supply as well as on many other factors. The state of the self-representation at any moment was referred to as the "actual" self. The existence of a discrepancy between actual self and ideal self, at any point in time, was regarded as providing a motivating force for appropriate adaptive ego activity. If the gap between actual self and ideal self is too great, then it is experienced as pain of one sort or another (Joffe and Sandler 1965; Sandler and Joffe 1965).

The representational approach allows us to see the close relationship between the various mechanisms of defense and the ideal shape of the self. The mechanisms operate to bring about a change in the self-representation so that it becomes one that is more acceptable to the individual, arouses less conflict and unpleasure, and is more consistent with his internal standards (which may or may not be related to his superego introjects). The mechanism of reaction formation, seen in this way, clearly involves an identification with an ideal—in the example given it is the ideal of being clean and tidy.

Ideal shapes of the self can be simply states of instinctual wish fulfillment or may be shapes of the self that the individual regards as being most desirable to his objects or to his introjects. So the shape reflecting the "good child" desired by the parents at any one time may be quite different from the shape of the self that represents the fulfillment of an instinctual wish of one sort or another. Indeed, we can look at psychic conflict, as unconsciously sensed by the ego, as being conflict involving different ideal shapes of the self, the ego being motivated to identify with different ideal self-representations. This is well illustrated by the frequent conflicts that exist for the ego (Sandler 1974) in regard to reaching an ideal state of instinctual satisfaction (the "instinctual" ideal) and reaching an ideal shape of the self that is felt by the ego as being held up to it by an introject. Much of the ego's activity can then be seen as being concerned with the finding of compromise representational solutions so that, as far as possible, the conflicting tendencies will be satisfied. We can also look at the changes that occur in therapy, from a representational point of view, in terms of discrepancies between actual and ideal self-representations. If, for example, we are dealing with someone who is depressed, who has had a depressive reaction to a painful gap between his actual self (as he sees it) and his ideal self, then we can think in terms of therapeutic interventions that predominantly affect his (conscious or unconscious) view of his actual self and those that affect his ideal self (e.g., impossibly high standards of conduct or attainment associated with "strict" superego introjects).

At any one time we have a whole system of ideal selves that are derived from different sources. One may be closely related to the aims of an unconscious instinctual wish, another may be linked to superego standards, others with the ideals of the real parents or of the group of which we are a part, and so on. The ideal we fashion from all these self-representations will be a function of many forces. Above all, the roles played by sources of well-being and self-esteem are highly significant. It has often been said half-jokingly that the superego is that part of the mental apparatus that is soluble in alcohol, and the truth in this statement comes from the fact that alcohol (like many other drugs) provides an alternate feeling of well-being so that the need to appease the superego—that is, to identify with the ideal self felt to be held up by the superego, the need to gain the feeling of internal parental approval—is temporarily diminished or absent.

One way of looking at the superego (Sandler 1981) is to see it as referring to phantom companions who exist in the unconscious part of the representational world. These are companions who are unconsciously treated and reacted to as if they were really present but who do not normally appear in recognizable form above the threshold of normal perception. Having a superego is like living with such phantom companions, who are tolerated because they are not only felt to criticize but also felt to provide approval and support. Of course, if we can embody such phantoms in external figures or in external institutions, we will do so and will relate to these institutions and figures as if they were the superego introjects. In therapy we see such processes of externalization occurring over and over again, and these may provide one of the avenues for the therapeutic intervention to find an effective way into the mind of the patient. The analyst or therapist then becomes a source of new ideal shapes of the self, and it is probable that every psychoanalytic interpretation carries with it a new ideal, even if that ideal only reflects the view that it is permissible to tolerate and even enjoy all sorts of wishes in fantasy, even if they are not appropriately translated into action. The therapist who says to his patient, "Well, of course you would like to kill me because you are angry with me," conveys an ideal to the patient that it is permissible to have such a wish, permissible in the area of wishes and fantasies, the "child" part of oneself as a normal state of affairs.

Psychoanalytic theory has traditionally placed enormous emphasis on the role of the instinctual drives and drive derivatives in its theory of motivation. The part played by such drives in mental life is central to psychoanalytic thinking, but more and more noninstinctual factors are being admitted into our understanding of the way people function. For example, it seems to be very clear now that, whatever the role of urges toward instinctual drive satisfaction may be, an overriding consideration for the individual is to preserve a feeling of safety. If the threat to his safety is too great, he will give up the striving toward the gratification of his drives (Sandler and Joffe 1969). Freud was aware of this when he wrote of the self-preservative drives of the ego (Freud 1910), and Anna Freud (1936) has written of the need to preserve the integrity of the ego as a motive for defense.

In addition to instinctual drive satisfaction and the need to preserve a background feeling of safety (Sandler 1960), there has been increasing emphasis in recent years on the individual's need to regulate his supplies of well-being (Joffe and Sandler 1967).

If we pick up on the formulation of Anna Freud (1936), in *The Ego and the Mechanisms of Defense,* that the motives for defense are neurotic anxiety, superego anxiety (guilt), realistic (reality-based) anxiety, and threats to the integrity of the ego, we can develop a basis for a psychoanalytic theory of motivation that puts feeling states at the center of the stage (Sandler 1972). The drives can be regarded as stimuli that disturb the basic feeling state and mobilize instinctual wishes, but there are also wishes of other sorts, prompted by other factors, that have to take their place as important psychological motives. We can think in particular here of wishes to apply one or another mode of defense, such wishes being stimulated by the motivating power of unpleasant affective states referred to by Anna Freud. Narcissistic imbalance brought about by wounded self-esteem can provide the affective basis for the creation of unconscious wishes of one sort or another.

The striving for pleasant feelings of all sorts must be given the same weight as the avoidance of unpleasure in the psychoanalytic theory of motivation. In this context, a differentiation has to be made between the erotic satisfaction gained in the process of instinctual drive gratification and the "after-satisfaction" experienced as a result of the instinctual gratification. The two are substantially different. The baby sucking at the breast obtains an erotic satisfaction gained in the process of instinctual drive gratification and the "after-satisfaction" experienced as a result of the instinctual gratification. The two are substantially different. The baby sucking at the breast obtains an erotic oral satisfaction, but the blissful feeling experienced by the child after his feed is a satisfaction of a vastly different quality. I do not want to dwell too long on the possibilities for a revised psychoanalytic theory of motivation, except to say that, in my view, a model of the sort I have mentioned seems to be a necessary consequence of the line of thought initiated by Freud's revision of the theory of anxiety in *Inhibitions, Symptoms and Anxiety* (1926).

It is possible to understand more of the complexities of object relationships by taking the view that wishes involve not only self-representations but also object representations and representations of the interaction between self and object. Again, these wishes need not be only instinctual but may be motivated by factors such as the need to preserve feelings of safety and to redress narcissistic wounds. From very early in his life, the interaction between the child and his mother provides feelings of safety and security. Margaret Mahler (1978) has described how the child manages to develop a capacity for separateness from the mother via the process of "checking back to mother," in which he allows himself to move away from her, while constantly turning back in order to gain supplies of reassurance and affirmation. The obtaining of what Mahler has called "refueling" remains as an essential part of object relationships, and this process continues into our social life, where, by unconscious convention, we normally provide one another with minute signals of affirmation and reassurance. In general, it is now not difficult for us to make a link between the concept of the wish, instinctual or otherwise, and the concept of object relationship (Sandler and Sandler 1978).

It has been pointed out that the wish contains representations of self, object, and the interaction between the two. As wish fulfillment comes about when the wished-for state is reached, what is gained is not only a particular state of the self-representation but a state in which self and object interact. The *aim* of a wish is a wished for interaction, involving a response of the object as well as an activity on the part of the subject. The individual will do all he can to satisfy his wishes in a direct or indirect way, and he will do so through a process of actualization (Sandler 1976a, 1976b; Sandler and Sandler 1978). He will attempt to change the external world or himself so that he can bring about a situation in which the wish is satisfied. A very large part of the process of actualization involves the manipulation of objects so that they conform to the role implicit in the wish. A great deal of "trying out" of what has been called the individual's "role-responsiveness" (Sandler 1976a) occurs as part of normal social life. The process of actualization, as it relates to unconscious wishes and the associated object relationships, can best be seen in the psychoanalytic situation, where transference is now generally regarded as involving more than the distortion of the patient's picture of the analyst, including as well attempts on the part of the patient to manipulate the analyst into playing a particular role (Sandler, Dare, and Holder 1973). The effect of this manipulation can be felt and assessed in the countertransference (Sandler 1976a).

To turn now to the topic of identity, we may first observe that bringing about an identity of perception between a wish and an actual state of affairs is a means of gratifying wishes. This description frames wish and gratification as part of a feedback loop or signal system rather than in energic terms.

To discuss the concept of the identity of an individual, I should like to go back to something touched on earlier, that is, the parallel between self and object. I am convinced that the most useful way to look at the notion of self is to maintain the strictest possible parallel between the ideas of self and object and to examine, as far as we can, the parallel between the two in different contexts. So, for example, we can understand the concept of identity relatively easily in relation to an object, for the object has a name, endures in time, and is perceived by us again and again. We recognize objects as existing, not only in space, but also in time, and because of this we can abstract a notion of identity in relation to the object. We do not have a problem saying, "This is Mr. Smith. We know things about him because we know his past, and he is not Mr. Jones." If we then transfer this concept of identity to the self, it becomes clear that whatever we can say about the object with regard to identity can also be said about the self (Sandler 1977). It is as if the self-representation is the representation of a companion, an object we have grown up with, one that shows relatively slow changes over time and is immediately recognizable. The self is our oldest and closest object, and because of this its identity is normally well known to us.

REFERENCES

Freud, A. 1936. *The Ego and the Mechanisms of Defense.* London: Hogarth, 1954.

Freud, S. 1910. The psycho-analytic view of psychogenic disturbance of vision. *Standard Edition* 11:209–218. London: Hogarth, 1957.

Freud, S. 1923. The ego and the id. *Standard Edition* 19:3–66. London: Hogarth, 1961.

Freud, S. 1926. Inhibitions, symptoms, and anxiety. *Standard Edition* 20:77–178. London: Hogarth, 1959.

Hartmann, H. 1939. *Ego Psychology and the Problem of Adaptation.* New York: International Universities Press, 1958.

Hartmann, H. 1950. Comments on the psychoanalytic theory of the ego. *Psychoanalytic Study of the Child* 5:74–96.

Head, H. 1926. *Aphasia and Kindred Disorders of Speech.* New York: Macmillan.

Jacobson, E. 1954. The self and the object world: vicissitudes of their infantile cathexes and their influence on ideational and affective development. *Psychoanalytic Study of the Child* 9:75–127.

Joffe, W. G., and Sandler, J. 1965. Notes on pain, depression, and individuation. *Psychoanalytic Study of the Child* 20:394–424.

Joffe, W. G., and Sandler, J. 1967. Some conceptual problems involved in the consideration of disorders of narcissism. *Journal of Child Psychotherapy* 2:56–66.

Mahler, M. 1978. *The Psychological Birth of the Human Infant.* New York: Basic.

Sandler, A.-M. 1977. Beyond eight-month anxiety. *International Journal of Psycho-Analysis* 58:195–207.

Sandler, J. 1960. On the concept of superego. *Psychoanalytic Study of the Child* 15:128–162.

Sandler, J. 1962. Psychology and psychoanalysis. *British Journal of Medical Psychology* 35:91–100.

Sandler, J. 1972. The role of affects in psychoanalytic theory. In *Physiology, Emotion and Psychosomatic Illness.* Ciba Foundation Symposium 8, n.s. Amsterdam: Elsevier/Excerpta Medica.

Sandler, J. 1974. Psychological conflict and the structural model: some clinical and theoretical implications. *International Journal of Psycho-Analysis* 55:53–62.

Sandler, J. 1976a. Countertransference and role-responsiveness. *International Review of Psycho-Analysis* 3:33–42.

Sandler, J. 1976b. Dreams, unconscious fantasies and "identity of perception." *International Review of Psycho-Analysis* 3:33–42.

Sandler, J. 1981. Character traits and object relationships. *Psychoanalytic Quarterly* 50:694–708.

Sandler, J.; Dare, C.; and Holder, A. 1973. *The Patient and the Analyst.* London: Allen & Unwin.

Sandler, J.; Holder, A.; and Meers, D. 1963. The ego ideal and the ideal self. *Psychoanalytic Study of the Child* 18:139–158.

Sandler, J., and Joffe, W. G. 1965. Notes on childhood depression. *International Journal of Psycho-Analysis* 46:88–96.

Sandler, J., and Joffe, W. G. 1969. Towards a basic psychoanalytic model. *International Journal of Psycho-Analysis* 50:79–90.

Sandler, J., and Rosenblatt, B. 1962. The concept of the representational world. *Psychoanalytic Study of the Child* 17:128–145.

Sandler, J., and Sandler, A.-M. 1978. On the development of object relationships and affects. *International Journal of Psycho-Analysis* 59:285–296.

21 IMPINGEMENT OF CULTURAL FACTORS ON IDENTITY FORMATION IN ADOLESCENCE

STANLEY SCHNEIDER

It is very difficult to know people and I don't think one can ever really know anyone but one's own countrymen. For men and women are not only themselves; they are also the region in which they were born, the city apartment or the farm in which they learnt to walk, the games they played as children, the old wives' tales they overheard, the food they ate, the schools they attended, the sports they followed, the poems they read, and the God they believed in. It is all these things that have made them what they are, and these are the things that you can't come to know by hearsay, you can only know them if you have lived them. You can only know them if you are them. And because you cannot know persons of a nation foreign to you except from observation, it is difficult to give them credibility in the papers of a book. [W. Somerset Maugham 1944]

The point is that it is almost impossible (except in the form of fiction) to write in America for Americans. You can, as an American, go to the South Sea Islands and write upon taking leave; you can, as an immigrant, write as you get settled; you can move from one section of this country to another, and write while you still have one foot in each place. But in the end you always write about the way it feels to arrive or leave, to change or to get settled. You write about the process. [Erik Erikson 1950]

Erik Erikson (1950) in his eight ages of man viewed the developmental stage of adolescence as "identity verses role confusion." The adolescent is trying to progress developmentally in an effort to discover "Who am I?" (Erikson 1950, 1968). The terms "role confusion," "identity diffusion," and "identity confusion" are concepts that Erikson wrestled with in order to try and understand how the adolescent progresses through the emotional growth process leading to an eventual formation of identity.

We know that the process of identification involves internalization of parental values and ideals, its most significant movement taking place during the adolescent period. Here, we find the adolescent shifting from previously internalized rigid and moralistic views of right and wrong to a more flexible view that is based on the values and ideals found not only in his own parental world but also in the adult and social world around him. This helps lay the foundation for the development and establishment of the ego ideal, on which identity can be formulated (Sandler 1960). In this chapter, I focus on cultural factors and how they affect the formation of identity in adolescents.

Culture, Identity, and Adolescence

Erikson (1950) noted the following: "I have focused on the problem of ego identity and on its anchoring in a cultural identity because I believe it to be that part of the ego which at the end of adolescence integrates the infantile ego states and neutralizes the autocracy of the infantile superego." What is this "cultural identity"? Rakoff (1981) proposes "a model for the role of custom and history in personal psychological development analogous to Winnicott's (1953) transitional objects." Rakoff feels that, without an understanding of a contextual issue called "a continuing history," the individual may not know where he or she has come from, where he or she is or is going to. "His selfhood and identity have not been liberated, but truncated" (Rakoff 1981). Winnicott (1959) defined the third "area of existing or area of living" as an important area that complements the previous areas that he had mentioned: the individual psychic or inner reality and external reality. This third area of experiencing and its relation to the cultural life of the child is an important factor in our understanding of the concept of transitional objects and transitional space. While we can begin to understand the framework that Winnicott (1960) provided for us regarding the concept of the holding environment, this transitional space can be extended beyond the mother-infant relationship and beyond the therapeutic environment to include the cultural context as well. This sameness of customs, language, dress, and other sociological phenomena allows the individual to identify, develop, and enhance his or her identity formation. As long as the cultural issues remain the same, the individual seems to be able to have a relative period of quietude (if one can call adolescence, at any point in time, a relative period of quietude) in developing one's identity. It is only when changes take place that one can sense the potential disruptions in identity equilibrium. Since the adolescent is, by definition, going through a relatively difficult period of disequilibrium in developing and enhancing his or her identity, cultural disruptions may complicate a tenuous identity balance.

In distinguishing the lives of human beings from the animal world, Freud (1927, 1930) viewed culture as being something that allowed the individual to progress to a higher mode of functioning and understanding. He even defined psychoanalytic therapy as culture: "Where id was, there ego shall be. It is a work of culture—not unlike draining of the Zuider Zee" (Freud 1933a; cf. Devereux 1953). We are, as Freud (1915) stated, susceptible to culture: "We need not deny susceptibility to culture to all who are at the present time behaving in an uncivilized way, and we may anticipate that the ennoblement of their instincts will be restored in more peaceful times."

While the adolescent is growing up and is faced with a period of cultural stability, the identity formation process can proceed in a relatively uninhibited manner. However, if there is cultural upheaval, the potential possibilities of difficulties in adolescent identity formation are there; the issues of role confusion and identity confusion may arise. Lowenfeld and Lowenfeld (1972) felt that the permissive society in which adolescents are presently growing up seriously impairs superego formation by allowing for the release of uncontrolled aggressive and infantile drive impulses that run counter to the demands of civilized life. As they state, "The task of 'reconciling man to civilization' is not made easier through the liberation of drives. . . . in a period of cultural stability, the infantile, rational demands of the superego could be worked-out in the analytic process. . . . the present cultural chaos confronts psychoanalysis with entirely new tasks." Freud (1933b) stated, "The psychical modifications that go along with the process of civilization are striking and unambiguous. They consist in a progressive displacement of instinctual aims in a restriction of instinctual impulses. . . . Of the psychological characteristics of civilization two appear to be the most important: a strengthening of the intellect, which is beginning to govern instinctual life, and an internalization of the aggressive impulses, with all its consequent advantages and perils.'' Freud viewed these modifications as a type of ''evolution of culture.'' The individual grew within the cultural context. However, this was a cultural context that one grew up in and was living in. One needs to address the question of individuals who leave their cultural context and move on to other areas. How does this affect the psychical apparatus? For our purposes, how will it affect the adolescent's identity formation?

Migration

Grinberg and Grinberg (1989) look at the phenomenon of migration and exile in terms of the various types of anxieties that may be awakened: persecutory anxieties in the face of change, depressive anxieties in which one mourns for others left behind and for the lost parts of the self, and confusional anxieties over the inability to distinguish between the old and the new. The Grinbergs feel that the essential factors relating to an understanding of the psychological aspects of migration and exile are in an understanding of normal and pathological mourning. As Grinberg (1973) had stated, the ''social aspects of identity . . . [are] based on the relationship parts of the self and external objects, a relationship mediated by the psychic mechanisms of projective and introjective identification.''

While there have been studies done on psychiatric complications that ensue from migration (Bar-El, Kalian, Eisenberg, and Schneider, in press), there have been studies by others (Mirsky and Kaushinsky 1989; Schneider and Rimmer 1988) that have tried to show how the migration process for adolescents may serve not only as a negative factor but also as a positive growth experience. Poland (1977) has written about pilgrimage as a healthy phenomenon; the personal pilgrimage is viewed ''as representing a pattern of action that can serve as an organizer for resolving conflict and psychic growth.''

In working with adolescents and young adults who are emotionally disturbed, we have found that Israel specifically can function as a therapeutic catalyst for adolescents who are experiencing developmental and environmental difficulties. In our psychiatric residential treatment facility in Jerusalem, we treat Israelis and non-Israelis who come to Israel for psychiatric treatment. It is interesting to note that we have found that the non-Israeli is able to utilize the identification process of identifying with Israel in a much more extreme and healthier manner than his Israeli counterpart (Schneider and Rimmer 1988). If we follow Erikson's dictum that "the adolescent mind is essentially a mind of the moratorium, a psychosocial stage between childhood and adulthood, and between the morality learned by the child and the ethics to be developed by the adult," it would seem that the adolescent could utilize a time-out period during this stage of emotional development. A different culture might be able to offer less pressure than the home environment. Removal from the country of origin to Israel could allow for a potential regression. However, this regression would be in the service of the ego. The adolescent is learning to utilize healthier aspects of his or her ego: learning a new language, learning how to transact in a foreign currency, learning how to deal with another culture, learning to interact with other adolescents who are from many nations of the world, etc. (Schneider and Rimmer 1988). This "regression" would allow the adolescent to draw on the healthier parts of his or her internal psychic structure in order to move ahead therapeutically. The adaptation of the adolescent to a new environment would enable him or her to draw on reserves in the psychic structure, which has up until now potentially been in a state of psychic disequilibrium, and bring it upward into a healthier equilibrium.

While we understand that mental health values are culturally specific (Moses and Kligler 1966), we have shown (Schneider and Moses 1982) "that an emotional illness, pathology, and treatment are determined and affected by culture. Just as mental health values are culturally determined and specific, so too is the diagnosis and treatment of emotional illness." While studies have shown that uprooting and cultural changes can bring about intense anxiety and alienation, for the less healthy and weaker adolescent it may provoke an emotionally tumultuous crisis that could lead to emotional decompensation and the expression of serious pathological behavior. However, if these changes take place in the framework of a protective, supportive, and therapeutic placement, the results could be quite different. The inner shifts that take place within the adolescent when he or she is moved into a different sociocultural atmosphere can be used as a growth-promoting experience.

Identity Formation

In writing about identity formation, theoreticians have stated how the individual might have to experience a "crisis" in order to provoke a heightened sense of identity. Erikson (1956) has stated, "Crisis is used here in a developmental sense to connote not a threat of a catastrophe, but a turning point, a crucial period of increased vulnerability and heightened potential." Arnstein (1979) viewed this as a need for young people; in order for them to develop in a healthy manner, they must achieve and experience wholeness. He states, "The wholeness to be achieved at this stage I have called a sense of inner identity." Josselson (1987, 1989) and Looney (1979) have written about the crises adolescents may go through in order to help them forge their identity during the stage called the moratorium. During this stage, adolescents become more aware of choice, and, while they may be "stuck" in knowing what types of choices to make, their being a part of strong family and/or cultural systems can help them in this quest. As Josselson (1987) has stated, "Fortunate life circumstances, external events that offer identity-forming possibilities, have a significant ameliorative effect on identity diffusion." The cultural system functions as a collective group identity that allows the adolescents' identity to coalesce.

We need to stress again the fact that, when adolescents are involved in cultural shifts, the need for a warm and nurturant environment is crucial as this is already a very difficult period for them psychologically. Being in a different culture increases the individual's sense of separateness, which "develops in parallel with the increasing complexity of his personality development" (Denford 1981). As Sandler and Sandler (1978) state, "The urge to re-experience important subjective aspects of object relationships from the first years of life constantly recurs and persists [i.e., represents unconscious wishes] particularly when our feelings of security or safety are threatened, as they constantly are." This would it is hoped come out in the transference relationship. However, the need for having a stable figure relates not only to the therapist but also to the emotional/cultural environment.

We have found that adolescent populations that have difficulty in identity issues do well in our residential treatment facility in Jerusalem.

Adopted adolescents, second-generation Holocaust-survivor adolescents, and learning-disabled adolescents seem to be able to attach themselves to a cultural identity in Israel that enables them to find or repair a lost or damaged identity (Schneider 1978a, 1978b, 1980, 1981, 1986, 1988; Schneider and Rimmer 1985; Schneider and Schneider 1986). We know that the sense of peoplehood and community (in addition to family) is very crucial in the development and enhancement of the adolescent's self-image, self-esteem, and feelings of belonging. In Israel, the adolescent finds more meaning and outlets for expression. This may be because Israel, being under a constant threat of war, galvanizes the adolescent into utilizing his or her healthier ego parts in order to be able to face the external threat to Israeli society. While he or she may not be directly affected by the Israeli political process, one is nonetheless able to derive an inner strength from separateness and difference, which is enhanced by being in Israel. Israel respects the value of each individual to contribute to a society, taking into account all individual differences. One can even look to the kibbutz culture as an example of integration of various different groups of people. While the kibbutz culture may be an exclusionary one, which does not easily allow for the infusion of foreign cultures, nonetheless they too can provide an understanding of cultural venues and serve as an example for others in Israel and in other countries as to the importance of a supportive environment that can enhance nurturance (Doron 1977).

Identity formation can be viewed as a creative process, where the cultural shifts and nuances that take place can help push one toward further growth. For the adolescent, this is especially true if he or she does not feel that the doors to return to his or her country of origin are closed. Thus, the "claustrophobic anxiety decreases" (Grinberg and Grinberg 1989). Foreign adolescents who come to Israel for treatment can even apply for citizenship in Israel; in effect, they can be an adolescent with two countries. For, under the "Law of Return," Jews who come to Israel can apply for immediate citizenship. This, in effect, gives them two cultures, two worlds, and the ability to know that there is always a country in the world (i.e., Israel) that can accept them for who they are. As an example, for the adolescent adoptee, the fact that one is having difficulty in identity formation and does not know much regarding past roots, having a country that will welcome one with open arms irrespective of who one is provides a sense of collec-

413

tive identity that could not occur anywhere else. Also, the second-generation Holocaust-survivor adolescent, whose parents have had difficulties with their own identity and its transmission to their children, is able to find new meaning and expression in Israel. Holocaust survivors and their adolescent children have been able to find meaning in life and rebuild psychic structure because the country of Israel has allowed them to mourn for family and self.

Hanna Segal (1952), building on the work of Melanie Klein, shows how one can deal "with loss and infantile depression, and its relationship to later reparation and restoration through sublimation and creativity" (Pollock 1978). As Segal states, "It is only when the loss has been acknowledged and the mourning experienced that re-creation can take place." One can view moving to another culture as a creative process, which can enable a push toward growth. As Segal states, "In a great work of art the degree of denial of the death instinct is less than in any other human activity. . . . It is expressed and curved to the needs of the life instinct and creation." Pollock (1978) feels that "at times the creative product is not the end result of the mourning process, but represents an attempt at mourning work through creativity." Creativity and change allow the adolescent to separate from internal representations of objects and from the self that may be linked to his or her previous cultural background. Thus, the mourning for one's previous culture and past is a necessary ingredient for enhancement of the identity process. As Grinberg (1978) has stated, "Faced with the loss of an object, one rushes to the mirror to find out what has become of one's image [since,] in every significant experience of object loss, we should take into account not only the mourning for the object but also the mourning for the lost parts of the self."

Creativity allows the adolescent to move in new directions, which aids the self in cohesion and in identity formation. This creativity is in the guise of "change," movement, for not to move at all during adolescence leads to stagnation. Movement, even with regressions and ups and downs, is change—and change means growth.

In discussing how both creativity and neuroses can help resolve internal conflicts, Noy (1979) makes the distinction that one attempts to deal with neuroses by reworking old patterns of behavior. In creativity, one can resolve internal conflicts by utilizing new ways of understanding and coping.

When a person comes to a new culture, he can either adapt in a defensive manner (wear the same clothing, follow the same customs, etc.) or adapt immediately, as a fish takes to water. This is done with little forethought or defensive operation. Adolescents often seek immediate identification and adaptation. This "creative process" propels them. One may view this direction as a reaction formation, as a defense against internal anxiety. We feel that the "running away" may in fact be part of the creative-growth-change process.

Conclusions

I can sum up this chapter with a quote from the Talmud (Rosh HaShana 16b): "Rabbi Isaac said: Four things cancel the doom of man, namely, charity, supplication, change of name, and change of conduct . . . some say a change of place." Maimonides states, "The essence of this Talmudic passage is to awaken man to change his actions . . . and if the awakening and change can take place by an external movement then that is of great benefit to one's soul." Change *can* provide a healthy growth process.

REFERENCES

Arnstein, R. L. 1979. The adolescent identity crisis revisited. *Adolescent Psychiatry* 7:71–84.

Bar-El, I.; Kalian, M.; Eisenberg, B.; and Schneider, S. In press. Tourists and psychiatric hospitalization with special reference to ethical aspects concerning management and treatment. *International Journal of Medicine and Law.*

Denford, J. 1981. Going away. *International Review of Psycho-Analysis* 8(3): 325–332.

Devereux, G. 1953. Cultural factors in psychoanalytic therapy. *Journal of the American Psychoanalytic Association* 1:629–655.

Doron, N. 1977. Kibbutz adolescent identity (in Hebrew). In *The Kibbutz,* vol. 5. Tel Aviv: Federation of Kibbutz Movements.

Erikson, E. H. 1950. *Childhood and Society.* New York: Norton.

Erikson, E. H. 1956. The problem of ego identity. *Journal of the American Psychoanalytic Association* 4:56–122.

Erikson, E. H. 1968. *Identity: Youth and Crisis.* London: Faber & Faber.

Freud, S. 1915. Thoughts for the times on war and death. *Standard Edition* 14:275–302. London: Hogarth, 1957.

Freud, S. 1927. The future of an illusion. *Standard Edition* 21:5–56. London: Hogarth, 1961.

Freud, S. 1930. Civilization and its discontents. *Standard Edition* 21:64–145. London: Hogarth, 1961.

Freud, S. 1933a. Dissection of the personality and anxiety and instinctual life—new introductory lectures on psycho-analysis. *Standard Edition* 22:57–111. London: Hogarth, 1964.

Freud, S. 1933b. Why war? *Standard Edition* 22:197–215. London: Hogarth, 1964.

Grinberg, L. 1973. Identity and ideology. *Adolescent Psychiatry* 2:424–434.

Grinberg, L. 1978. "The Razor's Edge" in depression and mourning. *International Journal of Psycho-Analysis* 59(2–3): 245–254.

Grinberg, L., and Grinberg, R. 1989. *Psychoanalytic Perspectives on Migration and Exile.* New Haven, Conn.: Yale University Press.

Josselson, R. 1987. Identity diffusion: a long-term follow-up. *Adolescent Psychiatry* 14:230–258.

Josselson, R. 1989. Identity formation in adolescence: implications for young adulthood. *Adolescent Psychiatry* 16:142–154.

Looney, J. G. 1979. Adolescents as refugees. *Adolescent Psychiatry* 7:199–208.

Lowenfeld, H., and Lowenfeld, Y. 1972. Our permissive society and the superego: some current thoughts about Freud's cultural concepts. In S. C. Post, ed. *Moral Values and the Superego Concept in Psychoanalysis.* New York: International Universities Press.

Maugham, W. S. 1944. *The Razor's Edge.* London: Heinemann.

Mirsky, J., and Kaushinsky, F. 1989. Migration and growth: separation-individuation processes in immigrant students in Israel. *Adolescence* 24(95): 725–740.

Moses, R., and Kligler, D. S. 1966. A comparative analysis of the institutionalization of mental health values: the United States and Israel. *Israel Annals of Psychiatry* 4:148–161.

Noy, P. 1979. Form creation in art: an ego-psychological approach to creativity. *Psychoanalytic Quarterly* 48:229–256.

Poland, W. S. 1977. Pilgrimage: action and tradition in self-analysis. *Journal of the American Psychoanalytic Association* 25(2): 399–416.

Pollock, G. H. 1978. Process and affect: mourning and grief. *International Journal of Psycho-Analysis* 59:255–276.

Rakoff, V. 1981. A reconsideration of identity. *Adolescent Psychiatry* 9:22–32.

Sandler, J. 1960. On the concept of superego. *Psychoanalytic Study of the Child* 15:128–162.

Sandler, J., and Sandler, A.-M. 1978. On the development of object relationships and affects. *International Journal of Psycho-Analysis* 59:285–296.

Schneider, S. 1978a. Attitudes toward death in adolescent offspring of Holocaust survivors. *Adolescence* 13(52): 575–584.

Schneider, S. 1978b. A model for an alternative educational/treatment program for adolescents. *Israel Annals of Psychiatry* 16:1–20.

Schneider, S. 1980. A proposal for a network of psychiatric treatment services for adolescents. *International Journal of Therapeutic Communities* 1:5–14.

Schneider, S. 1981. A proposal for treating adolescent offspring of Holocaust survivors. *Journal of Psychology and Judaism* 6:68–76.

Schneider, S. 1986. The adoptee: interface between psychiatry, law, and ethics. *Medicine and Law* 5:441–444.

Schneider, S. 1988. Attitudes toward death in adolescent offspring of Holocaust survivors: a comparison of Israeli and American adolescents. *Adolescence* 23(91): 703–710.

Schneider, S., and Moses, R. 1982. A therapeutic community program for a multi-cultural adolescent population. *Israel Journal of Psychiatry* 19:81–92.

Schneider, S., and Rimmer, E. 1985. Adoptive parents' hostility towards their adopted children. *Children and Youth Services Review* 6:345–352.

Schneider, S., and Rimmer, E. 1988. Treatment by temporary culturectomy. *International Journal of Adolescent Medicine and Health* 3(3): 225–232.

Schneider, S., and Schneider, A. 1986. A modified therapeutic community program for learning-disabled adolescents. *International Journal of Therapeutic Communities* 7(2): 111–119.

Segal, H. 1952. A psycho-analytical approach to aesthetics. *International Journal of Psycho-Analysis* 34(2): 89–97.

Winnicott, D. W. 1953. Transitional objects and transitional phenomena. *International Journal of Psycho-Analysis* 34(2): 89–97.

Winnicott, D. W. 1959. The fate of the transitional object. In C. Winnicott, R. Shepherd, and M. Davis, eds. *Psycho-Analytic Explorations*. Cambridge, Mass.: Harvard University Press, 1989.

Winnicott, D. W. 1960. The theory of the parent-infant relationship. In *The Maturational Processes and the Facilitating Environment*. London: Hogarth, 1985.

22   I, ME, MYSELF:

THE SUBJECTIVE ASPECT OF IDENTITY

ANA-MARIA RIZZUTO

Erikson's work has illuminated the process and the difficulties of becoming oneself in the course of life, particularly in adolescence. His
notions of identity crisis and identity diffusion as common characteristics of troubled adolescents and young adults have guided our clinical
work. Erikson insisted that we attend to the total person and not only
to the conflictual aspects of pathology. Erikson's phenomenological
description accurately portrays the nature of the adolescent's task of
self-integration as well as the failure to achieve it.

The beginning of adolescence offers the first opportunity to experience a sense of identity. "I have tried to demonstrate," says Erikson,
"that the ego values accrued in childhood culminate [in adolescence]
in what I have called a sense of ego identity" (1959, p. 89). Erikson
locates the sense of identity as coming from "the sum of childhood
identifications" and one's own drives, endowments, and past opportunities synthesized now as "the accrued confidence that one's ability to
maintain inner sameness and continuity (one's ego in the psychological
sense) is matched by the sameness and continuity of one's meaning
to others" (p. 89). Such confidence is essential for psychic existence
because, "in the social jungle of human existence, there is no feeling
of being alive without a sense of ego identity" (p. 90).

In this chapter, I survey the subjective aspect of the sense of identity
in order to attempt to integrate its conceptual meaning with other aspects of analytic theory. I examine the significance of the personal
pronouns in the process of self-apprehension as well as their relation

to a psychoanalytic theory that uses the nominalized pronoun "I" (ego) as the foundation of psychic structure. The point in question is one of the most difficult in psychoanalytic theorizing: how to talk about a living mind in process without mechanizing its structures and functions. Freud's apparatus had no theory for the full living being. Erikson attempted to solve the problem by attending to the full individual's sense of identity in a concrete social environment. Erikson succeeded in making us aware of the problem, but he could not avoid a mechanistic concept of identity as something that acts within the subject and gives it identity.

I hope that my reflections may contribute to our understanding of the processes involved in the adolescent's awareness of being a unique individual.

Para vivir no quiero
islas, palacios, torres.
!Que alegría más alta:
vivir en los pronombres!

To live I do not desire
islands, palaces, towers.
How much deeper the joy
of living in pronouns!

Quítate ya los trajes
las señas, los retratos;
yo no te quiero así,
disfrazada de otra,
hija siempre de algo.
Te quiero pura, libre,
irreductible: tú.
Sé que cuando te llame
entre todas las gentes
del mundo
solo tú seras tú.

Rid yourself of your garments,
your features, your resemblances;
I do not desire you thus,
masquerading as another,
daughter always of someone.
I want you free, unalloyed,
constant, immutable: you.
I know that when I may call you
from among all the people
of the world,
only you will be you.

Y cuando me preguntes
quién es el que te llama,
el que te quiere suya,
enterraré los nombres,
los rótulos, la historia.
Iré rompiendo todo
lo que encima me echaron
desde antes de nacer.

And when you may ask me
who is he that calls you,
who is he that desires you,
I shall bury all names,
labels and history,
and, breaking away from all
that has been thrown over me
since before I was born,

Y vuelto ya al anónimo	back again to the eternal
eterno del desnudo,	namelessness of the naked,
de la piedra, del mundo,	of the stone, of the world,
te diré:	I shall say:
"Yo te quiero, soy yo."	"I love you, I am I."

Pedro Salinas [1940]

Freud acknowledged that poets preceded psychoanalysts in their insights into the human psyche. In agreement with Freud, I suggest in this chapter that the core experience of identity as subjective self-recognition occurs in Salinas's "deeper . . . joy of living in pronouns." I shall present the metapsychological difficulties of the concept of identity, a clinical theory about the significance of pronouns for the affective component of the sense of identity, and my own theoretical overview about the conceptualization of the subjective experience of identity.

Freud's psychoanalysis—its theory and its technique—aimed at creating a science of subjective experience. Psychoanalysis originated a comprehensive method and a theory to understand the subtlest of human psychic processes. The theory, however, did not attend to the subjective experience of personal identity and did not have a term for it. The theory, nonetheless, offered a key concept for the conceptualization of the human subjective sense of identity: the notion of progressive genetic processes aimed at the formation of a stable psychic structure where dynamic phenomena kept the past of the individual present. Personal continuity in time is established in the unified synchrony of unconscious dynamic processes originating in diverse moments of development and their partial manifestations as the person's conscious subjective experience. The uniqueness of each individual's developmental processes furnishes the particular elements to account for his objective and subjective exclusive singularity.

Identity as a concept entered the analytic lexicon when Erikson published *Childhood and Society* (1950). Erikson suggested that "this sense of identity provides the ability to experience one's self as something that has continuity and sameness, and to act accordingly" (p. 42). Erikson was eager to attend to the components of a living experience, the somatic, the societal, and the personal, without "actively dissolving its total living situation in order to be able to make an isolated section of it amenable to a set of instruments or concepts" (p. 37).

Erikson's existential description of identity did not include any attempt to integrate it with the body of psychoanalytic theory, in particular its metapsychological points of view. Freud had said explicitly that, in dealing with psychical processes, "we have no other aim but that of translating into theory the results of observations" (1915, p. 190). Erikson's concept of identity became a parallel notion, unintegrated with the main body of psychoanalytic theory. Its descriptive power and clinical relevance, however, prompted many analysts to accept it without questioning its theoretical status. Authors that made significant contributions to psychoanalysis (Eissler, Greenacre, Jacobson, Mahler) incorporated it into their vocabularies without any significant effort to connect it with the main body of psychoanalytic theory. Other writers such as Blos (1962) and many self psychologists use the term as self-evident. Lichtenstein (1961, 1963, 1977) made some attempts to connect identity with the structural theory without resolving the inherent metapsychological difficulties of two different frames of reference.

The absence of theoretical clarity has had a double effect. It has produced an extensive and clinically relevant literature that cannot be integrated into Freudian theory. Abend (1974) and Spruiell (1981) have discussed the theoretical difficulties of the term and the many confusions that it adds. Simon (1978) concludes that the term is tantalizing but "amorphous" in its analytic connotations: "It encompasses the subjective and the objective, the conscious, the preconscious and the unconscious, the social and the intrapsychic, as well as the ego ideal and the 'ideal self'" (p. 460).

The term, nonetheless, is here to stay. Patients use it. Analysts resort to it when they are describing their patients' "crises of identity" or their "confused identities." Trying to eradicate it would affect this very communication. The choice left to us is to study the phenomena supporting the concept, their emotional value, and attempt to find a way of conceptualizing it in accordance with psychoanalytic theory.

Freud's Translation of Observation into Theory

Freud's detailed clinical observations culminated in a key conclusion: "The division of the psychical into what is conscious and what is unconscious is the fundamental premise of psycho-analysis; . . . it alone makes it possible for psycho-analysis to understand the pathological processes in mental life" (1923, p. 13). Freud's conclusion was based on what patients said to him, which in turn depended on the patients' verbalization of what occurred to them, in the privacy of their minds. Freud assumes that whatever they were saying had something to do with them as the subjects of what occurred to them and as the speakers of their sentences. Freud's knowledge of their private worlds "is invariably bound up with consciousness" (1923, p. 19) on the part of the self-observing and reporting patient. The conscious awareness of mental processes is an act of internal perception similar to external perception: "In psycho-analysis there is no choice for us but to assert that mental processes are in themselves unconscious, and to liken the perception of them by means of consciousness to the perception of the external world by means of sense-organs" (Freud 1915, p. 171).

Freud conceives of consciousness as an act of perception that opens a slit of light in the middle of two dark and essentially unknowable realities: "Psycho-analysis warns us not to equate perception by means of consciousness with the unconscious mental processes which are their object. Like the physical, the psychical is not necessarily in reality what it appears to us to be" (1915, p. 171).

The essential words that people use in analysis and in life to refer to their discoveries in inner reality and in the world are only three pronouns: "I," "me," and "myself." Whatever Freud learned about his own private world or the inner life of his patients had to pass through the narrow gate of the three pronouns. There is no other way to reveal private experience. The unexpectedly happy Miss Lucy said it well and succinctly to the surprised Freud: "'It is just that you don't know me. . . . After all, I can have thoughts and feelings to myself'" (1893–1895, p. 121).

"I" is the key word for all perceptions, external and internal, which occur "as if they came from without" (Freud 1923, p. 23). Words are indispensable for capturing elusive mental processes: "By their interposition internal thought-processes are made into perceptions" (p. 23). A conclusion seems to follow by itself. "I," the pronominal word, is the indispensable mediator for all intrapsychic knowledge. What is not "I" has to be perceived as external to it by the mediation of "I" itself. Analytic theory comes here to a convergence of the multiple roles of "I," a play of mirrors, in which the perceiver is his own means, his own object, and the structurer of all conscious perception. Freud's patients could do nothing but use "I" as a pronoun to refer to themselves as the subjects of their experiences and to use "me" and "myself" to describe themselves as the object of their perception.

Freud's aim was to transform the patients' observations into theory. He could not escape the powerful presence of "I," the indispensable pronoun. To make "I" into theory, Freud carried out a grammatically forbidden act: he placed an article in front of the pronoun, and *Ich* became *das Ich,* an entity, an agency of the mind, not a subject, but an object suitable for theoretical discourse. Much was gained in the move, but something also was lost. What was lost was the speaking subject, who became blurred and confused with the agency of the mind. In spite of Hartmann's (1950) efforts, we have not to this day found a suitable way of talking about "I," the pronoun, representing the living subject. Freud himself, however, never completely excluded the pronominal usage of "I." On the contrary, he "exploits traditional usages . . . plays on the ambiguities thus created, so that none of the connotations normally attaching to 'ego' or 'I' ('Ich') is forgotten" (Laplanche and Pontalis 1973, pp. 131–132).

Freud selected another pronoun made into a name, *das Es,* "the it," which in Strachey's translation became the latinized id, to designate the unconscious part of the mind. He was following Groddeck, who had observed (in *The Book of the It,* 1923) the passive way in which we live some experiences: "There was something in *me* at that moment that was stronger than *me*" (my italics; quoted by Laplanche and Pontalis 1973, p. 197). The it, id, and "me," as the passive subject of experience or the object of self-discovery and -recognition, seem to have a direct relation to each other.

Freud's id "contains the passions" (1923, p. 25), is "the great reservoir of libido" (p. 30), and seeks love objects. Freud presents a most illuminating paragraph about the relations between the ego and the id at the time of transformation of object libido into narcissistic libido: "This transformation of an erotic object-choice into an alteration of the ego is also a method by which the ego can obtain control over the id and deepen its relation with it—at the cost, it is true, of acquiescing to a large extent in the id's experiences. When the ego assumes the features of the object, it is forcing itself, so to speak, upon the id as a love-object and is trying to make good the id's loss by saying: 'Look, you can love me too—*I* am so like the object'" (p. 30).

This paragraph presents the fascinating return of the stubborn pronouns, which seem to insist on being used to refer to loving and loved people. Freud's theory has completed a circle: the ego insists on saying "I" to the loving id, presenting its wish by saying, "Love me."

Am I playing with words, or am I touching on an essential aspect of analytic theorizing? The answer is twofold: analysis is a play of words because what is to be analyzed, a living person, is always far more complex than the words we have for the task. I am touching on an essential and difficult aspect of psychoanalytic theorizing. Freud's structural theory and his masterful efforts to create a mental apparatus whose predictable mechanisms would permit us to understand the private processes of the minds of living people, even those unknown to them, became, unfortunately, a one-person psychology, a self-sufficient entity. It can describe only how the person is put together psychologically, the gears that move the machinery of a particular mind. It can say nothing about what people feel most strongly about themselves, that is, what they are, the "I" and "me" of Miss Lucy, so simply eloquent about her present and past sense of being herself in spite of her neurosis.

It is at this point that we can see what was lost when Freud created the structural theory. The personal pronouns, "I," "me," "myself," and "you," are very special words. They have no synonyms. As Salinas says, not even the name of the person is a synonym for them. The referent of a personal pronoun is always subjectively specific. The affect experienced by a person at a given moment must pass through the narrow door of the pronoun. In fact, there are no other words that carry a heavier load of affect than "I," "me," and "you." We do live, love, and die "in pronouns"—or, as Salinas puts it, "How much deeper the joy of living in pronouns!"

Freud overlooked a simple fact: the patients were not only talking about themselves; they were talking to him. What he overlooked his patients forced him to consider. Dora made him realize that his patients were saying to him what was to become his 1923 formulation of the ego speaking to the id ("Look, you can love me too") while they were doing their best to show their affections for him. The living patients wanted dialogue, love, attention, interaction. Freud wanted scientific knowledge. It is a great tribute to his genius that he managed to learn so much about the patients and their unconscious processes without being drawn into a direct personal relation with them. The double effort to learn the unknown and to keep the process within therapeutic boundaries did not allow for further elaboration of the personal use the patients were making of the pronouns "I" and "me" to refer to *whom* and *what* they felt themselves to be.

Erikson responded to the lack of attention to the living speaker in his concrete circumstances by focusing on the person's sense of identity. Unfortunately, the definition of the term has the same theoretical difficulties as Freud's conceptualization of the ego. It is a sort of an entity within the subject, not the subject itself. It is the sense of identity, Erikson says, that "provides the ability to experience one's self as something that has continuity and sameness, and to act accordingly" (1950, p. 42). The living subject has once more been displaced by a sense of identity that gives identity to the person. This is a petitio principii, an instance of circular logic.

Is there a way out of the theoretical dilemma? Do we analysts have to give up our structural concepts to save the living subject, or must we keep our theories and let the living subject take care of itself?

The way out, in my opinion, is found in two sources. The first is Freud's epoch-making discovery and description of the genetic development of the human mind in the course of time. A mind is its own historical representative, the narrator of the vicissitudes it has undergone, the loves and hatreds it has encountered, the successes and the injuries it has faced, and the written record of a sentient developing body and a learning intellect. The second is the detailed observation of the developmental transformations of the essential personal pronouns and their referents.

Clinical Theory about the Significance of Pronouns in Psychic Development

Pronouns are part of language, and language is the essential human matrix for the formation of the mind. The child's predisposition to speak depends on the adult's willingness to address him or her as a partner in spoken communication. The need for a parental wish to communicate with the infant is so indispensable that even before spoken language is possible a dialogue of bodies, rituals, gestures, and sounds must be established between the mother and the child if the infant (*in-fans*, "not speaking") is to survive emotionally. Such sensory exchanges register in the child's mind as affectively significative memorial processes. The memories, in turn, are the building blocks of psychic representations (Rizzuto 1990). At the time when language appears in development, these are potentially usable as the obligatory representational referents, in particular, affective referents, for newly acquired words (Rizzuto 1988). These earliest of memories carry with them the first and dominant patterns of object relatedness, modes of affective communication, forms of need satisfaction, and, most important for our subject, ways of feeling and perceiving oneself as the alternating dyadic subject and object of an inseparable pair.

Psycholinguistic research (Sharpless 1985) reveals that the first usage of pronouns occurs as part of learning to participate in a conversation without having as yet a consistent interpretation of their meaning and without an invariable referent. Before twenty-two months of age, during Mahler's rapprochement phase, the use of personal pronouns does not say much about the child's sense of self. After twenty-four months, at the end of the rapprochement phase, begins a second phase of personal pronoun acquisition, when first-person pronouns are mastered. Six months later, the child masters the second- and third-person pronouns. Sharpless draws significant conclusions from the observation that "over this half-year period the child masters the sense of each pronoun as well as its reference in different conversational contexts." These conclusions suggest that Mahler is "justified in employing I and You (and other person pronouns) as behavioral markers of identity formation at the end of the rapprochement crisis" and that "person pronouns constitute a valid, reliable index for drawing inferences about certain intrapsychic events" (1985, p. 881). We find here an assumed correlation between the epigenesis of the pronominal function usage and the dawning of the subjective sense of identity.

Sharpless sees more than identity formation in the mastery of the pronouns. She considers them also as psychodynamic signals of wishes in conversational roles, the desire "not just for the recognition of our individuality, but also our desire to assert ourselves through communication. By adopting the speaker role, *we place our viewpoint in the center of our psychic stage,* communicating this to all whom we address, ourselves included" (1985, p. 878; my italics). Self and other become simultaneously separate and interrelated in conversational roles and exchanges defined by the pronouns that later facilitate integration into a larger social milieu.

Sharpless does not attend to the affective component of the personal pronouns or to the specific psychic referent that may connect them to different uses in diverse personal contexts. She presents the pronouns as related to a global sense the speaker has of himself or of the person he addresses: "The referents for the person pronouns are self and other . . . as either intrapsychic or corporeal entities" (1985, p. 877).

I must make a distinction here. Linguistic competence and mastery of pronouns reveal only a basically normal epigenetic development, not interfered with by specific psychotic or neurological processes that affect language development. Such normal development says nothing about the affective and representational components of the pronoun's referent associated to the use of the pronoun in the mind of the speaker. The referents of the spoken pronouns are based on primary-process imagery and fantasies as well as on secondary-process beliefs and stories organized as conceptions people have about who and what they are and about what has happened to them. They also include their hopes and fears about other people's perceptions of them. Distress about any of these aspects of self-perception motivates patients to request analytic or psychiatric help. A young obsessive man described his dilemma: "I can't decide whether my girlfriend is the right woman for me. I might overlook a better woman. I need the best for me."

Language as a tool for cognitive and practical communication is a function that is altered only in neurological conditions, in schizophrenia, and during moments of acute psychotic confusion. The same cannot be said for the use of language at the service of inter- and intrasubjective communication (Rizzuto 1988). To talk with others and with ourselves as the object (Bollas 1982) of inner discourse ("I said to myself") requires the establishment of emotional contact, what Jakobson (Waugh 1976) calls the phatic function of language, illustrated by the question, Can you hear me? Here, "me" means the feeling subject.

In this chapter, I suggest that the sense of identity that has emotional weight and counts for the positive feeling of being oneself is that in which we can rest assured that we can have the "much deeper . . . joy of living in pronouns." The sense of identity lies in knowing that someone can recognize who we are and can say "you" and make us feel "that is me." It may be that the one who says "you" is the inner speaker in an act of self-recognition. The other side of this essentially pronominal identity is the certainty that if we say, "I love you, I am I," someone would respond, "I know." I am not playing with words.

I am saying that the sense of identity has two very uneven components. One is made of all the practical realities that locate us in society as part of a group, a social class, a religious denomination, and a member of a family. The other is composed of the elaboration of cumulative experiences of being the object of the love and recognition of another person, who in turn is a love object for us. The uniqueness of such experiences, the exquisite particularity involved in each of them, cannot be referred to by any other word than a pronoun. Names do not have sufficient linguistic specificity to carry out the task (Litowitz and Litowitz 1983). They can even bring confusion to the issue, as illustrated by a woman's complaint: "Julia is my mother's daughter, the name she gave me, but Julia is not me." "I," "me," and "you" can refer only to the specific members of the dialogue, as they feel themselves to be in a mutual act of validating recognition. Salinas said it well:

> And when you may ask me
> who is he that calls you,
> . . . .
> I shall bury all names,
> labels and history,
>
> . . . .
> I shall say:
> "I love you, I am I."

Identity, as a subjective experience, is, in my opinion, a matter of loving and having been loved. It is the cumulative result of the fantasized elaboration of the history of our loves, of the love (or lack of it) of others for us, and of our love (or lack of it) for them. It is the history of how we were loved when we were too small to take the initiative, of what we did with the manner in which we were loved when we were able to respond, of what measures we took to compensate for the rejection of our wishes to be loved or for the refusal of the love we offered. Identity is experienced not as a list of descriptive characteristics but as a relational narrative in the context of others. Identity is a description of oneself as a love object.

Brief quotations from a few analysands say it well, illustrating pedestrian or bizarre narratives. "That is my identity: a Hamlet, strong, tolerant, but why would they like me? All I am is a sullen rebellious boy," said a man who could not commit himself to his woman friend.

A homosexual woman insisted, "I don't want to have a gay identity. I want to be me. I am who I am. I used to make myself dizzy focusing on myself trying to see how my mother saw me." Another woman insisted, "The woman my husband loves is not me. I don't recognize her. I don't know her. She is a performer. I spent my childhood as a performer for my parents." A young man who was very attached to his mother insisted on their manner of remaining together: "I gave a penis to my mother and I made her into me. I am like my mother."

These narratives differ in remarkable ways from the secondary-process language of gender or personal identity that we employ to talk theoretically about identity and identity formation. Nonetheless, I believe that subjective identity formation occurs along the lines of these private, perceived, and fantasized narratives about the modes of relating to and being related to by the people who are indispensable for our psychic survival. In all cases, the narrative is an unconsciously organized construction that is ego syntonic and affect laden.

The question is how to integrate the essential phenomena of subjective narrative with the body of psychoanalytic theory without doing violence either to the patient's experience or to the accumulated knowledge gathered by classic Freudian concepts. I think that we can return to Freud's original concept of consciousness as the tool to perceive the two realities extrinsic to it: external and internal reality. Our innermost core, the psychic support of our being, is an it, id, something we cannot know directly. The source of our passions, the reservoir of the most precious memories of our first loves, the rejected aspects of ourselves prompted by earlier and later superego development, are extrinsic to our conscious awareness of who we are. We are what we do not know, and we feel certain we know who we are. Freud knew that he had inflicted a great narcissistic injury on us by demonstrating how little we know about ourselves. On the other hand, we know something of who we are. In conclusion, "identity" can be considered a relative subjective term, a functional description for the feeling that we know ourselves and for moments of self-recognition. It cannot be more than a flexible concept, without a fixed referent.

In chapter 7 of *The Interpretation of Dreams*, Freud suggests that "the aim of the first psychical activity [the hallucination of satisfaction] was to produce a 'perceptual identity'—a repetition of the perception which was linked with the satisfaction of the need" (1900, p. 566). Earlier, in the unpublished *Project for a Scientific Psychology*, he mentions "the sensation of identity" (1895, p. 329) and describes the manner in which such identity is attained (p. 361). Freud concludes, "The aim and end of all thought processes is thus to bring about a *state of identity.* . . . *Cognitive* or *judging* thought seeks an identity with a bodily cathexis, *reproductive* thought seeks it with a psychical cathexis of one's own" (p. 332).

Freud did not use the term "identity" again, but the concept it conveyed remained present in the description of the search for the satisfaction of wishes and the search for the object that provided the earliest satisfaction. Complex aspects of the notion of identity of experience reappeared in the conceptualization of transference and in the selection of love objects.

Freud's early "identity of experience" may appear far removed from the contemporary conceptualization of personal identity. I suggest that it can be of great use if understood in the context of the satisfaction not only of biological needs but also of the specific human needs for emotional contact and communication.

Freud's early example of identity of experience describes a simplified situation aimed at bringing about "the experience of satisfaction" of a particular need. However, living babies in their mothers' arms have a complex multitude of needs, each of which requires its own experience of satisfaction. What I consider important in Freud's description of the search for satisfaction and identity of experience is that he considers it an intrapsychic act, the earliest constitutive psychic act. If Winnicott and Freud had had the opportunity to discuss it long enough, perhaps they would have agreed that what Freud called "hallucination of satisfaction" Winnicott called "creation of the mother." I am sure that both would have concurred that the worst catastrophe for a child is the failure to attain what Freud describes as "the desired perceptual identity being established from the direction of the external world" (1905, p. 566). Winnicott says it concretely: "The mother places the actual breast just there where the infant is ready to create, and at the right moment" (1971, p. 11). Freud did not draw any conclusion about the affective component of the experience of identity for the formation of the subjective sense of being oneself. He did, however, call the searching hallucination "the first psychical activity."

A Theory about the Experience of Identity

I suggest that this first psychic process, whether we call it hallucination or creation, reveals that the child has a "knowledge" of what he or she needs to be psychically alive and seeks it actively in the environment. My clinical experience has convinced me that there are some essential components of that search that are the key elements in the formation throughout life of experience of personal identity. Even when they cannot be articulated into words at the beginning of life, they respond to the following questions addressed to the mother. Do you see me? Do you hear me? Are you emotionally in touch with me? Do you recognize my invitation, my spontaneous gesture toward you? Are you willing to respond to me? Do you want me with you? The affirmative response to these questions always produces from birth to death a pleasurable recognition of "identity of experience." The accent in each of the questions and in the experience itself is on the pronoun "me."

The infant does not speak and cannot say "me." Nonetheless, from the earliest moments of life children seem to be equipped with a capacity to discriminate authentic affective contact. Whether they recognize the affective proprioceptive messages of the maternal body, the emotional communicative value of pitch of voice, or perhaps subtle synchronization of the maternal actions and facial expressions, infants seem to be able to feel whether they are accepted and communicated with. I wonder if these earliest elements have something in common with Freud's bodily and psychic cathexis seeking identity of bodily satisfaction, most specifically the "psychical cathexis of one's own" (1895, p. 332). I interpret such cathexis of one's own as the capacity to seek emotional identity with the need to be in touch with oneself and with the maternal object, whatever form it takes at this early age. The child needs the mediation of the mother's attention to be constituted as her child, a love object.

These experiences of integration between the "creation" or "hallucination" of the wish to be perceived by the mother and the actual achievement of a moment of being in emotional contact with her, or their partial absence, are the essential affective representations of the total complex of self-representations that become, at the time of the conscious emergence of a certain sense of self, the basic referents for the pronouns "I" and "me." These pronouns condense not so much cognitive self-representations as the affect of specific modes of identity of perception between mother and child at the moment when satisfaction has taken place in some or all of the modalities wished for by the baby. The manner in which a child and her mother have found each other in their way to satisfaction registers as memorial processes of a developing relationship that becomes a gestural dialogue, if not yet a verbal commentary, about the "me" of the child as the object of maternal attention. Thus, an experience of satisfaction may be a composite of contradictory, complementary, or alternating feelings. A mother may have good conscious wishes toward her baby, but her body may reveal in her stiffness the fear of a "wild baby." She may look at the child tenderly, but her high-pitched voice may reveal worries about her competence as a tender person. She may feed the baby with adequate calm, but her abrupt movements, even if controlled, may reveal her impatience with a temperamentally slow baby.

These are ordinary observations anyone can make. They reveal that "the experience of satisfaction" has a remarkable complexity. Furthermore, they call attention to the infant's capacity for unconscious perception and registration of the maternal emotions. I reflect, following Freud, that, if the unconscious of the analyst is capable of communicating with the unconscious of the patient, it stands to reason that even infants must have unconscious, neurologically mediated ways of perceiving the maternal perception. We still know very little about unconscious modes of perceiving except that we analysts earn our living by counting on them.

The memorial processes of these experiences of satisfaction seem to find their main organizer and source of retrieval in the affect experienced rather than in other representational components. Litowitz and Litowitz point out that "the memory for persons is different from and developmentally earlier than abstract conceptual memory" (1983, p. 401). In my opinion, the difference rests in the assumption that these are memories of relational affects in the context of unconscious or conscious memorial processes about concrete exchanges with the parents. Later in development they are linked to the so-called episodic or personal memory (Tulvig 1972), which is always autobiographical.

The formation of self- and object representations is influenced by the composite affect of the different aspects of the experience of satisfaction. The representations accentuate some aspect of the perception of oneself or of the object, or of both, as a unity either in distress or in relative pleasure. The process of internalization from the earliest primary identification to late moments of development with representational separation between self and object is, in my opinion, regulated by the composite affects of the interaction. "Internalizations are complex forms of human action . . . a dynamic process, motivated and impelled" (Meissner 1981, p. 57). The motivation for internalization, I suggest, arises from the complex affect of the experience of satisfaction that prompts the individual to carry out psychic acts of incorporation, introjection, and identification, defensive maneuvers of avoidance, rejection, withdrawal, or other defense mechanisms. In all cases, be they self- or object representations, portrayed as dyadic interaction or as transformed self-representations through identification with the object, what remains as the point of reference for the sense of self is the affect of the experience of satisfaction. I like to insist that here experience of satisfaction is understood as a broad concept of the satisfaction experienced by the living child and not simply the satisfaction of a particular biological need.

A brief clinical example may illustrate my point. A patient may say, "My mother fed me on schedule. She took time to make sure I had the right stuff in me. But there was a vacuum in her. A sense of duty and doom, as though she had to save me from the poisons of the world. To eat was to fight a chemical war in a dangerous world. She loved me but she had no joy in life. I took it in. I can't let myself go." The internalization of the relationship has left the patient with an ego restriction, connected to an affectionate bond to the maternal perception of a dangerous world and of a fragile child.

The organization of "I" and "me" finds its essential referents in the affectively laden and organized self- and object representations of interactions and relations, as the example above illustrates. What counts is the interplay, in double mirroring, of the perceptions of mother and child acting in the world. The interplay gives the experience of satisfaction an exclusive particularity, which is specific for that mother-child pair.

The emergence of language occurs after the process described in the preceding paragraph has gone on for at least a year and the relational patterns have been well established. In their effort to help the child master language, the mother and other adults use baby talk and provide a "linguistic input for children in a way that differs radically from usage between adults. . . . For example, a mother often uses "we" to include both herself and the child in an activity that only one of them is performing. In this way, she signals that she and the child are a unit" (Litowitz and Litowitz 1983, p. 408). These efforts would bring about the child's mastery of language, what linguists call "linguistic competence." Only massive psychopathology would interfere with the child's learning to talk. Even in such cases, the child has learned to talk but refuses to do so. Psychological help usually permits the child to talk without difficulty at its own developmental level.

I have suggested elsewhere that "the same representational reality that modulates the emergence of affect is the essential and unavoidable referent for all spoken words" (Rizzuto 1988, p. 383). For the pronouns "I" and "me," the referent finds its final common pathway in the effect of the internalized relational moments of experiences of satisfaction. These moments are cumulative, and each new experience adds representational and affective complexity to the pronouns' unconscious referents.

The time when the pronouns acquire full psychic referential meaning coincides with the emergence of the capacity for conscious fantasy formation and transformation of relations with the parents. The child becomes a more separate individual, and relations are from now on progressively negotiated by language exchanges. Words become prevailing mediators of affective exchanges that were earlier regulated by bodily interactions. The latter never disappear. They persist as double registers of gestures and signals for transformation of self- and object representation. Among the gestures and signals, the maternal eyes and voice and their expressions become significant organizers of self-experience. They convey the perceived maternal and paternal judgment of the child. Language, however, becomes the dominant medium, the playground for the display of indispensable object relations.

The pronouns bring with them the previously absent capacity consciously to objectify oneself and the object. The child can now say, "That is me," or refer to himself or herself as the active subject of actions or of existence: "I am." The reflective power of the pronouns gathers now the entire affective heritage of previously experienced interactions and ways of perceiving and being perceived in them. This makes the pronouns "I" and "me" the two most affect-laden words in all language, followed immediately by the pronoun "you."

The objectification of oneself afforded by the pronouns permits complex processes of transformation and rearrangements of the conscious and preconscious aspects of their referents. Fantasies, defenses, and the telescoping of reinterpretations allow for many elaborations of previously held beliefs about oneself. One may say, "Well, I am not that bad. If my mother could not tolerate my being very active, it is not that I was no good. That was my mother." In fact, after the appearance of the pronouns, we spend the rest of our lives trying to objectify, correct, know better, and figure out who and what we really are. Each new relation brings out new angles of ourselves, and each change in our bodies requires a new elaboration of our bodily self. Both call for an inner search eventuating in the repeated internal sentences, "That is me," "That is not me." The resulting "me" is a construct formed from selected elements of the large reservoir of "me" memories to create the most apt "me" for the concrete relational circumstance.

Language has its limitations in its capacity to facilitate the expression of a sentient person. It can be used to avoid oneself, to isolate affect, to hide, and to refer to oneself as a thing. It can objectify the person not from the point of view of herself but from the point of view of the internalized object. The introjected eyes and words of the loved or hated object may prevail in directing the effort to objectify oneself. Neither "I" nor "me" are simple words. They carry with them an entire relational, fantasized, and interpretive history. To find out who is "me" in the spoken "me" requires careful introspection to discover from whose point of view the "I" speaks of "me." I have presented elsewhere (Rizzuto 1988) the case of an adult woman who had never said "I" with the feeling that she was herself. She always spoke from the point of view of an "imitation" of herself, devoid of affect as she felt her parents expected her to be. The pronoun obtained the capacity to refer to her after the moment when the joint analytic effort brought forth the shared recognition that she did not need to "imitate" herself and was allowed to feel what she felt. The patient recognized the defensive nature of her disaffected "I": "I wanted to be heard, to be known. I responded with a lifelong temper tantrum."

Conceptualization of the Sense of Identity: Conclusions

In view of the preceding considerations, I am now ready to draw my own conclusions about the sense of identity as the conscious, language-mediated, pronoun-mediated awareness of being a particular individual with unique characteristics. I agree with Loewald's conclusions: "The absolute validity of individual consciousness and will and their autonomy, in view of the knowledge we have gained of the unconscious and its fluid and permeable boundaries, is in serious doubt. Individuality and personal emancipation are no longer primary psychological facts for us, but resultants of a developmental process of uncertain outcome. . . . That I am, as an individual psychic entity, no longer can be taken for granted" (1984, pp. 174–175).

What I am and what is me can be described as today's slit of light between two unknowns: the unconscious and the world and its objects. The conviction we have about our sense of identity is based on the contextual experience of refinding aspects of our selves in the present-day situation. The feeling of identity finds its most intense power of conviction where self- and object representation, affect, and word form a unit of ego-syntonic meaning. To be oneself in this manner is always to be with another, either in life or in the inner world. It is in those moments that we experience a feeling of self-recognition, of inner wholeness, of personal unity, that permits us to say, "That is me," or, "I am I," as Salinas would say to his beloved. Those moments are rare in psychic life. Most of the time, we struggle to sort ourselves out while carrying a more obscure sense of knowing who we are. This sense of identity is the result of vastly complex memorial processes that include the chronicle of prevailing modes of relating to our historically more significant objects. Thus, a person can say with great conviction, "I am always the first to love," while another may conclude, "I am used to being loved. It always happens to me that way."

"Me" can never be spoken as a whole. Its complexities and historical roots cannot be fully grasped. The language of "me" is always metaphoric because it describes feelings and percepts with multiple referents. Patients say it well: "A part of me wants." They know that they cannot attend simultaneously to all aspects of themselves. The language of "I" has more precision. It does refer to the person who acts and speaks but says little about the motivation for the action. The man who falls in love does not know that in finding his beloved he is also refinding an early object. "Me" and "I" cannot be taken for granted. They always mean more than we know.

In conclusion, I propose that identity as conceptualized by Erikson and as it is frequently used in clinical theorizing is a vague descriptive concept without a specific referent. It has no technical or theoretical usefulness; it only adds confusion to our analytic terminology (Abend 1974). Clinically, accepting the description of "my identity" as explanatory may detract from the need to help the analysand be concrete about the recognition of aspects of himself or herself and about his or her own perceptions and feelings. The term "identity" can be accepted as a descriptive everyday word without specific theoretical connotations.

REFERENCES

Abend, S. 1974. Problems of identity: theoretical and clinical applications. *Psychoanalytic Quarterly* 43:606–637.

Blos, P. 1962. *On Adolescence: A Psychoanalytic Interpretation*. New York: Free Press.

Bollas, C. 1982. On the relation to the self as an object. *International Journal of Psycho-Analysis* 63:347–360.

Erikson, E. 1950. *Childhood and Society*. New York: Norton, 1963.

Erikson, E. 1959. *Identity and the Life Cycle*. Psychological Issues, vol. 1. New York: International Universities Press.

Freud, S. 1893–1895. Studies on hysteria. *Standard Edition* 2:3–305. London: Hogarth, 1955.

Freud, S. 1895. Project for a scientific psychology. *Standard Edition* 1:281–392. London: Hogarth, 1966.

Freud, S. 1900. *The interpretation of dreams. Standard Edition* 5:339–686. London: Hogarth, 1958.

Freud, S. 1915. The unconscious. *Standard Edition* 14:159–216. London: Hogarth, 1957.

Freud, S. 1923. The ego and the id. *Standard Edition* 19:1–59. London: Hogarth, 1961.

Hartmann, H. 1950. Comments on the psychoanalytic theory of the ego. In *Essays on Ego Psychology*. New York: International Universities Press, 1964.

Laplanche, J., and Pontalis, J.-B. 1973. *The Language of Psycho-Analysis*. New York: Norton.

Lichtenstein, H. 1961. Identity and sexuality: a study of their interrelationship in man. *Journal of the American Psychoanalytic Association* 9:131–142.

Lichtenstein, H. 1963. Dilemma of human identity: notes on self-transformation, self-objectification and metamorphosis. *Journal of the American Psychoanalytic Association* 11:172–223.

Lichtenstein, H. 1977. *The Dilemma of Human Identity*. New York: Aronson.

Litowitz, B. E., and Litowitz, N. S. 1983. Development of verbal self-expression. In A. Goldberg, ed. *The Future of Psychoanalysis.* New York: International Universities Press.

Loewald, H. 1984. Review of *The Selected Papers of Margaret Mahler. Journal of the American Psychoanalytic Association* 32:165–174.

Meissner, W. W. 1981. *Internalization in Psychoanalysis.* New York: International Universities Press.

Rizzuto, A.-M. 1988. Transference, language, and affect in the treatment of bulimarexia. *International Journal of Psycho-Analysis* 69:369–387.

Rizzuto, A.-M. 1990. The origins of Freud's concept of object representation ("Objektvorstellung") in his monograph "On Aphasia": its theoretical and technical importance. *International Journal of Psycho-Analysis* 71:241–248.

Salinas, P. 1940. *Truth of Two and Other Poems.* Baltimore: Johns Hopkins University Press.

Sharpless, E. A. 1985. Identity formation as reflected in the acquisition of personal pronouns. *Journal of the American Psychoanalytic Association* 33:861–885.

Simon, B. 1978. Review of *Dimensions of a New Identity: The 1973 Jefferson Lectures in the Humanities,* by E. Erikson. *Psychoanalytic Quarterly* 47:458–464.

Spruiell, V. 1981. The self and the ego. *Psychoanalytic Quarterly* 50:319–344.

Tulvig, E. 1972. Episodic and semantic memory. In E. Tulvig and W. Donalson, eds. *Organization of Memory.* New York: Academic.

Waugh, L. R. 1976. *Roman Jakobson's Science of Language.* Lisse, the Netherlands: de Ridder.

Winnicott, D. W. 1971. *Playing and Reality.* New York: Basic.

23 THE ADOLESCENT'S SARTORIAL DILEMMAS

ANA-MARIA RIZZUTO

Late adolescence is the moment of development when contemporary society expects an individual to fulfill certain tasks: to become independent of parents and to decide about fitting into one of the many social roles available. The young person has to declare sexual preference, class appertaining, select a way of earning a living, and make loyalties explicit. All this can no longer be done with words. It demands actions, integrated in the context of concrete situations. The decisions made at this point will provide lasting qualifiers for the individual: heterosexual, blue-collar worker, lower-middle class, Republican, Red Sox fan, nice-looking girl, etc.

These qualifiers reveal their personal meaning not in themselves but in connection with the inner context of previously experienced relations and ways of objectifying oneself. The inability to integrate whatever steps the adolescent takes into social life depends almost exclusively on the previously described sense of being a particular being and on the private narratives that give meaning to the vicissitudes of becoming such a being. The late adolescent's psychological task challenges self-definitions, identifications, and modes of relating to oneself, others, and the world. Yesterday's child has to wear adult shoes on equal footing with those who rule the universe.

Blos (1979) describes this transformation as "the second individuation process" in which "the developmental task . . . lies in the disengagement of libidinal and aggressive cathexes from the internalized infantile love and hate objects" (p. 179). I agree with Blos, but I prefer to describe key aspects of this second individuation task in a more concrete manner. The adolescent's task is to face again those early attachments and to tease out from them the contribution they make, through the power of the internal object, to the subjective elements we all employ to evaluate ourselves. These are the points of view of inner vision, voice, and self-judgment. The adolescent must try to find his or her own point of view, personal voice, and a personal style of self-judgment. Such a task requires an interplay between the internal transformational actions and the actual need for the real and internalized object, that is, a change of cathexis. A change of point of view implies that, where the feeling of being good or bad or having a certain characteristic depends on being seen by the object's eyes, it be replaced by the effort to look at oneself from one's own point of view, which must first be defined. A similar process is required for words. The inner voices of the internal objects need to be challenged to inquire if they are compatible with the adolescent's way of objectifying himself in the new context, as the *person in charge*.

Both processes, the acquisition of one's own internal vision of oneself and of an internal voice for self-reference, impose a very strenuous task on the young person. The new judgment, a superego function of a (secondary) narcissistic nature, aims at a subjective affirmation: "I see myself, I hear myself, and that is the way I am or I want to be." The adolescent must negotiate this new subjective perception with the old internal objects to obtain surrender of their internally felt view of him or her and of their voices to judge. The difficulty of the task is such that, as Blos points out, it may break the seams of the up-to-now contained sense of being oneself. If the task succeeds, the sense of self, of being a unique "me," obtains such powerful emotional value that it has to be defended at all costs. Its importance in giving meaning to life is so significant that death is preferable to losing that core sense of oneself, that voice won with such effort in the course of development. It goes beyond the concept of identity. It belongs to the notion of being, to the verb "to be," to existence itself. Perhaps this is what Shakespeare captured in Hamlet's immortal question, "To be or not to be?"

What the adolescent does not know in his passionate self-definition is that the task continues for as long as we live and cannot be completed. At each new turn in the spiral of life, we refind the old objects: their looks, their voices, their judgments, and, with them, old loves and hates. Once more, to refind and redefine ourselves, we have to go through the task of separating points of view, voices, and judgment to be able to say, "That is me," "That is not me."

The adolescent's process of separating the sense of self from the libidinal and aggressive attachments to the internalized objects completes, according to Blos (1979, p. 477), the resolution of hetero- and homosexual ties of the Oedipus complex. The reawakening of oedipal feelings, together with the intensification of sexual sensibilities, challenges the entirety of the adolescent's erotic life. The veiling and revelation of the sexually mature, socially significant body becomes an absorbing task. Fashion and clothing become the arena for a subjective, intrafamilial, and social discourse that goes without and beyond words. This discourse, the use of clothes and fashion in the process of differentiation from internal objects, their looking eyes, voices, and judgments, has been neglected in the literature. Clothing and bodily decoration are complex nonverbal languages to codify sex, age, class, and status in the social context and to regulate interpersonal messages about sexual and psychic closeness and distance. Clothes and decoration are signifiers of great subtlety, capable of revealing what is taboo to express in spoken words.

Clothes and grooming are well known as a critical battlefield between parents and adolescents. What is being fought on the sartorial field is who controls the messages given by the adolescent's clothes to the world, what clothing defines the body of the adolescent and who he is. The messages include assignments of sexual roles, sexual revealing or hiding, social status, appertaining to a particular group or clique, conformity or defiance, and, last but not least, attracting or repelling others. Each one of these functions of clothes and grooming may become a specific battle with the actual parents and with the internalized parental representation, be it to identify or to reject identification or both at the same time. A significant aspect of the battle is that the adolescent not only represents himself in his clothes but in a certain manner makes a statement about his parents, his family, his cultural group, by dressing one way or another. Peter Corrigan (1989), a sociologist from Dublin, has reported in a case study of an Irish mother her concerned opinions about what the dress of the older girl would reveal about her and her family if she were to wear a particular Christmas dress.

Shopping for clothes becomes an important personal task. The adolescent assumes responsibility for selecting and for rejecting available garments. Parents are no longer welcomed as shopping partners. The adolescent replaces them with peers as an overt signal that the young person's body no longer "belongs" to the parents. The body, as an object for decoration, is now presented as though it is located in the social space of the same age group. The adolescent, however, has one eye on the parents and the other eye on his peers and the fashions they propose. The task is to join the peers and separate from the parents. Present-day behavior, related to the industrial society offering a large variety of garments and objects of decoration, allows the adolescent to select from among a vast number of subtle sartorial messages. Most adolescents, however, choose to join a particular style, popular in the immediate surroundings, and follow it with obsessive dedication, attributing enormous meaning to each detail.

Adolescents, nowadays, seem to use clothes as a substitute for the absent social rites of initiation into adulthood. There is the same attention to the ritual of dressing and the taboos to be avoided as there has been in the past for tribal rituals of initiation. The difference is that the object tie offered by the community is mediated only by anonymous or high fashion adult designers, who have no direct involvement with the adolescent or the immediate group to which he or she is linked by personal ties. The adult master and mentor for the initiation rites is nowhere to be found. For our mass society, this is the ritual initiation into impersonal, vague, and diffuse sexual and role identifications mediated through media manipulation and its pervasive subliminal influence. Not much is to be regretted about the mode of initiation because it is compatible with the society the adolescent must adapt to.

A recent article in the trendy London monthly *Face* (reported in *World Press Review,* January 1990, p. 50) seems to support my point. It reports that "in the style capital of Africa—Kinshasa, Zaire—there exists a new religion. . . . Its disciples worship at the altar of high fashion. . . . Dressed to kill, they are the *sapeurs*." A Congolese sociologist concluded "that the subculture is a substitute for traditional initiation rites that have not survived in the city. Those who cannot dress well do not belong. Or as the local king of the sapeurs says, 'Those who can't be *sapeurs* we call them the living dead.' " American adolescents seem to have kept their tribal inclinations or their wish to be initiated into adulthood in their own compelling fashions. In both cases, the emotionally absent adult designer rules from a distance, deciding what the young person must wear to belong. It is a remarkably enlightening exercise to look at magazines where the fashion commandments are written for all of us. In the 1990s, a young male must look casual, distant, uninvolved, serenely holding his hands in his pockets while looking far away. His clothes, casual or formal, must be "simply elegant," while trying to convey the sense that he does not care much about them. A young woman must present herself as unisex, with pants, jackets, and sweaters conveying sportly casualness. Her clothes alternate between pointing directly at her genitals and breasts and hiding them under oversized garments. She too must appear distant, with wild hair, a cultivated simplicity, a low-key sensuality. This is what I found in my perusal of the March issue of several magazines. What the adolescents decide to do with it becomes now a matter of the encounter between personal psychodynamics, separation from the real and the internal parents, and the efforts to be integrated in present-day society.

The normally developing adolescent can negotiate with varied degrees of friction the multiplicity of issues involved in declaring and hiding a sexual body in front of the parents, conveying to them that they are no longer needed and very much needed while trying to negotiate similar issues with sexually interested peers. The normal fights about clothes and grooming provide an optimal ground to test one's own appearance and inner sense of self without having to declare publicly the concerns about bodily adequacy. They also permit adolescents to obtain disguised sexual gratification from parental figures while declaring them hopeless old-fashioned types who do not understand sartorial matters of urgent significance. Last, but not least, the adolescent experiences a need to create a sexual gap mediated by fashion between a sexually mature child and his or her parents. One of my male patients said it well: "My mother does not understand a thing about male clothes. They don't mean anything to her."

The troubled adolescent may use extreme measures to separate from excessive preoedipal or oedipal attachments to parents, by becoming slovenly, bizarre, and a misfit. To be ugly, dirty, and repulsive is a well-known defense against incest in adolescence, as illustrated by Perrault's story "Donky-skin" (1961), about a young princess who escapes her father's sexual proposals by wearing the skin of a donkey.

Other adolescents may need to go to the opposite extreme. Worried about their adequacy as independent beings and their maturing sexual bodies, they indulge in an excess of grooming and in an obsessive dedication to the slightest details of the latest fashion as a desperate effort to convince themselves that they are as grown up as they are supposed to be. They want to prove to themselves that they are capable of decoding the mysteries of being an adult and proclaim their conviction with a fanatic attention to sartorial detail. A critical comment about their grooming may bring their confidence tumbling down like a castle of cards.

There are many more observations to be made about the significance of clothing and grooming in adolescence, one of the areas in which the adolescent has to define his or her own sense of identity by acquiring a view of the body and a personal sartorial voice to declare social stance and convey sexual messages. The judgment that the adolescent is passing is, frequently, written in garments worn, hairstyle, and other details of grooming. Attending to the overt and subtle messages of the personal clothing system and helping the adolescent to decode and articulate this nonverbal language may prove a fruitful way of having access to otherwise neglected aspects of the historical components, of the sense of identity, the "I" and "me" of the moment. To get dressed, after all, is always to dress oneself, to package oneself for others with the hope that, by looking, they can find the person we want to show, our favorite public persona, inside the clothing. Dressing codes, however, have as many unconscious slips of the garment as spoken language has slips of the tongue. No one is capable of dressing carefully enough to hide the indiscretions of the unconscious.

Clinical Example:
Oedipal Competition and Sex Appeal

Mariela, a nineteen-year-old woman, came to psychotherapy because she had difficulties with being in college, apart from her family. She was lonely and socially awkward, feeling that men were not attracted to her and that she would never "make it." Her relationships with female classmates were restricted by the feeling that they had "something" that she did not, which permitted them to attract their male counterparts. She had retreated into artistic contemplation of nature and meditation as her way of feeling superior to those driven by carnal concerns.

When she came to the first hour, I noticed that she was slightly overweight and literally hidden under her clothes and hair. She informed me in the first few minutes that a man would never make love to a fat girl. That is the way men are. She had not had sexual relations because the only boyfriend she had in the past was not responsive to her. Everybody else she knew was having a sexual relation, but nobody wanted her. It became clear to me that she was involved in a complex dilemma of wanting to have sex and not wanting to have sex. She was quite attractive, blonde, tall, and articulate and had a good sense of humor.

After a few rather intense sessions, we put her dilemma into black and white: to sleep or not to sleep with a man. The next session she looked like a new person: her eyes were bright, her hair was pulled up, giving her a womanly look, her pants were tight, and she was wearing a top with a logo at the level of her breasts. This and the next few sessions were devoted to the history of love affairs in her family. Her mother and father had fallen in love head over heels at the age of twenty and had remained in love ever since. The paternal grandparents had a similar story. Both narratives were legend in the family. She told the stories with great excitement and after some hesitation conveyed her suspicion that the parents had had a wonderful premarital sexual experience and had conceived her, their first child, out of wedlock. She considered such a possibility an exciting event, a proof of their passionate sexual love, but confessed that she had never had the courage to ask her parents about it.

The drift of the conversation focused on what an exciting story a love such as her parents' makes for the next generation. We then discovered that she wanted her first sexual experience to be just like her mother's, an earthshaking, life-lasting, story-making type of affair that she could tell with equal excitement to her children! We calculated that she was living her potential first sexual affair in the year 2005 when she could tell her children about it.

Several sessions later, after much talking, she became aware that she did not want to have sex with a man who would not provide the conditions for the love tale. No man she knew qualified. She returned to the baggy clothes, and the hair veiled her face once more. After much work about the oedipal rivalry with the mother and the deidealization of what the first act of intercourse had to be like, she began to see that she could have a personal and sexual relation that was less than a fairy tale for the next century. Her clothes and looks changed again. The hair went up once more, and she declared that she had noticed that fat girls have boyfriends too. Her mother, however, had always been slender and very good looking. Mariela went shopping and bought expensive, elegant clothes (like her mother's), following the fashion of the day. For the first time, she wore a pendant. Two weeks later, she had a boyfriend, with whom she made out for the first time in her life. Her first action after the event was to call up her mother to say that she had a boyfriend. The mother approved and repeated some portion of her own love story.

The relation with the boyfriend did not last. He sensed her driven need to get him to enact some relational event (identification with the mythical images of the grandmother and the mother) that he did not understand, and he gently pulled out of the relationship. She had no time to mourn. The rejection prompted her to refuse to reenact the family tradition. She decided that she was going to be involved in a sexual relation with a man as her peers were (a new identification with her equals). She talked now about the need to accept the man and the relation he offered not so much as she dreamed it but as it could evolve. Her posture changed. She was now walking tall, with bright eyes and a newly acquired sense of "this is me" and "I don't have to be like the others in my family." Her clothes enhanced her figure, and her carriage advertised that she was available. Two months later, she became involved with a classmate, and in a few weeks they were engaged in a quiet, by no means spectacular, personal and sexual relationship. She concluded, "Now I am like the other girls. I did not have to be like my mother and grandmother." Her clothes had silently narrated her evolution from avoidance of an impossibly idealized sexual encounter, to a rejection of her mythical family role, to a partial identification with her mother as a well-dressed, appealing, sexual woman, to end in describing her personal way of being sexual in the way her peers were.

REFERENCES

Corrigan, P. 1989. Troublesome bodies and sartorial dopes: motherly accounts of teenage daughter dress practices. *Semiotica* 77:369–392.

Blos, P. 1979. *The Adolescent Passage: Developmental Issues.* New York: International Universities Press.

Perrault, C. 1961. *Perrault's Complete Fairy Tales.* New York: Dodd, Mead.

24   BEYOND IDENTITY: INVENTION, ABSORPTION, AND TRANSCENDENCE

CHARLES P. FISHER

I have two aims in presenting this chapter. The first is to honor the work of Erik Erikson—in particular his development and application of the concepts of identity, identity crisis, and identity diffusion. My second aim is to describe some areas in which it is useful to ask, What is beyond identity? I accept this concept of identity as a useful one, provided that we understand what it does *not* do.

Erikson and some of his coworkers, including Emanuel Windholz and Joseph Wheelwright, first used the term "identity crisis" to describe the plight of certain World War II soldiers seen at the Mount Zion Veterans Rehabilitation Clinic (Erikson 1968). These soldiers returned from war having lost "a sense of personal sameness and historical continuity." As we know, Erikson later developed the term to describe a normative crisis of late adolescence and young adulthood, leading to the consolidation of identity or the peril of role confusion. "Identity diffusion" describes a condition, which may be mild or malignant, in which the individual has lost a sense of inner coherence and experiences confusion about sexual, social, and cultural roles. In contrast to the painful difficulties of identity crisis and identity diffusion, Erikson uses uplifting language to describe identity formation as "an evolving configuration—a configuration which is gradually established by successive ego synthesis and resynthesis throughout childhood. It is a configuration gradually integrating constitutional givens, idiosyncratic libidinal needs, favored capacities, significant identifications, effective defenses, successful sublimations, and consistent roles" (1968, p. 163). This integration sounds so comprehensive that it is easy to take for granted—and it may seem presumptuous to ask what lies beyond it. To do so, I will borrow a method used often by Erikson—that of considering the question within the context of another culture.

The people of the Luwu District on the Indonesian island of Sulawesi maintain a complex and hierarchical society that has been strongly influenced by Buddhist and Hindu religious traditions. The elite of this society are a highly philosophical and intellectual group. One of their major concerns is the effort to obtain a "clean soul" by overcoming *pamrih*. The concept of *pamrih* refers to "the distortions of perception and affect that a person brings to [interpersonal] situations due to his prejudices and attachments to previous situations that may be irrelevant to what is at hand" (Errington 1988; see also Errington 1989). *Pamrih* is what we would call transference. Overcoming it is not only a spiritual and psychological matter but in Luwu is also considered to be essential for proper behavior, particularly for leadership.

In order to overcome *pamrih,* these people practice a form of meditation that bears certain resemblances to psychoanalysis. Its technique resembles free association, and its immediate aim of visualizing and rehearsing emotion-laden situations corresponds to working through. Interpretation must be supplied by the meditator himself. Full affective experience is considered highly desirable in order to facilitate awareness, understanding, and mental rehearsal or visualization.

In contrast to psychoanalysis, the goal of this meditation is the dissolution of all attachment, insofar as possible. Nonattachment means not withdrawal from social life or relationships with loved ones but rather the effort to disinvest oneself from all of the unique and idiosyncratic configurations that we think of as constituting personal identity. Identity is thus equated with *pamrih,* as an impediment to obtaining a clean soul and as an obstacle to the clear and careful consideration of new situations. In Luwu, personal identity is seen as an impediment to emotional growth. I propose that we ask ourselves whether there are comparable ideas anywhere within our own tradition.

In fact, we do not have to look very far to find such ideas, or ones that are closely related. Erikson himself has pointed out a variety of ways in which it is important to look beyond identity. Before detailing his ideas on this topic, I quote two of the various definitions of identity that he has offered. In *Childhood and Society* (Erikson 1950, p. 261), he spoke of identity as "the accrued confidence that the inner sameness and continuity prepared in the past are matched by the sameness and continuity of one's meaning for others, as evidenced in the tangible promise of a 'career.' " Some years later (Erikson 1968, p. 22), he described identity as "a process 'located' in the core of the individual and yet also in the core of his communal culture, a process which establishes, in fact, the identity of those two identities." These definitions are social as well as psychological ones. Note that, in the first definition, a social dimension is enfolded within a psychological construct. Identity is *the accrued confidence* (psychological) of a match between one's inner sameness and the sameness and continuity of one's meaning for others (social). If one's meaning for others changes, what happens to one's identity? Rapid social change within one's environment or emigration to another society can be accompanied by profound shifts in this kind of identity. I am not saying that inner character change can occur so simply. I am saying that identity is not the same thing as character and that identity as described by Erikson can sometimes change quickly. Because identity is in part a social phenomenon, we usually cooperate with one another to confirm, support, and mutually acknowledge each other's ongoing sameness. But this need not always be the case. The fact that identity can be reinforced or dislocated by social factors is one implication of Erikson's definition.

I turn now to some of the ways in which Erikson himself has indicated that it is important to look beyond identity. An obvious example is his use of the term "beyond identity" to refer to phases of the life cycle past late adolescence. He describes crises of intimacy versus isolation, generativity versus stagnation, and integrity versus despair in connection with early adulthood, mid-adulthood, and old age. If all goes well, these crises lead to the virtues of love, care, and wisdom (Erikson 1982, pp. 32–33).

In his clinical writing, Erikson describes an "identity resistance" (Erikson 1959, p. 135; Erikson 1968, p. 214), which consists of the patient's fear of losing his or her own identity and having it replaced by that of the analyst. This description points to the possibility that, under some circumstances, one's identity and one's attachment to it may be an impediment to emotional growth and change. This is close to the Luwu idea.

Erikson has described a related idea in a social context. He has spoken and written passionately about the notion that individuals in different nations and religious and ethnic communities may lose sight of their common humanity. He introduced the term "pseudo-speciation" to refer to this phenomenon (1968, p. 41). To the extent that identity is a social as well as a personal concept, it reflects attachment to a particular economic and cultural role "at the expense of the denial of major aspects of existence." This aspect of identity promotes pseudo-speciation. Erikson referred to this feature of identity as an "inner arrest" (1970, p. 758).

Most significantly, identity itself is a kind of illusion, albeit a useful one. Erikson speaks of identity as entailing the adult's ability to "selectively reconstruct his past in such a way that, step by step, it seems to have planned him, or better, he seems to have planned *it*" (1958, p. 112). He adds, "Psychologically we *do* choose our parents, our family histories, and the history of our kings, heroes, and gods." From this point of view, identity involves both the illusion of freely choosing what we have in fact been given without alternative and the even greater illusion of having caused the events that shaped us. This reinvented past is a useful tool for coping with life, but it is also quite plainly a "personal myth," of the kind described by Ernst Kris (1956). The late adolescent must reinvent his past in order to take responsibility for himself and for his life. But such an invention is a creative act, not an act of discovery. It is a myth in the sense of a useful and organizing narrative, and it is potentially deceptive when it confuses the creation of serviceable stories and metaphors with the observation of facts. I do not mean to suggest that historical truth cannot be discovered—through psychoanalysis, or in other ways. I mean that identity—insofar as it presents a single and coherent story that seems to lead inevitably to the individual as he is at the present moment—is in the realm of myth. I am not sure whether Erikson understands it this way as well, but he has gone so far as to state that "there are 'pseudo' aspects in all identity which endanger the individual" (1968, p. 42). In the same passage, he speaks eloquently of enabling "the individual to *transcend* his *identity*—to become as truly individual as he will ever be, and as truly beyond all individuality."

Despite the fact that identity concepts are quite central to Erikson's work, he speaks of stages of the life cycle beyond identity, of an identity resistance, of pseudo-speciation as reflecting one way in which identity may become an "inner arrest," of identity as a creative reorganization of the past, and of the need to transcend identity to find and

451

pass beyond individuality. It would be hard for the philosophers of Luwu to ask for more. And yet there *is* more.

If we remove the explicitly social aspects of Erikson's definitions of identity, some important phrases are left: "the inner sameness and continuity prepared in the past" and "a process 'located' in the core of the individual." But, if we look more closely at these concepts, the sameness and continuity at the core of the individual's experience of self turn out to have a somewhat illusory quality as well. While aspects of a person's character are stable, *experiences* of self have an evanescent and ever-changing quality. Instead of simple continuity and sameness, we find a fluid interplay among self- and object representations. When we look past the stabilizing social aspects of identity to what is within a person, we find constantly changing configurations of inner experience involving fantasies, identifications, memories, wishes, and affects—all tied to a repertoire of inner characters derived from past and present relationships, both actual and imagined. This changing inner scene is evoked nicely by Joyce McDougall's (1985) metaphor "the theater of the mind."

Erik Erikson has addressed this inner diversity in his sketch of the internal structure of identity. He describes "the sense of 'I' that is the individual's central awareness of being a sensory and thinking creature endowed with language, who can confront a self (composed, in fact, of a number of selves)" (1982, p. 85). This confrontation between "I" and self is the basis of identity (1982, p. 73). "The self" that Erikson describes is composed of a number of selves. But his concept of identity portrays these multiple selves—or identifications—as organized into a stable configuration like atoms that make up a molecule. In McDougall's metaphor, our inner selves move about as freely as characters on a stage. While a sense of identity seems to be a highly valued aspect of the way people conceptualize themselves, it is the theater metaphor that more accurately captures the way people experience themselves. I now provide some examples, beginning with some experiences of people in groups.

Consider the concept of inspiration. An inspiring speaker or performer not only engages an audience in an interpersonal way but also evokes a special kind of internal dialogue within each audience member. The individual who is inspired experiences a complex and vivid inner sense of being better, nobler, more energetic, or more tranquil than she usually feels herself to be. The experience is like discovering a new character within oneself—one that is familiar in some ways but wonderfully transformed in others. The person who is inspired unconsciously constructs a new version of herself, using familiar bits and pieces—and then consciously steps back and admires it. A significant part of this response is a sense of pleasant surprise—"I didn't know I had it in me." What I wish to emphasize is the sense of surprise about a change in one's self-experience.

One could equally well describe examples that are very different in tone—the transformations experienced by individuals in an unruly mob or, for that matter, in a small unstructured group such as a Tavistock group. A clinical example might be seen in a therapist's experience of countertransference irritation, anger, or rage in response to a patient's projective identification. In these experiences, we surprise ourselves when we discover what we are capable of. This experience of surprise implies that we are not simply experiencing strong feelings but rather encountering ourselves in unfamiliar ways and thereby creating new internal relationships.

If this is the case, then a sense of identity, defined as inner sameness and continuity, is like a snapshot of a system that is in constant motion. It captures features that are characteristic and familiar but creates an illusion that we are organized in a more static way than we really are.

Some related ideas appear in contemporary cognitive science. There is considerable evidence (Baars 1988) that our minds function as parallel processors in many ways. This simply means that we carry out many thought processes at the same time or in parallel rather than sequentially. Most of this parallel processing is unconscious. In fact, while human consciousness has a very powerful effect, it is quite limited in its scope. We are able to be conscious of only a few things at a time. This limited span of consciousness is a feature of cognition that is quite distinct from the concept of a dynamic unconscious, with its implication that certain thoughts and feelings are excluded from awareness altogether. When I speak of a limited span of consciousness, I am referring to the size of the window through which we may peek into our own minds. While consciousness is a narrow span, unconscious thought is vast in its scope, involving multiple processes that go forward in ways that are parallel, complementary, contradictory, or essentially unrelated. Because we look through a small window into a highly complex inner world, seeing only a bit at a time, we tend to minimize how complex, contradictory, and fluid we actually are. Thus, the illusion of a relatively static organization of the mind is made possible by an artifact of consciousness.

Identity is thus a historical myth, in that it reinvents the past in a creative and useful way, and also a kind of structural illusion, in that it emphasizes inner consistency and stability above variety, contradictoriness, and change. It is an important, perhaps an essential conceptual tool for the late adolescent and often for the adult, but, in many circumstances, it is to our great advantage to move beyond it by detaching ourselves from static self-concepts.

I turn now to some examples of ways in which we make good use of our capacities to experience ourselves in novel ways. A rather obvious one is the process of psychoanalysis. Both the patient's free association and the analyst's free-floating attention reflect processes of detachment from ordinary identity and thought. In the patient's role, the purpose of this detachment is to experience thoughts and feelings that are ordinarily rejected from awareness. In the analyst's role, the purpose of this detachment is to attune oneself to another person.

Invention, or creativity, provides another category of examples. It is well known that artists may describe experiences in which creative work seems to come from outside themselves. A writer friend describes creating characters who then seem to act on their own to carry forward a plot. These seemingly spontaneous events reflect the creative person's ability to give voice or shape to inner characters that are not part of his usual personal identity. Phyllis Greenacre has written on this theme: "Every artist is at least two people, the personally oriented self and the artistic one. The relationship between these two (or more) people in one body varies enormously. Sometimes they are on good speaking terms with each other; sometimes the identities are relatively separate and in extreme cases may be quite dissociated one from the other" (1958, p. 528). This striking passage, from a paper entitled "The Relation of the Impostor to the Artist," conveys the notion of the artist's successful use of a certain fluidity of self-concept. In "Creative Writers and Day-Dreaming" (1908, p. 150), Freud described this process in quite active terms, referring to the writer's ability "to split up his ego, by self-observation, into many part-egos, and, in consequence to personify the conflicting currents of his own mental life in several heroes."

While artists and writers have a special ability to make images and characters come to life, similar processes occur in most people's dreams. A patient reported a dream in which he encountered a clever friend who told a story that was both amusing and wise. In the dream, the patient had appreciated the story and had also had the thought, "I could never think up a story like that! It's hard to understand how anyone is able to do that." In the morning, the patient enjoyed the sudden realization that he *had* in fact concocted the amusing and wise story in the dream. However, he could not overcome the feeling that the story had *seemed* to come from somewhere outside himself. This rather frequent occurrence in dreams illustrates what I take to be a fundamental property of the human mind—the ability to substitute object representations for self-representations freely, and vice versa. This ability is reflected in defenses such as projection, introjection, identification, and turning passive into active. It appears in the dream I just mentioned when the dreamer experiences a part of himself as foreign and intrudes into waking life when he reclaims only a portion of what had been projected in the dream. The ability to take subject as object and object as subject, in relation to any of a large number of wishes and fears, imparts a highly variable quality to the individual's experience of himself—a variability that is employed and expressed in the ordinary creativity of dreams and the extraordinary creativity of the artist.

A slightly more complex version of this theme of variable self- and object representations appeared in a dream reported by another patient, Mr. K., who had recently become the father of a young son. In the dream, Mr. K. experienced himself as a spectator in a gallery. Onstage, in the dream, he observed two men—one a young man who performed an amazing sexual feat, the other an old man who was no longer the man he once had been. All three characters—the spectator, the young man, and the old man—represented the patient. In the manifest dream, he identified himself with the spectator. In associating to the dream, he implicitly identified with the young man whose stunning performance was witnessed by his elderly father. At the same time, he defended against seeing himself as an "old man" who was now being upstaged by an infant son. As the patient told me his dream and his ideas about it, it was clear that I played a maternal role in the transference. As analysts and therapists, we are quite familiar with dreams like this that involve multiple self-representations, contradictory roles, and reversals. I mention it here to call attention to the complex internal relationships and shifting experiences of self that occur in such a dream and that persist unconsciously in waking life.

The state of absorption provides another example in which day-to-day identity is left behind. In a collection of essays entitled *Actual Minds, Possible Worlds* (1986), Jerome Bruner approaches literature by inquiring "how and in what ways the text affects the reader," seeking to "provide an account of the processes of reading and of entering a story" (p. 4). Bruner describes the process of reading fiction as one in which the reader "must write for himself what he intends to do with the actual text" (p. 24). So the reader "receives [a narrative] . . . by composing it." "Literary texts initiate '*performance of meaning*' " in the minds of readers. That is, the reader "performs" the meaning of the text by way of shifting imaginative identifications with the characters, the narrator, and the author and with inner characters who are carried within the unconscious mind of the reader. Once again, this is possible because of the reader's ability to experience himself in an altogether novel way, if only temporarily.

Bruner goes on to describe some of the ways in which skillful writers work—for example, various techniques for triggering presupposition in the mind of the reader. These techniques work because of the reader's ability to decompose his own identity so as to find some aspect of himself that is capable of entering the fictional world.

Such literary adventures can have enduring effects. Jay Martin, a psychoanalyst and literary scholar, has written a book entitled *Who Am I This Time? Uncovering the Fictive Personality* (1988), which describes the effects of fictions, including literary fictions, on individuals' lives, demonstrating that identifications with fictional characters can revise and enrich one's inner repertoire of self- and object images. This seems to have been the case with a late-middle-aged patient in my practice, a man who grew up in a tiny and rather backward town in rural California, the only child of a coarse and foul-mouthed mother and an immigrant father with a very limited education. I was unable to understand how he became the rather thoughtful and well-spoken person I saw in my office until I learned about his intense involvement with Shakespeare during his adolescence. His early fascination with Shakespearian texts, and particularly with phonograph recordings of the plays and sonnets, had evolved into a brief career as an actor specializing in Shakespeare. Many years later, he could still quote extensively from the plays, and, in times of emotional distress, he recited favorite passages to himself and sometimes to me. An identification with Shakespeare himself, symbolized by my patient's ability to reproduce the words of Shakespeare's characters, provided my patient with an image of a person who had risen above obscure origins to create original work. For my patient, who had quite serious difficulties, becoming his own man seemed so daunting a project that it compared in scope and difficulty to the creative work of Shakespeare. It seemed to him—and with some reason, given his early relationship with his mother—that only a man of extraordinary inner resources and determination could escape from endless repetitions of the primary relationship. No less a figure than Shakespeare would suffice for the task. For my patient, then, his adolescent fascination with Shakespeare was a serious, even desperate, effort to absorb needed qualities into himself, in contrast with the more playful states of absorption that characterize most people's relationships with literature and art.

Finally, I take up the issue of what can be meant, concretely, by the idea of transcending one's identity. A late adolescent, Mr. G., began seeing me in a state of considerable agitation. His father had died in a car accident approximately a year earlier. His mother, who had been driving at the time, had been injured but was now in good physical health. Mr. G. blamed her for causing his father's death and also criticized her for *saying* that he blamed her since he had never told her that. An older brother had recommended that Mr. G. seek therapy because of his agitation and difficulty in concentrating on his studies in his junior year of college. Mr. G.'s mother agreed to pay for his treatment. In his initial hours with me, he cried almost continuously about his father's death. He was surprised to find that the anniversary of the death was almost as painful as the event itself had been.

Within a few weeks of beginning treatment, Mr. G. decided to take the following year off from school in hopes of regaining his equanimity somewhat before completing his degree and applying to graduate schools. He obtained a very desirable scientific job—a kind of internship position—in a field closely related to his studies. For the first time in his life, he supported himself on his own salary, except for the fact that his mother sent him money with which to pay for therapy. This was necessary because his salary was quite modest. I neither supported nor opposed this plan of his, but, while the arrangements were being made, I pointed out on several occasions that he seemed afraid to confront the issue of how and whether he would be able to pay for therapy. With some anxiety, he brought himself to discuss the issue first with me and then with his mother, asking her to continue to send him the money for therapy, although he was otherwise self-supporting. He predicted rather fearfully that she would use this issue to try to control him. By this time, he felt that the therapy was very important to him. He also felt that attempting to pay for it himself on a salary that barely covered living expenses would result in a fee so low as to be rather unfair to me. It was with these considerations in mind that he brought himself to ask for his mother's help despite his fears.

As a matter of fact, she did use the money as a means of controlling him in a variety of small ways. Invariably, her check to him was late, and he had to ask for it. She often procrastinated or forgot to send it for some time, until various conditions were met. Mr. G. became angrier and angrier at his mother for these conditions. I pointed out that he was also angry at me for presenting bills and discussing them with him. This configuration reproduced Mr. G.'s conscious anger at his mother for depriving him of his father and his unconscious anger at his father for having allowed his mother to drive the car despite her poor driving record.

In response to my interpretations, Mr. G. became more aware of his anger toward his father and seemed to proceed through a mourning process. He became closer to his girlfriend and asked her to move in with him. This created a new crisis, in that Mr. G. felt sure that his mother would strongly object to his new living arrangements. He anticipated that she would respond by refusing to pay for therapy any longer. He believed that he could conceal the new arrangement from his mother, but he resented the notion that his mother would withhold her assistance from him if he told her the truth. He also felt proud of his deepening relationship with his girlfriend and wanted to announce it to his entire family.

As he made plans for a holiday visit to his mother, Mr. G. implicitly invited me to tell him what he ought to do. I said that I thought he was concerned about what we would do about therapy and the fee if his mother were to withdraw her financial help. He readily agreed that this was the issue and turned to me again. I said that I thought we should continue meeting, with the understanding that the fee would depend on what he could afford. He then said that he thought it was most likely that his mother would angrily withdraw her support for a while and then resume giving it later.

With this, there seemed to be a marked change in Mr. G.'s perspective. In place of fear and resentment, he seemed to feel confidence and courage. His time perspective shifted from the immediate to the long term. He composed a letter to his mother, which he sent prior to his visit. As he read the letter to me, I experienced a feeling of awe. The letter was stunning in its eloquence and simplicity. It seemed to have been written by someone I had never met. He described the situation from a point of view that seemed to take all sides into account— making contact with the needs and wishes of both generations and both sexes involved in a complex problem. Without being entirely explicit, the letter reflected an appreciation of his mother's values and of her need to be in control of something following the loss of her husband. At the same time, the letter conveyed a sense of his own needs and values, including his respect and love for his girlfriend and an appreciation of his therapy with me.

While Mr. G.'s courage and perspective were derived in part from a temporary identification with me, his response so far surpassed anything I anticipated that something more had to be at work. I believe that the "more" involved Mr. G.'s temporarily transcending the limitations of his personal identity in a way that enabled him to empathize both evenly and in depth with all of the parties to a conflict. One might describe the turning point in this vignette as an identity crisis of late adolescence—a point of discontinuity resulting from a significant decision, a reorganization resulting in a new identity. Such language places these events within a context of ordinary processes of identity and identity formation. But, if this is the case, then the ordinary processes of identity formation and reorganization in late adolescence involve episodes in which the adolescent transcends the level of personal identity. The same may be true in later developmental phases as well.

In the case of Mr. G., the episode of transcendence, which seemed so dramatic to me, may have been augmented by an identification with an idealized image of his dead father and perhaps with an "external" point of view. But I would propose that this is a particularly lucid instance of a way in which adolescents and adults acquire and express values beyond identity.

REFERENCES

Baars, B. 1988. *A Cognitive Theory of Consciousness*. Cambridge: Cambridge University Press.

459

Bruner, J. S. 1986. *Actual Minds, Possible Worlds*. Cambridge, Mass.: Harvard University Press.

Erikson, E. 1950. *Childhood and Society*. New York: Norton, 1963.

Erikson, E. 1958. *Young Man Luther*. New York: Norton.

Erikson, E. 1959. Identity and the life cycle. *Psychological Issues* 1:1–171.

Erikson, E. 1968. *Identity, Youth, and Crisis*. New York: Norton.

Erikson, E. 1970. Autobiographic notes on the identity crisis. *Daedalus* 99(4): 730–759.

Erikson, F. 1982. *The Life Cycle Completed*. New York: Norton.

Errington, S. 1988. Meditation in Luwu. Typescript.

Errington, S. 1989. *Meaning and Power in a Southeast Asian Realm*. Princeton, N.J.: Princeton University Press.

Freud, S. 1908. Creative writers and day-dreaming. *Standard Edition* 9:141–153. London: Hogarth, 1959.

Greenacre, P. 1958. The relation of the imposter to the artist. *Psychoanalytic Study of the Child* 13:521–540.

Kris, E. 1956. The personal myth: a problem in psychoanalytic technique. *Journal of the American Psychoanalytic Association* 4:653–681.

McDougall, J. 1985. *Theatres of the Mind: Illusion and Truth on the Psychoanalytic Stage*. New York: Basic.

Martin, J. 1988. *Who Am I This Time? Uncovering the Fictive Personality*. New York: Norton.

PART V

ADOLESCENT
SUBSTANCE
ABUSE

EDITOR'S INTRODUCTION

HARVEY A. HOROWITZ

This section contains four chapters that are the first reports from an ongoing adolescent psychopathology research project at the Institute of Pennsylvania Hospital. The project is studying hospitalized adolescents from the perspective of developmental psychopathology, that is, from the perspective that current symptomatology and maladaptive behavior patterns may be understood as the organization and expression of a complex of biological and psychosocial risk factors. Among the contributing factors identified for analysis within this project are (1) early relational experiences and their internalizations, (2) cognitive development and its sequelae, and (3) patterns of family interaction as manifested in the practicing family.

In the four chapters to follow, the authors focus on a sample of hospitalized adolescents with comorbid substance abuse disorders and another major psychiatric disorder. The first chapter presents data that suggest that there is stability to the pattern of comorbidity in adolescence among substance abuse, conduct, and mood disorders. The authors propose a model of the pathogenesis of this comorbidity that rests on the centrality of the development of self-regulation in the first three years. In this model, comorbid conditions and their behavioral symptomatology—affective instability, impulsivity, and nonreflectivity—are seen as the manifestation of a disorder of self-regulation of affect, behavior, and cognition.

The second chapter focuses on the internal world of the comorbid adolescent, the domain of the organization of subjective experience. Using a methodology grounded in attachment theory, a sample of dually diagnosed adolescents was given a semistructured interview and a resultant attachment classification. This classification is thought to reflect what Bowlby called internal working models of self and other (primary caregiver). The possible relations of this attachment classification as a reflection of organization of subjectivity and clinical patterns of dysregulation of affect, behavior, and cognition are then explored.

The third chapter looks at the family as a primary regulatory context in adolescence and describes a methodology for investigating the regulatory functioning of the families of comorbid adolescents. The authors discuss the methodological issues presented by family and adolescent research conducted from a developmental perspective where two theoretical positions and designs need to be included. These two theoretical views construct two families, what David Reiss has called the represented or internalized family and the practicing or interactive family.

It is suggested by the authors that a research strategy that investigates the connections between attachment, cognition, family interaction, and individual psychopathology will also begin to clarify the relationship of practicing and represented aspects of family process, particularly of regulatory processes. In presenting a protocol for the investigation of the practicing family of comorbid adolescents, the project moves toward an understanding of the relation between the family's and the adolescent's regulatory competence.

The fourth chapter looks at cognitive development and how a particular form of thinking, formal operational thought, may play a role in regulating the affect and behavior of the adolescent. Following a brief review of the ontogenesis of formal or reflective thought and its effects on adolescent thinking, the authors look at formal operational thought and self-regulation. Particular attention is paid to the development of the "observing ego" and how the emergence of reflective thought provides the adolescent with a greater capacity to contain affects and impulses, to reflect and then to act. It is emphasized that the acquisition of reflective thought makes personality change possible during adolescence by providing for reflection on existing internal working models of relationship, which guide affect regulation, and by providing for the renegotiation of the adolescent's status within the family context.

25 COMORBID ADOLESCENT SUBSTANCE ABUSE: A MALADAPTIVE PATTERN OF SELF-REGULATION

HARVEY A. HOROWITZ, WILLIS F. OVERTON, DIANA ROSENSTEIN, AND JOHN H. STEIDL

Psychiatric comorbidity—the coexistence of major psychiatric disorders and syndromes and the cooccurrence of their symptoms—has recently emerged as a focus of substantial empirical research and a topic of fundamental clinical and theoretical importance. The phenomenon has been extensively studied in clinical samples of adults where affective and anxiety disorders are commonly found to coexist (Maser and Cloninger 1990). In clinical populations of children and adolescents, affective disorders, conduct disorders, and substance-abuse disorders are reported to occur together (Bailey 1989; Bukstein, Brent, and Kaminer 1989).

The emergence of the phenomenon of comorbidity is a reflection of change in our system of classification. Unlike its predecessors, DSM-III-R (American Psychiatric Association 1987) rejects the basic assumption that mental disorders are discrete, discontinuous, and mutually exclusive; rejects the use of exclusionary hierarchical rules; and encourages the clinician to "give multiple diagnoses where multiple syndromes occur together in one episode of illness" (p. xxiv). These modifications not only represent change in classification system and nosologic practice but, more important, reflect a critical reexamination

The authors wish to express appreciation to the members of the Epistemology, Development, and Psychotherapy Seminar at the Institute of Pennsylvania Hospital, where many of the ideas in this chapter were first expressed and worked through.

of our underlying theories of psychopathology, particularly the dominant Kraepelinian biomedical view of discrete disease entities linked to biological etiologies in simple linear causal chains. Psychiatric comorbidity calls for a theoretical model of psychopathogenesis that can accommodate the greater complexity of circular causality, common vulnerability, and multiple interactive risk factors as well as accounting for the overlap and commonality of the clinical presentation of comorbid conditions.

While psychiatric comorbidity raises these fundamental questions concerning our theories of psychopathology, the available data indicate that the coexistence of psychiatric syndromes is neither random nor artifactual. In reviewing the literature and reporting their findings from the Washington University Clinic Study, Cloninger, Martin, Guze, and Clayton (1990) maintain that certain syndromes and symptoms tend to occur in particular and predictable patterns in the same individuals and in the same families. For example, in clinical populations of adults with chronic anxiety disorders, there is a significant risk of secondary depression, while patients with antisocial personality disorders infrequently present depressive or anxiety syndromes. Cloninger concludes that psychiatric comorbidity has a stable empirical structure.

Empirical stability has also been reported in studies of conduct and affective disorders in children and adolescents. In a study of major depression in a clinical sample of forty-three prepubertal boys referred for outpatient psychopharmacologic treatment, Puig-Antich (1989) found that one-third also fit criteria for conduct disorder. In a study of comorbidity in a sample of hospitalized children and adolescents, Woolston, Rosenthal, Riddle, Sparrow, Cicchetti, and Zimmerman (1989) reported greater than 50 percent prevalence of both anxiety/affective disorders and behavior disorders.

The comorbidity of substance abuse and other psychiatric disorders in adolescents shows stability despite greater diagnostic variability and clinical heterogeneity. Empirical research reviewed by Bailey (1989) and by Bukstein et al. (1989) suggests a major role for substance abuse in the pathogenesis of affective disorders, anxiety disorders, and the behavior disorders, including conduct disorder, antisocial personality disorder, and attention deficit hyperactivity disorder. Conversely, this same spectrum of psychiatric disorders appears to contribute to increased vulnerability to and risk of substance-abuse disorder in adoles-

TABLE 1

PATTERNS OF COMORBID SUBSTANCE ABUSE IN A SAMPLE OF EIGHTY-FOUR
HOSPITALIZED ADOLESCENTS

	AFF + SA	CD + SA	CD + AFF + SA	SA + Other	N
Female.........	18	2	7	2	29
Male............	16	16	18	5	55
Total...........	34	18	25	7	84
	(40)	(21)	(30)	(8)	

NOTE.—AFF = affective disorder; CD = conduct disorder; SA = substance-abuse
disorder; Other = schizoaffective disorder (3) and Axis II personality disorders (4).
Numbers in parentheses are percentages.

cents. Results from our sample of eighty-four hospitalized adolescents
with comorbid substance abuse (summarized in table 1) are consistent
with these reports and confirm a general pattern of comorbidity. This
general pattern of comorbidity includes four groups: (1) coexisting conduct disorder and substance abuse (21 percent); (2) coexisting affective
disorder and substance abuse (40 percent); (3) coexisting affective,
conduct, and substance-abuse disorders (50 percent); (4) substance
abuse coexisting with either Axis II personality disorders or schizoaffective disorder.

Despite these diagnostic distinctions, the population of comorbid
adolescents in our study presents with a commonality of symptoms
and a consistent pattern of maladaptive behaviors (summarized in table
2). This presentation features a clinical triad of affective instability,
behavioral impulsivity, and cognitive nonreflectivity. This triad is more
fully described as (1) affective instability, with two typical forms characterized by (a) liability of affect with frequent sudden, intense, and
reactive changes in mood and affect, most commonly depression, agitation, and anger, or (b) volatility of affect, with less frequent but
highly reactive episodes of explosive anger and rage associated with
shame, frustration, deprivation, and a perceived threat of loss of control, cohesion, connection, or esteem; (2) behavioral impulsivity and
"acting out," including delinquency, noncompliance, hyperaggressiveness, hypersexuality, hyperactivity and recklessness, social intru-
siveness, and self-destructiveness; (3) cognition compromised by nonreflectivity, egocentrism, globality, poor judgment, and immature,
externalizing defenses.

Impressed with the related phenomena of stability in the structure

467

TABLE 2
CLINICAL PRESENTATION OF COMORBID ADOLESCENT SUBSTANCE ABUSE

A. Affect dysregulation
   1. Affective instability
      a. Lability and mood swings
      b. Volatility and explosiveness
   2. Inability to self-modulate
      Inability to tolerate distress
      Inability to terminate affective event
      Inability to self-soothe
   3. Affective dyssynchrony: inability to regulate affect within a relationship via communication
B. Behavioral dysregulation
   1. Impulsivity
   2. Noncompliance
   3. Hyperactivity
   4. Hyperaggressiveness
   5. Hypersexuality
   6. Heightened risk taking
C. Cognitive dysregulation
   1. Nonreflectivity
   2. Globality
   3. Egocentrism
   4. Instability of self-concept, self-esteem
   5. Poor judgment
   6. Prominence of immature defenses
   7. Lack of empathy
   8. Disturbance of boundaries

of adolescent comorbidity and the consistency and commonality of the clinical presentation across diagnostic categories in our sample, we then turned our attention to questions concerning the developmental psychopathology of comorbid adolescent substance abuse and to a search for underlying psychodynamic mechanisms and developmental processes contributing to a common vulnerability of comorbid conditions. Returning to the clinical data—the triad of affective instability, impulsivity, and nonreflectivity—we constructed a working model of comorbidity. This working model views comorbidity as the affective and behavioral expression of a disorder in the development of self-regulation. Disturbances in the capacity to regulate affects, behavior, and thinking are, within the model, at the center of the development of comorbid conditions. In the next four sections, we will describe the nature of our working model by tracing the path from (1) the basic assumptions that define our developmental perspective, (2) the domain of developmental psychopathology that emphasizes linkages between early experience and later disorders, (3) infancy and early childhood research that suggests an approach to the ontogenesis of adaptive self-regulation, leading to (4) a model of the development of comorbid adolescent substance abuse from a matrix of disordered relational regulation and disordered self-regulation.

The Developmental Perspective

The model described here is grounded in a developmental perspective that views development as a process of directed change, of competencies and adaptive patterns emerging from the reorganization of previous patterns, structures, and competencies. According to Werner (1957), this process "proceeds from an initial state of globality and lack of differentiations to increasing states of articulation, differentiation and hierarchical integration." The developmental perspective is defined by a number of basic assumptions. (1) Development is a dynamic process that embodies both structure and process, organization and activity, differentiation and integration, continuity and discontinuity, stability and change (*dialectical and paradoxical*). (2) Development proceeds within a relational matrix; it is interactive and contextual. In human development, the individual is seen as emerging or differentiating from within this matrix and remaining interdependent within relational contexts throughout the life span (*relational and contextual*). (3) Development is a coconstruction of meaning and knowledge through a coordination of actions, affective communication, language, awareness, and shared experience. All human categories, including "reality" and "objectivity," are metaphoric, constructed from experience, constrained by biology, and finding stability in the consensual domain of human meaning systems (*constructivist and metaphoric*). (4) Development is a living process with systemic and holistic properties embodying complex circular causality, self-reference and self-generation (autopoiesis), coherence, and integration (*cybernetic and recursive*).

The Domain of Developmental Psychopathology

The domain of developmental psychopathology focuses on individual patterns of adaptation and maladaption and the complex developmental transformations that link earlier adaptation to later psychopathology. From an organizational perspective (Sroufe 1979, 1985), behavior, development, and personality are viewed as related and dynamic aspects of an underlying organization or pattern, an essential coherence over time and across contexts. This essential coherence is also referred to as the person or the self. The continuity of development, of personality, and of the self lies, not in isomorphic manifest behavior, but in the stability of pattern and the coherence of the organization of behavior over time. Sroufe and Rutter (1984) write, "The proposition is that individual functioning is coherent across periods of discontinuous growth and despite fundamental transformations in manifest behavior."

The links between early experience, early adaptations, and later disorder require a complex developmental view of the person-experience-environment interaction such as those proposed by epigenetic theorists, including Erikson (1963), Piaget and Inhelder (1969), Sander (1962), Sroufe (1979), and Werner (1957). These developmentalists propose a lawful sequence of salient developmental, adaptive issues that are integrative and include the affective, cognitive, and social domains. Furthermore, the outcome of the negotiation of issues at one period is seen as laying the groundwork for subsequent issues in subsequent periods as well as being of continuing and central relevance throughout the life span.

Thus, to construct a model of comorbid adolescent substance abuse as a disorder of self-regulation from the domain of developmental psychopathology, it is necessary to seek patterns beneath the plastic and manifest behavior described in the clinical presentation. An understanding of disordered self-regulation must include an account of the course of development of self-regulation, its relation to development of the self, and the factors that mediate and modify that course, thus contributing to later maladaptive functioning.

The Development of Self-Regulation

The emergence of self-regulation described here and central to the construction of our model of dysregulation rests on the psychoanalytically informed observational infancy and early childhood research of Emde (1984, 1989), Sander (1962, 1975), Sroufe (1979, 1989), Stern (1985), and others. The focus of this body of work has been the dyadic infant-caregiver system. We view the dyadic context as central and as mediator of the larger and more complex family and social systems in which the dyad is embedded. These larger systems have substantive and long-term effects on the developing individual. In the first stages of model construction, we will focus on the dyadic system as mediator in the development of self-regulation.

Sander's (1975) work begins with a commitment to the organic biological systems view of the living organism as actively self-organizing and self-regulating while, simultaneously and necessarily, existing in continuous intimate exchange with its surround. From this perspective, and with a deep awareness of its paradoxical nature, Sander proposes an epigenetic sequence of the adaptive issues negotiated over the first three years in the interactions between infant and caregiver. This epigenetic sequence describes the movement from dyadic organization and regulation within the infant-caregiver system toward self-regulation and inner organization—an ontogeny of self as a differentiation of basic self-regulatory mechanisms from a relational matrix. This movement is viewed as the central adaptational task of early development and reflects a commitment to a relational model shared by developmental and psychoanalytic theorists. Sroufe (1989) writes, "The developmental account, thus, traces the origins of the inner organization (self) from the dyadic organization—from dyadic behavioral regulation to self-regulation" (p. 73).

The phases in the development of self-regulation are schematically presented in table 3 and described below.

PHASE 1: BIOLOGICAL REGULATION

In the first three months of life, the infant's state, communicated to an available, responsive, and intervening caregiver, leads to the establishment of the regulation of biological functions such as feeding, sleeping and waking, and elimination. The dyadic regulatory system establishes "phase synchrony," a rhythmicity to the periods of relative activity and quiescence. Infant state and caregiver intervention become coordinated, a reciprocal or bidirectional coordination of actions about which Sander comments, "One of the features most idiosyncratic in the first three months is the extent to which the infant is helped or compromised in beginning to determine aspects of his own regulation" (1975, p. 137). It is in the development of biological regula-

471

TABLE 3

DEVELOPMENT OF SELF-REGULATION WITHIN A RELATION SYSTEM

Phase	Age (Months)	Infant Functions	Caregiver Functions	Adaptive Organization
Biological regulation.........	0–3	Arousal Affect Signal	Availability Coordination	Coordination of biological rhythmicity Modulation of state, affect Phase synchrony
Modulation of affect.........	3–9	Affect Activity Sociability	Attunement Availability Responsiveness Reciprocity	Coordination of action, affect, subjectivity Differentiation of affective, subjective self with capacity for affective sharing, tolerance of distress, self-soothing
Control of behavior..........	9–18	Attachment Exploration Locomotion Intentionality Contingency Symbolization	Secure Base Containment Prohibition Consistency Language	Internalization of relationship Differentiation of action, intentional self Coordination of actions, language Impulse control mediated by parental containment Compliance mediated by languaging of parental expectations, prohibitions Tolerance of delay, frustration Behavioral autonomy—connectedness
Monitoring of self	18–36	Representation Recall Recognition Language	Constancy Continuity Clarity Complexity Flexibility	Structuralization, internalization Differentiation of self-, shared awareness Constancy of self-, other representations associated with stable self-esteem Coherence: integration of recall memory, affective and action self-schemas Cognitive autonomy: capacity to regulate affect, behavior mediated by operations on internal, psychological structures Autonomy—interdependence

tion that the earliest patterns of psychological regulation may be seen in the capacity to structure, order, or "schedule" life.

PHASE 2: MODULATION OF AFFECT

From months 4–9, the infant-caregiver system facilitates the early development of the capacity for self-modulation in two steps. During months 4–6, the appearance of social smiling and infant vocalization in the context of caregiver responsiveness leads to more active reciprocal and coordinated behavioral exchanges, punctuated by the sharing of positive affects. Sander writes of these interactions, "The affect of joy or delight becomes established as a criterion for precision in the matching of interpersonal reciprocations" (1975, p. 145).

From month 7 through month 9, an increasingly active and goal-directed infant initiates interactions with the caregiver, challenging the dyadic system to accommodate and further coordinate behavior in highly complex affective and behavioral exchanges such as greeting sequences. At the same time, the infant's emerging intentionality brings "a first active bifurcation in the direction of the child's initiative: toward her and away from her" (Sander 1975, p. 138).

It is also during the seven- to nine-month period that the infant develops what Stern (1985) calls the sense of a subjective self, the discovery that he or she has a mind and that others have minds as well. With this "working notion" of separate and distinct minds, intersubjectivity—the sharing of subjective experience—becomes possible for the infant, who now enters the new domain of intersubjective relatedness. At this stage, "for the first time one can attribute to the infant the capacity for psychic intimacy—the openness to disclosure, the permeability or interpenetrability that occurs between two people" (Stern 1985, p. 126). This emergence of intersubjectivity may be viewed as the beginning of the private and social worlds, defining what can be shared and what cannot. Affective experience, the core of subjectivity, enters the intersubjective domain by a process that Stern calls affect attunement, the sharing of affective states or communing between mother and infant. Attunement as a recasting or restatement of subjective state by way of nonverbal metaphor or analogue is seen as midway in the developmental progression from behavioral imitation to symbolic and linguistic forms of affect communication. As such, it is central to the development of affect regulation in verbal and nonverbal forms.

473

These developments, the coordination of complex, infant-initiated affective and behavioral exchanges, affect attunement, and the "bifurcation" brought on with intentionality, reflect movement toward greater reciprocity within a more genuine relationship. Sroufe (1989) writes that these developments "point to a coordination of affect and cognition (the emergence of affectively toned schemas) marking the beginnings of an inner organization of experience." The infant's experiences of reciprocity and coordination, attunement, and "bifurcation" within the dyadic relational matrix are internalized, leading to the earliest differentiation of self and other. This structuralization of the affective self and the available or unavailable caregiver contributes to the capacity for affective sharing, self-soothing, and self-modulation, all essential to the self-regulation of affects.

PHASE 3: CONTROL OF BEHAVIOR

This phase, encompassing months 9–18, is marked by three changes in the relational system having to do with exploration/attachment, locomotion/containment, and language/prohibition, all of which contribute to the emergence of self-control.

By providing a "secure base" (Ainsworth 1973) or "home base" (Mahler, Pine, and Bergman 1975), the caregiver facilitates the exploratory behavior of the curious ten- to thirteen-month-old and the regulation of affects associated with encounters with the novel, the insurmountable, and the threatening. Emde (1989) has described this interaction as social referencing, the affective communication between infant and caregiver that functions in novel situations to resolve the uncertainty and thereby regulate affect and exploratory behavior. Sander emphasizes the focalization of need-meeting demands by the infant on the mother in an effort to determine her availability: if "her availability is certain he can turn to greater novelties; if she tries to run away, he is demanding; if she reacts to threat by aggression, his demands may provoke her attack or surrender" (p. 139).

Bowlby (1973), focusing on the central organizing and regulatory function of the attachment relationship during these months, describes the emergence of "internal working models." Bowlby suggests that, at one year, the working models may be thought of as an internalization of the infant's experience of a caregiving relationship, of an attachment figure affectively colored as available and responsive or unavailable and unresponsive, and of a self seen as worthy or unworthy of maternal attention. Such internal working models are enacted in the patterns and affective quality of exploratory and attachment behavior, thus contributing to affective and behavioral regulation.

With the development of locomotion, conscious intentionality, and early means-ends thought, the infant asserts himself and widens the determination of his own behavior, frequently in opposition to caregiver's expectations. The caregiver, by providing protective containment and consistent limit setting while continuing to be emotionally available to the ambivalent toddler, facilitates the development of autonomy and impulse control.

The appearance of language adds a powerful new mode of mediation of impulse control and compliance balanced with initiative and autonomy. The languaging of parental prohibitions, expectations, and rules and the articulation and coordination of action and language within the relationship and within the toddler make possible a qualitatively different level of control.

By the end of this third phase at approximately eighteen months, the toddler has differentiated an affective and intentional self, asserts behavioral autonomy within a relational connectedness reflecting an enduring pattern of attachment, and demonstrates the beginnings of impulse control, compliance, and frustration tolerance.

PHASE 4: SELF-MONITORING

From eighteen to thirty-six months, the emergence of the symbolic capacity, language, recall memory, and representational thinking—secondary process functions—contribute to the toddler's recognition of self. Self-awareness, the recognition and communication by the toddler of his own state, perceptions, intentions, thoughts, and feelings as his own, and shared awareness, the "realization that another can be aware of what one is aware of within one's self" (Sander 1975, p. 142), are differentiated. This differentiation is facilitated by caregiving that provides an experience of empathic constancy, clarity, and continuity, yielding a coherence of the self and the self-regulatory core. This coherence, in Sander's view, is facilitated by the experience of restoration and reversibility following the toddler's intentionally initiated aggressive disruptions of the relationship. Psychological autonomy—the capacity to self-monitor and self-regulate affect and behavior through cognitive operations—is made possible by awareness of self and other that emerges in the context of the coordination of awareness and the conservation of relatedness. The emergence of this capacity to self-monitor further establishes adaptive patterns of self-regulation.

At thirty-six months, the child has developed an integrated, coherent self-structure that conserves the self as the active organizer of experience and differentiates a symbolic self that provides the reflective frame for increasingly complex and increasingly integrative levels of self-regulatory processes. Thus, self-regulation at this stage represents an integration of the epigenetically earlier capacities of self-modulation and self-control, an integration providing for greater flexibility of the self-regulation of affects and behavior across the many contexts of environmental challenges.

With this brief summary of the contribution of the infancy and early childhood literature as context, we now turn to the comorbid adolescent with the understanding that the nature of interactive regulation and organization will be embodied in the self-regulation and that this self-regulation and self-organization will organize later experience.

The Development of Self-Regulatory Vulnerability

In the following account of the pathogenesis of comorbid adolescent substance abuse, the manifest symptomatology is understood as an expression of an underlying vulnerability in the regulatory and adaptive activities of the self. This vulnerability evolves within the relational matrix of the infant-caregiver system and is embodied in the self-system of the child and adolescent. Ineffective dyadic regulation is thus a developmental link to the vulnerability of the self-system of the child. From this perspective, psychopathology expresses and reflects an organization of personality lacking the flexibility and mobility of functions necessary to meet the challenges of an increasingly complex internal and external environment.

More specifically, our model proposes that the clinical presentation in adolescence is the symptomatic outcome of patterns of relational dysregulation transformed to maladaptive patterns of self-regulation in the first three years—patterns that are maladaptive in that they are not adequate for the biological and psychosocial challenges of adolescence. The symptomatology—the triad of affective instability, impulsivity, and nonreflectivity—is developmentally linked to vulnerabilities emerging from the phase-specific tasks of acquiring self-modulation, self-control, and self-monitoring. The paths that link early relational patterns to later disorder are described here and schematically summarized in table 4.

1. The symptoms that reflect dysregulation of affects—affective instability—are linked to the development of self-modulation occurring in the dyadic context. Following this trajectory, ineffective dyadic regulation of affective states, particularly states of distress, compromises the differentiation of an affective self and compromises the internalization of an available and attuned caregiver. The experience of misattunement contributes to disturbances in the capacity for affective sharing and the self-modulation of the dysphoric affective states of agitation, rage, shame, hurt, and loneliness. This compromised capacity for self-modulation is expressed as an intolerance of distress and dysphoria, an inability to dampen the affective state or to contain and terminate the dysphoric event. In addition, there is little expectation of empathic responsiveness from others, from within-familial relationships where the communication of painful affects is integral to connectedness, trust, and the sense of well-being. In Erikson's (1963) schema, there is an absence of basic trust.

The experience of overwhelming affect in the adolescent with limited capacity for self-modulation and relational modulation—affective sharing—is likely to trigger fragmentation and disorganization. It is from this self-state that the adolescent will act to conserve and defend the self with the many forms of "acting out," including substance abuse.

Difficulty with the self-modulation of affects, described as affective instability in our sample of adolescent polysubstance abusers, is also observed by Khantzian and Schneider (1986) in their studies of adult narcotic addicts and defined as a disturbance of affect and drive defense. Writing from a psychoanalytic perspective, they suggest that drugs are used to compensate for defective ego mechanisms of defense. Krystal (1982) also views deficits in the tolerance of painful affects, particularly in the capacity to self-soothe, as a major component of the personality structure vulnerable to drug dependence. In Krystal's schema, these developmental deficits can be attributed to

TABLE 4
Vulnerability Contextualized: From Dyadic Dysregulation to Maladaptive Behavior Patterns in Adolescence

Regulatory Function ⇄	Relational System Dysregulation ⇄	Self-Regulatory Vulnerability ⇄	Contexts of Adolescence ⇄	Symptomatology: Behavioral Expression of Vulnerability
Modulation of affect	Misattunement Nonresponsiveness Unavailability	Compromised self-modulation affective instability: 1. Labile 2. Volatile	Family	Inability to tolerate limits; relational volatility; verbal, physical abuse; delinquency (lying, stealing); alienation, isolation, running away
Control of behavior	Ambivalent containment Ambiguous prohibitions Inconsistent limit setting	Compromised self-control behavioral impulsivity	School	Authority conflicts, disciplinary problems; noncompliance; lateness; truancy; academic failure
Monitoring of self	Ambiguous-indistinct attributions of self and other	Compromised self-monitoring nonreflectivity: 1. Ambiguous 2. Rigid	Community	Antisocial behavior, violence, vandalism, stealing; legal difficulties
	Rigid and concrete attributions of self and other		Peer	Drift toward drug using, delinquent, and/or peripheral "outsider" peer culture; instability of friendship patterns; isolation; heightened risk-taking behaviors, diminished play
			Substance availability	Persistent desire, preoccupation, seeking and use of substances, frequently to intoxication, in the face of failed attempts to control, and the face of family, peer, educational, vocational, and legal problems related to substance abuse

"infantile psychic trauma," a dissonance between the infant's needs and the caregiver's interventions, leading to overwhelming infant distress.

2. The symptoms that reflect dysregulation of behavior—behavioral impulsivity—are linked to the development of self-control in the dyadic context. Following this trajectory, ineffective dyadic regulation of exploratory activity, intentionality, and aggression compromise the differentiation of an active, intentional self and the internalization of a protecting, containing caregiver. Conflicts in the infant-caregiver system concerning issues of control, compliance, and aggression contribute to the experience of the attachment figure as unavailable. The uncertainty of availability compromises the development of exploratory behavior and the early forms of relational autonomy—an engagement with the novel in the context of a secure relationship. Caregiver inconsistency in the containing and protecting of the willful toddler, in the setting of limits, and in the languaging of prohibitions and expectations contributes to a vulnerability in containing, controlling, and protecting the self. These vulnerabilities, the structural limitations in the capacity for self-control, challenged by the developmental tasks of adolescence, are expressed in the impulsivity, hyperaggressiveness, noncompliance, and self-destructive risk taking of adolescents predisposed to a maladaptive comorbid outcome. Khantzian and Schneider (1986) also observe disturbances in self-control in their studies and attribute these disturbances to inadequacies in the ego functions responsible for self-care and self-protection.

3. The symptoms that reflect a dysregulation in cognition—nonreflectivity—are linked to the development of self-monitoring in the relational context. Following this trajectory, ineffective dyadic coordination and regulation of awareness, affect, and internal representations compromise the differentiation of affectively positive, complex, and coherent self and other schemas. This lack of differentiation of a fundamentally good and lovable self and a good and loving other renders self-esteem unstable. The compromised developmental trajectory has two forms, an ambiguous/indistinct and a rigid/remote articulation. Ambiguity within the toddler-caregiver relationship—the inability clearly to articulate the complexity of affects, of shared and personal awareness, and of the fundamental continuity of a mutually empathic relationship—disrupts the development of constant and complex cate-

479

gories of self and other and leads to instability in the maintenance of psychological boundaries, diffusion, and enmeshment.

Rigidity, concreteness, and emotional distance in the relational system—the inflexibility and global articulation of fundamentally negative affective experiences of relationship—disrupt the development of coherent, complex, and essentially positive categories of self and other and lead to forms of relatedness that are egocentric and exploitative. Moreover, where ambiguity or rigidity distort the articulation of the reflective self and preclude the validation of affective experience, there follows the development of a distorted understanding of the distinctions between "good" and "bad" behavior—a part or an aspect of an afffectively interactive moment—and "good" (acceptable) or "bad" (unacceptable) person, where the affective referent is the whole person or relationship. Thus, it is a fragile, inflexible, and inauthentic coherence of self, what Winnicott called a "false self," that is gained by the child, and it is the "false" self and false other, both representations of an invalidation of the child's affective experience, that compromise the development of cognitive autonomy—the capacity to regulate affect and behavior by self-monitoring processes mediated by internal operations on psychological structures.

These vulnerabilities, the ambiguity and fragility of a self-system, instability of self-esteem, and the lack of cognitive autonomy in a context of continuity of empathic relatedness, are expressed in the nonreflectivity, globality, egocentrism, lack of empathy, and boundary difficulties that characterize the comorbid adolescent.

From Vulnerability to Diagnosis

An understanding of the developmental path from the vulnerable self-regulatory core to the complex patterns of maladaptive behaviors, which constitute the diagnostic criteria for comorbid conditions, rests on an appreciation of the adolescent at risk. The at-risk adolescent experiences the stress and disequilibria of adolescence with a personality structure that embodies an organization of compromised capacities to modulate affect, control behavior, and monitor the self. It is this vulnerable self-regulatory core interacting with the varied and complex contexts of developmental challenge that makes manifest the sympathetic behaviors that characterize the comorbid diagnoses.

From this view, symptoms are adaptational capabilities challenged and vulnerability contextualized. Thus, the adolescent with a disturbance in self-regulation in the context of the family may have affective storms and rage reactions in response to parental authority, limit setting, and discipline. Affective instability may lead to verbal and/or physical abuse of family members, lying and stealing from family, and increasing isolation, alienation, and running away. The same adolescent will be symptomatic in school, where teachers report disciplinary problems, academic failure, lateness, and truancy, and in the community, where varied forms of delinquency surface, including stealing and shoplifting, vandalism and violence. Adolescent substance abuse—the persistent desire, preoccupation, seeking, and use of substances, frequently to intoxication, in the face of failed attempts to control, and in the face of family, peer, educational, vocational, and legal problems related to substance use—reflects the vulnerable adolescent's self-destructive and failed attempt to cope with affective disequilibrium, to self-medicate dysphoric affects, to belong in the face of alienation and isolation, to articulate an identity in the face of confusion and ambiguity, and to experience competence in the face of inadequacy.

Conclusions

The model of adolescent substance abuse offered here begins with a relational and adaptational view of development, focusing on the vicissitudes in the structuralization of self-regulation as a significant aspect of vulnerability in the pathogenesis of comorbid conditions. Based on this model, we have generated three lines of empirical inquiry that focus on three domains of adolescent development. (1) In the domain of the organization of the subjective experience of the adolescent, we explore attachment classification, a reflection of Bowlby's internal working models, and examine its relation with patterns of dysregulation of affects and behavior. (2) In the domain of the family context, we explore individual and internal self-regulatory functions as reflected in attachment classification in relation to global family functioning and specific features of the family's organization and regulation of affects. (3) In the domain of reasoning and abstract thinking, we investigate relations among formal operational thinking, disturbances in individual and internal self-regulatory functions, and family organization. The following chapters in this section will address theo-

481

retical and methodological issues in these areas and will offer preliminary data.

REFERENCES

Ainsworth, M. D. S. 1973. The development of infant-mother attachment. In B. Caldwell and H. Ricciuti, eds. *Review of Child Development Research,* vol. 3. Chicago: University of Chicago Press.

American Psychiatric Association. 1987. *Diagnostic and Statistical
Manual of Mental Disorders.* 3d ed., rev. Washington, D.C.: American Psychiatric Association.

Bailey, G. W. 1989. Current perspectives on substance abuse in youth.
*Journal of the American Academy of Child and Adolescent Psychia-
try* 28:151–161.

Bowlby, J. 1973. *Attachment and Loss.* Vol. 2, *Separation, Anxiety,
and Anger.* New York: Basic.

Bukstein, O. G.; Brent, D.; and Kaminer, Y. 1989. Comorbidity of
substance abuse and other psychiatric disorders in adolescents.
American Journal of Psychiatry 146:1131–1141.

Cloninger, C. R.; Martin, R. L.; Guze, S. B.; and Clayton, P. J. 1990.
Empirical structure of psychiatric comorbidity and its theoretical
significance. In J. D. Maser and C. R. Cloninger, eds. *Comorbidity
of Mood and Anxiety Disorders.* Washington, D.C.: American Psychiatric Press.

Emde, R. N. 1984. The affective self: continuities and transformations
from infancy. In J. D. Call, E. Galenson, and R. L. Tyson, eds.
Frontiers of Infant Psychiatry, vol. 2. New York: Basic.

Emde, R. N. 1989. The infant's relationship experience: developmental and affective aspects. In A. J. Sameroff and R. N. Emde,
eds. *Relationship Disturbances in Early Childhood: A Developmental Approach.* New York: Basic.

Erikson, E. H. 1963. *Childhood and Society.* 2d ed. New York:
Norton.

Khantzian, E. J., and Schneider, R. J. 1986. Treatment implications
of a psychodynamic understanding of opioid addicts. In R. E.
Meyer, ed. *Psychopathology and Addictive Disorders.* New York:
Guilford.

Krystal, H. 1982. Adolescence and the tendencies to develop substance dependence. *Psychoanalytic Inquiry* 2:581–618.

Mahler, M. S.; Pine, F.; and Bergman, A. 1975. *The Psychological Birth of the Human Infant: Symbiosis and Individuation*. New York: Basic.

Maser, J. D., and Cloninger, C. R. 1990. *Comorbidity of Mood and Anxiety Disorders*. Washington, D.C.: American Psychiatric Press.

Piaget, J., and Inhelder, B. 1969. *The Psychology of the Child*. New York: Basic.

Puig-Antich, J. 1989. Depression and conduct disorder in prepuberty. *Journal of the American Academy of Child and Adolescent Psychiatry* 28:118–128.

Sander, L. 1962. Issues in early mother-child interaction. *Journal of the American Academy of Child Psychiatry* 1:141–166.

Sander, L. 1975. Infant and caretaking environment: investigation and conceptualization of adaptive behavior in a system of increasing complexity. In E. J. Anthony, ed. *Explorations in Child Psychiatry*. New York: Plenum.

Sroufe, L. A. 1979. The coherence of individual development. *American Psychologist* 34:834–841.

Sroufe, L. A. 1989. Relationships, self, and individual adaptation. In A. J. Sameroff and R. N. Emde, eds. *Relationship Disturbances in Early Childhood: A Developmental Approach*. New York: Basic.

Sroufe, L. A., and Rutter, M. 1984. The domain of developmental psychopathology. *Child Development* 55:17–29.

Stern, D. N. 1985. *The Interpersonal World of the Infant: A View from Psychoanalysis and Developmental Psychology*. New York: Basic.

Werner, H. 1957. The concept of development from a comparative and organismic point of view. In D. Harris, ed. *The Concept of Development*. Minneapolis: University of Minnesota Press.

Woolston, J. L.; Rosenthal, S.; Riddle, M. A.; Sparrow, S.; Cicchetti, D.; and Zimmerman, L. D. 1989. Childhood comorbidity of anxiety/affective disorders and behavior disorders. *Journal of the American Academy of Child and Adolescent Psychiatry* 28:707–713.

26 FAMILY INTERACTION AS REGULATORY CONTEXT IN ADOLESCENCE

JOHN H. STEIDL, HARVEY A. HOROWITZ, WILLIS F. OVERTON,
AND DIANA ROSENSTEIN

The Interacting (Practicing) Family

Recently, Piercy and Frankel (1989) presented a model for both the treatment of and research in family therapy for substance-abusing adolescents. They addressed the question, Why use family therapy with substance-abusing adolescents? Among the data presented were (1) reports of current clinical practice that indicate some form of family intervention in over 90 percent of drug treatment programs; (2) family correlates of adolescent substance abuse that have been documented despite the fact that there may be a genetic predisposition to substance abuse and despite the demonstrated influence of a drug-using peer group; and (3) considerable research that indicates positive outcomes with adolescent substance abusers when family interventions are used. If adolescent substance abuse is a disorder of regulation, and if one views the family as a primary regulatory context for the adolescent, how do we integrate the perspective of family interaction with other modes of thinking about adolescents and their difficulties?

Recently, Reiss (1989) presented two contrasting perspectives on the family and its relation to individual development: the "represented" family and the "practicing" family. The "represented family" is a descriptor for a viewpoint in which family relationships are absorbed or internalized in the developing individual (Ainsworth, Blehar, Waters, and Wall 1978; Main and Cassidy 1984). The "practicing family" is a descriptor for a viewpoint that directly examines the current organization of the family (Beavers and Voellner 1983; Minuchin 1974; Reiss 1981; Stanton and Todd 1982). In talking about family interaction as regulatory context, we are in the domain of the practicing family in terms of research data. However, practicing is, in part, an enactment of the pattern of relationships between family members over time, which are stored in the represented family.

While Reiss has been an investigator of the practicing family, he points out the gaps in the research agendas of both perspectives and notes that these perspectives can and need to be reconciled because the actual world has represented as well as practiced aspects. Making a similar point, Sroufe (1989) points out that the social support available to the parents from spouses and others predicts the quality of infant care and that decades of research have confirmed links between parenting, parental relationship variables, and child behavior problems, with an especially strong link between parental disharmony and conduct disorders. Reiss concludes by arguing for a research strategy that seeks a clearer picture of the relative power of internal models and common practices to predict sustained patterns of both competent and maladjusted social relationships. It is this kind of thinking that has led us to look for connections that would allow us in a beginning way to follow Reiss's lead: connections between cognition, attachment, and family data, between these and individual psychopathology, and between these and outcome.

A Model for Investigating the Practicing Family

There are certainly a number of ways that one can go about investigating the family correlates of individual dysregulation in the practicing family. Any model for representing the complexities of the family as a relational context has built into it criteria for assessing disturbances and health (Fishman 1988; Minuchin 1974; Olson 1986).

We are using the methodology developed by the group at the Timberlawn Foundation, for whom W. Robert Beavers has been the primary theoretician (Lewis, Beavers, Gossett, and Phillips 1976). This is a model for assessing and treating families that has been developed from general systems theory and its notions about entropy and negentropy. That is, organisms and their processes can be viewed on a continuum from chaos (entropy), through more or less rigid structure, to structure with flexibility sufficient to adapt to changing conditions and circumstances (negentropy).

This is a model that admittedly addresses/assesses family functioning on the continuum of health and pathology. The assumption, supported by previous research data (Lewis et al. 1976), is that family pathology is associated with individual pathology and that the two are isomorphic in the sense that, the more pathological the family, the more pathological the offspring are likely to be. If the family is well structured and in addition is flexible enough to change with changing circumstances (the most negentropic), the offspring are likely to be free of overt symptoms and subjective distress. In effect, the adolescent has a holding environment that is predictable (structured), responsive (flexible), and, therefore, secure. If the family is highly but rigidly structured so that such flexibility is not currently available, its members are compromised in their ability to deal with the changing circumstances inherent in adolescence. In this situation, the adolescent is blocked in the changes required by his or her developmental tasks and is likely to become symptomatic. However, since the family functioning is at least consistent in its rigidity and therefore predictable, the adolescent is likely to be less disturbed or distressed than were the family context inconsistent and chaotic. In the latter situation, the most entropic and, hence, the most pathological adolescent will likely present with the most disabling psychopathology.

Many of the parameters of family functioning can be investigated along such a continuum, with implications for healthy or pathological functioning and, in the case of some of the parameters, with implications for the regulation and dysregulation of affect, behavior, and cognition that we see clinically. It is along this continuum that the Beavers model investigates such parameters as global health pathology, leadership and control, coalitions and alignments, degree of closeness and respect for individuality, ability to take responsibility for one's own past, present, and future actions, generational boundary integrity, problem solving, openness to feedback, expression of thoughts and feelings, and mood and tone of family interactions.

While the Beavers model is not specifically organized to rate families on the regulation of behavior, affect, and cognition, the scales can be clustered within these factors. For example, one might take the family power and control structure (family functions such as limit setting) as a measure of behavioral regulation and hypothesize that a chaotic control structure would predict a behaviorally dysregulated adolescent. Or one might take grossly inappropriate responses to feelings in the family as a measure of affective regulation and hypothesize that such chaos in affective responsiveness would predict an affectively dysregulated child. One might thus begin to look at the predictive power of the instrument in relation to the specific areas of dysregulation in the offspring.

The Family Research Protocol

Our research protocol involves the family in investigating whether there are areas of family functioning that are connected in some way with the adolescent's problems with regulation. Hence, it is enormously useful clinically. While families are aware that they are participating in a multifaceted research project and give informed consent, they also understand it as an important part of the workup for their child. The family, defined as broadly as possible, is asked to spend an hour and a half early in the hospitalization doing a series of tasks and talking with the treatment team and investigators. The tasks are apparently simple, but they are designed to evoke patterns of interaction that are diagnostic of family functioning. They are modified from those used by Minuchin, Montalvo, Guerney, Rosman, and Schumer (1967) in the Wiltwyck Project and subsequently used by Steidl, Finkelstein, Wexler, Feigenbaum, Kitsen, Kliger, and Quinlan (1980) in investigating families of hemodialysis patients and by Kosten, Hogan, Jalali, Steidl, and Kleber (1986) in investigating the effects of family treatment in a heroin-addicted population.

The tasks include (1) planning a limited-choice menu together; (2) identifying the various roles that family members fulfill, such as troublemaker, crybaby, the one who gets away with murder, the one who fights the most, etc.; (3) discussing in detail a recent family argument; (4) offering positive and negative feedback to each other; and (5) identifying changes that members would like to see in the family. Most families will perform these tasks in roughly half an hour, and, usually, by the time they have finished, they will have identified and be talking about the major areas of family difficulty that they connect with the adolescent's difficulties. Also by the time they have finished, experienced raters will have scored them on the Beavers-Timberlawn Family Evaluation Scale. One of the experienced clinician-raters will then orchestrate a thirty- to sixty-minute exploration of the primary areas of difficulty exposed by the family's participation in the tasks, moving toward a consensus with the family about family patterns that appear to be related to the adolescent's difficulties. A protocol for follow-up at twelve months posthospitalization is also in effect.

Discussion

The project in its entirety is an attempt to think about, as David Reiss suggests, the predictive power of the "represented" and "practicing" family in relation to adolescent functioning, specifically in relation to the adolescent's regulation of behavior, affect, and cognition. It assumes that systemic thinking about the many variables involved in adolescent substance abuse, or any other disorder, needs to take into account (1) the patterns developing in a family over time, patterns in both the "represented" family and the "practicing" family, and (2) the interaction of these patterns with the affective, behavioral, and cognitive development and regulation of offspring in that family. In this section of the project, we are investigating the "practicing" family, specifically, its regulatory competence in relation to the adolescent's regulatory competence.

If, in fact, individual and family patterns of dysregulation tend to be isomorphic, one would expect that a significant percentage of the families of dysregulated adolescents would score on the more pathological end of the spectrum, with the most dysregulated adolescents living in the most dysregulated (i.e., chaotic) environments.

To be more specific, in terms of the triad of behavior, affect, and cognition, one would expect adolescents to have problems with the regulation of behavior in a context of chaotic or rigid parental control as well as in the context of a weak parental coalition. One might also hypothesize that vague or ambiguous disclosure of thoughts and feelings within the family would be associated with dysregulation of behavior via a mechanism of the adolescent having to depend on acting out thoughts and feelings since verbal expression is not supported.

One would expect adolescents to have problems with the regulation of affect in a regulatory context marked by amorphous, vague, and indistinct boundaries, such that contagion of affect is likely. Further, problems in the expression of feeling or grossly inappropriate responses to feelings in the regulatory context might be expected to be associated with the dysregulation of affect in the adolescent.

Finally, one would expect adolescents to have problems with the regulation of thinking in a context marked by vague or ambiguous verbal expression and incongruencies between the family's concept of how it functions and that of a group of experienced observers.

REFERENCES

Ainsworth, M. D. S.; Blehar, M. D.; Waters, E.; and Wall, S. 1978. *Patterns of Attachment: A Psychological Study of the Strange Situation*. Hillsdale, N.J.: Erlbaum.

Beavers, W. R., and Voellner, M. N. 1983. Family models: comparing and contrasting the Olson circumflex model with the Beavers systems model. *Family Process* 22:85–98.

Fishman, H. C. 1988. *Treating Troubled Adolescents: A Family Therapy Approach*. New York: Basic.

Kosten, T. R.; Hogan, I.; Jalali, B.; Steidl, J.; and Kleber, H. 1986. The effect of multiple family therapy on addict family functioning: a pilot study. *Advances in Alcohol and Substance Abuse* 5(3): 51–62.

Lewis, J. M.; Beavers, W. R.; Gossett, J. T.; and Phillips, V. A. 1976. *No Single Thread: Psychological Health in Family Systems*. New York: Brunner/Mazel.

Main, M., and Cassidy, J. 1984. Predicting rejection of her infant from mother's representation of her own experience: implications for the abused-abusing intergenerational cycle. *Child Abuse and Neglect* 8:203–217.

Minuchin, S. 1974. *Families and Family Therapy*. Cambridge, Mass.: Harvard University Press.

Minuchin, S.; Montalvo, B.; Guerney, B. G.; Rosman, B. L.; and Schumer, F. 1967. *Families of the Slums*. New York: Basic.

Olson, D. H. 1986. Circumflex model VII: validation studies and FACES III. *Family Process* 25(3): 337–351.

Piercy, F. P., and Frankel, B. R. 1989. The evolution of an integrative family therapy for substance abusing adolescents. *Journal of Family Psychology* 3(1): 3–17.

Reiss, D. 1981. *The Family Construction of Reality*. Cambridge, Mass.: Harvard University Press.

Reiss, D. 1989. The represented and practicing family: contrasting visions of continuity. In A. J. Sameroff and R. N. Emde, eds. *Relational Disturbances in Early Childhood*. New York: Basic.

Sroufe, L. A. 1989. Relationships and relationship disturbances. In A. J. Sameroff and R. N. Emde, eds. *Relational Disturbances in Early Childhood*. New York: Basic.

Stanton, M. D., and Todd, T. C. 1982. *The Family Therapy of Drug Abuse and Addiction*. New York: Guilford.

Steidl, J. H.; Finkelstein, F. D.; Wexler, J. P.; Feigenbaum, H.; Kitsen, J.; Kliger, A.; and Quinlan, D. M. 1980. Interactions between medical condition, adherence and family functioning in chronic dialysis patients. *Archives of General Psychiatry* 37:1025–1027.

27   ATTACHMENT AND INTERNALIZATION:
RELATIONSHIP AS A REGULATORY
CONTEXT

DIANA ROSENSTEIN, HARVEY A. HOROWITZ, JOHN H. STEIDL,
AND WILLIS F. OVERTON

The concept of attachment as it is manifest in adolescents, particularly substance-abusing adolescents, is a relatively unexplored area. It is easy to understand the importance of attachment relationships for the well-being of infants and small children. However, if we think of adolescence as a period of increased separation from parents and family of origin, direct and immediate parental influence is less apparent. The attachment model provides a lens through which we can view the continuing influence of internalized, abstract, organizational features of attachment relationships and the relationship between attachment figures and the self. These internal working models of attachment are the basic regulators of affect and behavior in relationships throughout the life span.

The term "attachment" is often used loosely to describe any close, emotionally involved relationship. The term, as first used by the British psychoanalyst John Bowlby (1958), was intended to refer to a specific form of affective relationship. That relationship is an enduring and deep emotional bond between one human and another. The attachment figure provides protection, soothing, comfort, and help, leading to physical security in the very young but also to the experience of emotional security and well-being. This is not a model for describing any interpersonal relationship, nor is it the description of relationships only in infancy. As development proceeds, attachment behaviors are reorganized to include newly acquired skills that express the underlying, stable attachment organization. The mechanisms by which the attachment organization retains its stability and the behavioral manifestations of that attachment organization in adolescence are what we hope to describe further. The central organization of attachment remains the same throughout the lifespan, barring severe trauma or deliberate attempts to change the organization, for example, through psychotherapy. The attachment relationship, the dyadic organization, is dyadic regulation.

In infancy, the burden of assessing the need for and providing security rests with the caretaker. Sensitive, consistent care leads to expectations that security needs will be met and hence to a secure attachment. Ainsworth, Bell, and Stayton (1974) have shown that the quality of mother-infant attachment can be predicted from aspects of their interaction as early as the sixth week of life. Three main attachment classifications exist, one secure and two types of insecure attachment—ambivalent and avoidant. The standard assessment of attachment in infancy is the Ainsworth-Wittig Strange Situation procedure (Ainsworth and Wittig 1969). In a series of short episodes, an infant and its mother are brought together in a laboratory, joined by a friendly stranger, and then separated from one another. The infant is left with the stranger, and then alone, and finally reunited with its mother. Observation of both separation and reunion behaviors determines attachment classification. Secure infants may or may not protest maternal absence but greet the mother with pleasure on reunion. If distressed, the infants are calmed by the mother's return or ministrations, such as holding or reassurance. These infants have a working model of the mother as sensitively responsive to their needs. The term "sensitively responsive" refers to the caretaker's capacity to understand the needs of the child accurately and to respond to those needs. This model is not to be thought of as a conscious, reflective representation, as it may become in adolescence or adulthood with the advent of formal operational thought. Rather, the model is embedded in the behavior of the infant. Securely attached infants expect that their mothers will see their distress and also will see and respond to their signals about how to end their distress.

The second classification, the ambivalent-insecure attachment, is characterized by cyclical efforts to gain security from the attachment figure and avoidance of the attachment figure. On reunion, infants clamor to be picked up, only to push their mothers away, and then again ask to be held. They fail to be soothed and appear to be in unending conflict with the attachment figure. This is the rarest organization in infancy (less than 10 percent) and is often associated with severely disordered relationships and sometimes with neurological compromise in the infant. These are infants who have experienced inconsistent sensitivity from their mothers. At times, these mothers will hold and comfort their distressed infants; at other times, they will leave their infants unattended for hours. The infants' inconsistent adaptation reflects the mothers' inconsistent caretaking.

By contrast with their ambivalent counterparts, insecure-avoidant infants rarely show overt distress over separation. On reunion they are indifferent to mother's return and literally avoid interaction with her. Like the other two attachment organizations, infant avoidance reflects the relational history of the mother-infant dyad. These infants have relational histories that include emotional and physical rejection, particularly in times of distress. The infant has created an adaptational strategy to deal with rejection and to regulate its affective response to this rejection. The rejection of attachment behavior leads to anger and anxiety within the infant. Avoidance serves to cut off interaction, which might arouse attachment behavior, thereby avoiding the arousal of negative affect as well.

Main (1981) further views the function of avoidance as maintaining the attachment relationship. Avoidance is a compromise between alienating the attachment figure with angry demands for attention and maintaining an angry, rejected position in the absence of a comforting attachment figure. Avoidance serves to cut off the affective arousal before it is experienced as distress. This allows the infant to regulate its affect, thereby maintaining its organization during times of distress, and to maintain some comforting physical proximity to the attachment figure. The presence of such a complex strategy in an infant as young as twelve months speaks to the early, organized, effective and adaptive nature of internal working models.

If one expects that the infant behavior in the Strange Situation procedure is based on an internal working model, which is in turn based on a relational history, it would stand to reason that the internal working model would remain stable so long as the context from which it emerged remained stable. Empirical evidence supports this idea. Attachment classification is quite stable through at least the first six years of life (Main, Kaplan, and Cassidy 1985). Internal working models are solidified in the preschool years and are difficult to change without conscious effortful reflection on one's behavior and experience. In what Sroufe (1989) calls a "sophisticated sensitive period hypothesis" (p. 85), Bowlby (1973) claims that internal working models are difficult to change (1) because early prototypes of inner organization are not readily accessible to conscious awareness and continue to operate out of awareness and (2) because of a tendency to form new relationships that are congruent with earlier models and hence tend to reinforce the validity of those models. The latter point embodies the concept of recursion in development.

Observations of toddlers and young school-age children show the enduring and widespread effects of attachment organization on many aspects of their functioning, not just on emotional or social functioning (Arend 1984; Matas, Arend, and Sroufe 1978; Sroufe, Fox, and Pancake 1983; Sroufe and Rosenberg 1980). Preschoolers with secure attachment histories as infants are more positive in their affect, more enthusiastic, confident, and persistent in problem solving, and better able to use adults effectively when distressed or needing assistance. They seem more confident and flexible in managing impulses, feelings, and desires. Socially, they are more engaged and empathic. Children with insecure attachment histories show the converse behaviors. Affect is often angry, frustration tolerance low, and social competence poor. Adults are avoided angrily or clung to. Peer relationships are characterized by negative affect, lack of empathy, and shallowness. Behavior disorders are more common in this group, as is childhood depression. Follow-up of these children is still in process in two longitudinal studies at the University of Minnesota, directed by Alan Sroufe, and at the University of California, Berkeley, led by Mary Main.

In our work, we are trying to describe what these children may look like as adolescents. To do so, we rely on the scant literature on adult and adolescent attachment. George, Kaplan, and Main (1985) have developed a semistructured interview that can be used to classify an adolescent's or adult's state of mind with respect to attachment. Keep in mind that this interview does not purport to capture the quality of the literal attachment relationship when the now adult was an infant but rather looks exclusively at components of the adults' current representation of attachment. The adult's current state of mental organization, rather than his or her history, is being assessed. This interview has been successfully used with several other groups of adolescents, but to our knowledge this is its first use with any psychopathological population. The interview asks questions regarding the basic structure of the family, about quality of caretaking and affective tone, about security operations, and about experience of loss. It is designed so that the subject is asked to support through memories or anecdotes the generalizations put forth earlier in the interview about the quality of relationships with each of the parents. Classification parallels the infant classification scheme, though it is obviously based, not on the observation of behavior, but of the use of language in the interview and in the content of the interview. The adult's or adolescent's coherency and consistency of description of attachment-related experiences form the core of the classification scheme.

The classification derived from this interview embodies the four principles of development central to a self-regulatory system. (1) It has structure and process in that both the content of the individual's narrative regarding his childhood and the process by which that narrative is put into language are considered. (2) It is relational and contextual. The focus of the interview is on a description of the quality of relationships with parents. (3) It is constructivist. The meaning made by the individual of his childhood experiences is the information of interest. (4) It is cybernetic and recursive. The process by which the narrative of childhood is constructed reflects an abstraction and reintegration of processes inherent in the relationship itself. The internalization of the organization of earlier relationships is demonstrated in language in the interview.

From the Adult Attachment Interview, three major classifications can be made of adult attachment: one secure and two forms of insecure. The analogue to the secure infant is an autonomous adult/adolescent. These individuals value attachment relationships and regard attachment-related experiences as influential. They are relatively independent and objective regarding any particular experience or relationship. The interview is coherent and consistent. The generalized description of relationships with parents is supported by specific memories. The parents are differentiated from one another. Discourse is fluent, relaxed. The individual seems at ease with the topic and therefore able to reflect on experience with parents objectively. He or she is largely free of idealization or angry preoccupation with unsupportive or incompetent parents. The individual's narrative is believable to a listener or reader.

The histories of these individuals include parents who served as a secure base in an ongoing way or who have had considerable productive reflection on the reason for parental failings and are now resolved regarding their disappointments in the relationship. The autonomous organization requires considerable effort and insight and requires the acquisition of formal operational thought. Moreover, most of these individuals possess what Main (in press) has termed "metacognitive monitoring" or the capacity to monitor, report on the processes of their thinking, and recall as they speak. They are able to put their current thought processes in the context of their habitual ways of thinking, comment on their biases and distortions, and recognize that others have viewpoints differing from their own. This metacognitive monitoring is the hallmark of cognition in an autonomous adolescent or adult. Since the internal working model of the self is the complement of the internal working model of the attachment figure, these individuals have a balanced view of self and others, valuing interdependence, and have a clear sense of identity.

Not always are they models of mental health, however. Many experience troubled periods in their lives and unsatisfying relationships. This is because the attachment function is only one of many functions of a relationship. Recall Bowlby's original definition of an attachment relationship as the regulatory function for the maintenance of security and the basis for confident engagement with the environment. One, however, would expect an overall psychological resilience and flexibility in adaptation absent from the insecure groups.

The parallel to the infant insecure-ambivalent category is called preoccupied in adulthood and adolescence. As the name implies, for these individuals the influence of parents and attachment-related experiences can be neither dismissed nor coherently stated and seems to preoccupy attention. They appear highly conflicted and in an ongoing cycle of fruitless reflection on relationships with parents and disavowal of interest in maintaining these relationships. Two distinct subtypes are found, an active and a passive. The actively preoccupied individual is marked by extreme anger that dominates his or her discourse. These individuals blame parents for their own difficulties yet exhibit placating attitudes toward parents. They are pseudopsychological, talkative, and ineffective in using their insight. Instances of role reversal or spousification with one parent are universal. Identity diffusion is common. These individuals have a history of enmeshed relationships with parents, with role reversal, and guilt-inducing efforts to control their behavior. The actively preoccupied individual in the extremes of personality disorder most closely resembles an individual with a borderline personality disorder.

The passively preoccupied individual can never settle on a characterization of his or her relationship with his or her parents. He or she may oscillate between a positive and a negative evaluation of parents or be so vague as to be incomprehensible. A sense of inchoate negativity about his or her relationships lingers, however. With respect to the self, he or she too exhibits identity diffusion. A third subtype can be classified on the basis of a response to trauma that leaves the individual overwhelmed and unable to construct a coherent overview of his or her childhood. The individual is either flooded with unintegrated memories or distressed by the lack of memory with respect to childhood. While this subtype is rare in a normal population, it is quite common in a psychiatric population and represents a poorly articulated area of the scoring system. However, we believe that individuals with essentially dissociative defenses or dissociative disorders will cluster in this category.

The third adult/adolescent classification is the one that we would like to focus on most closely because it is most commonly found in our population of substance-abusing adolescents, particularly the males. The adult parallel to an infant insecure avoidant classification is called dismissing. The individual either dismisses the importance of attachment or relationships or, if he or she does value relationships, dismisses the extent of their effect on him. There is an idealization of the parents or portrayal of negative experiences with the parents as normal. Frequently, these individuals lack memory for childhood, or, if negative memories do occur, they regard themselves as unaffected by them. Often, they highly value achievement, self-reliance, personal strength, or cunning. These qualities are sometimes cited as rationalizations for the lack of effect on self of negative experiences. In a study of older adolescents, Kobak and Sceery (1988) found that these individuals are the least likely of any attachment groups to avow internal distress. However, others view them as hostile and provocative, to act out their all-too-obvious inner disharmony and affective dysregulation.

This has proved true of our substance-abusing population as well. On a self-report measure of somatic and psychiatric symptoms, the SCL-90 (Derogatis 1977), the dismissing individuals see themselves as less symptomatic on all nine scales when compared to their preoccupied counterparts. They see themselves as less depressed, anxious, hostile, somatically and obsessionally preoccupied, sensitive, paranoid, phobic, or psychotic. The histories of these individuals include rejection by one or both parents and a pervasive lack of love and supportiveness. Since this description is identical to the description of the relational histories of avoidant infants, the question is raised whether the mothers of avoidantly attached infants do themselves have dismissing attachment organizations. Main et al. (1985) found this to be the case. There is a high correlation between maternal and infant attachment classification for all three attachment organizations.

At this point, we would like to return to a description of the defensive adaptation that is served by an avoidant organization. Recall that, for an avoidant infant, the adaption serves to regulate affective arousal (to diminish anger and anxiety) and to maintain an attachment relationship, albeit compromised. What are the reorganized expressions of these adaptive processes in adolescence? The dismissing adolescent defensively excludes from awareness any information that may evoke attachment behaviors and, hence, put himself in the position of being rebuffed and angered. For this individual, negative affects are not associated with ameliorative responses on the part of parents. Negative affects can be neither displayed nor tolerated in order to achieve mastery over threatening or frustrating situations. Hence, denial, repression, falsification of affective expression, or displacement of aggression is used as the primary defense of dismissing individuals. The lack of memory central to this organization serves to disengage the attachment system and reduce the experience of negative affect by screening from consciousness information that might elicit either attachment-seeking behavior or the anger over disappointment. Likewise, idealization serves an avoidant function in these individuals by also allowing selective ignorance of negative information relevant to attachment. Idealization also plays a part in what Bowlby (1980) calls "multiple contradictory models of attachment," that is, simultaneously holding contradictory ideas regarding the parent or attachment without awareness of the contradiction.

It is precisely this constellation of repressive defenses that we see in substance-abusing adolescents, both within the attachment interview and behaviorally. The widely observed affective regulatory function of substance abuse can be viewed from an attachment-theoretic perspective as a means to cut off awareness of negative affects surrounding attachment and as an effort to maintain an idealized view of attachment figures. These types of defenses are also likely to be the precursors to narcissistic and antisocial personality organizations, a connection that we are in the process of exploring empirically. This connection also stands to reason given the high rates of those personality organizations in comorbid adolescents. The antisocial character's affectionlessness, lack of empathy, disavowal of the importance of relationships, impulsiveness, and displaced aggression are all seen in dismissing individuals. Similarly, the idealization found in dismissing individuals may be a precursor of a narcissistic personality organization. If one thinks of the complementary models of the self that are generated from internal working models of attachment figures, then dismissing individuals should have idealized views of themselves and their capacities. In the extreme, this may take the form of the grandiosity and excessive self-centeredness of the narcissist.

Conclusions

In conclusion, questions regarding the cooccurrence of distinct personality organizations and attachment classifications are the direction in which we are taking attachment research with adolescents.

REFERENCES

Ainsworth, M. D. S., and Wittig, B. A. 1969. Attachment and the exploratory behavior of one-year olds in a strange situation. In B. M. Foss, ed. *Determinants of Infant Behavior,* vol. 4. London: Methuen.

Ainsworth, M. D. S.; Bell, S. M.; and Stayton, D. J. 1974. Infant-mother attachment and social development: "socialization" as a product of reciprocal responsiveness to signals. In M. P. N. Richards, ed. *The Integration of a Child into a Social World.* London: Cambridge University Press.

Arend, R. 1984. Preschoolers' competence in a barrier situation: patterns of adaptation and their precursors in infancy. Ph.D. diss., University of Minnesota.

Bowlby, J. 1958. The nature of the child's tie to his mother. *International Journal of Psycho-Analysis* 39:350–373.

Bowlby, J. 1973. *Attachment and Loss*. Vol. 2, *Separation, Anxiety and Anger*. New York: Basic.

Bowlby, J. 1980. *Attachment and Loss*. Vol. 3, *Loss, Sadness, and Depression*. New York: Basic.

Derogatis, L. R. 1977. *SCL-90 Administration, Scoring and Procedures Manual—I*. Baltimore: Johns Hopkins University Press.

George, C.; Kaplan, N.; and Main, M. 1985. An adult attachment interview: interview protocol. University of California, Berkeley, Department of Psychology. Typescript.

Kobak, R. R., and Sceery, A. 1988. Attachment in adolescence: working models, affect regulation and representation of self and others. *Child Development* 59:135–146.

Matas, L.; Arend, R.; and Sroufe, L. A. 1978. Continuity of adaptation in the second year: the relationship between quality of attachment and later competent functioning. *Child Development* 49:547–555.

Main, M. 1981. Avoidance in the service of attachment: a working paper. In K. Immelmann, G. Barlow, L. Petrinovich, and M. Main, eds. *Behavioral Development: The Bielefeld Interdisciplinary Project*. New York: Cambridge University Press.

Main, M. In press. Metacognitive knowledge, metacognitive monitoring, and singular (coherent) vs. multiple (incoherent) models of attachment: findings and directions for future research. In P. Marris, J. Stevenson-Hinde, and C. Parkes, eds. *Attachment across the Life Cycle*. New York: Routledge & Kegan Paul.

Main, M.; Kaplan, N.; and Cassidy, J. 1985. Security in infancy, childhood, and adulthood: a move to the level of representation. In I. Bretherton and E. Waters, eds. *Growing Points of Attachment Theory and Research. Monographs of the Society for Research in Child Development,* vol. 50, nos. 1–2, serial no. 209. Chicago: University of Chicago Press.

Sroufe, L. A. 1989. Relationships, self and individual adaptation. In A. J. Sameroff and R. N. Emde, eds. *Relationship Disturbances in Early Childhood*. New York: Basic.

Sroufe, L. A.; Fox, N.; and Pancake, V. 1983. Attachment and dependency in developmental perspective. *Child Development* 54:1615–1627.

Sroufe, L. A., and Rosenberg, D. 1980. Coherence of individual adaptation in lower SES infants and toddlers. Paper presented at the International Conference on Infant Studies, Providence, R.I.

28 FORMAL OPERATIONS AS REGULATORY CONTEXT IN ADOLESCENCE

WILLIS F. OVERTON, JOHN H. STEIDL, DIANA ROSENSTEIN,
AND HARVEY A. HOROWITZ

A major focus of the research project on adolescent psychopathology being pursued at the Institute of Pennsylvania Hospital has been on the construction of a developmental model of self-regulation (i.e., the self as a regulator of affect and impulses). The primary characteristics of this model are that it is relational (i.e., it asserts that regulation emerges from the ongoing interactions of self and other) and developmental (i.e., it asserts that self, as an organization, goes through a series of ontogenetic phases). In ontogenesis, the earlier forms or organizations are preserved and incorporated in later novel forms. This model is designed to account for psychological risk and common vulnerability in adolescence.

In other chapters, descriptions have been presented of the basic features of the model, the manner in which attachment theory understands the progressive internalization of a relational system (i.e., the infant-caregiver dyadic system) as the early relational precursor to self-regulation, and how family interaction functions as a context for regulation. The focus of this chapter concerns the way that cognition or, more specifically, a particular form of thinking called formal operational thought may play a role in regulating the affect and behavior of the adolescent.

Formal thought first emerges in adolescence, but it has its precursors in earlier types of thinking activities. Thus, in exploring formal thought as a regulator of adolescent affect and behavior, it is first necessary to consider the general developmental course of thinking and to use that ontogenetic sequence as a framework for further examinations.

Thinking

As a first approximation to considering the ontogenetic steps to formal thought, it should be noted that we are here describing a particular type of thinking, namely, logical thought or logical reasoning. Specifically, this is the type of thought usually understood as rational thought, thought whose main hallmarks are its coherence, its consistency, its precision, and its lack of contradictions. It is this logical thought that will be understood as relevant to the regulation of affect and behavior. We are not referring to a variety of other types of thinking such as fantasy thought, creative thought, and associative thought.

Jean Piaget's theory of cognitive development presents the most influential and most thoroughly empirically supported framework for considering the ontogenesis of logical thought on the scene today (see Piaget 1980, 1987; Piaget and Garcia 1986). This framework, along with a good deal of empirical work conducted in the Adolescent Reasoning Laboratory at Temple University, and also along with some theoretical contributions from the works of Heinz Werner, Harry Stack Sullivan, and Donald Winnicott, has provided the conceptual foundation for the formulation to be discussed.

With this background, we may briefly describe the steps on the way to formal operational or formal logical thought. First, beginning at birth and proceeding into the first year of life, there is no thinking and, hence, no logical thought. In this phase—which Piaget calls the sensorimotor phase—while the infant is cognitively alert, capable of discriminating signals, and fully attuned to the caregiver, he or she lacks a system of symbols detached from the objects symbolized. Because thinking is defined as the manipulation of symbols, there is no thought proper at this time. The mode of experience in the early part of this phase is like Sullivan's "prototaxic mode," Winnicott's "object relating" as distinct from the later "object use," and Werner's "things of action." The mode is also analogous to Freud's "primary process thinking" but should more appropriately be called "primary process experiencing."

Piaget's second phase—called preoperational thought—extends from somewhere around the eighteenth month up to five or six years of age. This phase begins when the child constructs the first detachable symbols. These are called protosymbols because they are composed of personal nonshared experience. Thought begins in this early period, but it is highly idiosyncratic, and objects of thought have a personalized, affectively imbued meaning. This early thinking is akin to Freud's "primary process thinking" and Sullivan's parataxic mode of experience.

As this phase proceeds, thinking, while lacking traditional signs of logic, becomes generalized and further detached from the original highly idiosyncratic meanings. Here, language comes to support generalized meanings. The child moves into the early arena of Freud's "secondary process thinking" and more solidly into Sullivan's parataxic mode. As Erikson (1980, p. 78) once noted about this period, language develops to the point that the child is capable of misunderstanding almost everything he hears. If you explore the child's thought in this period, you find a sort of illusion of logic. To the observer, there appears to be a logic, but, on close inspection, it is clear that this logic rides superficially on the syntax of language rather than being a structural feature of the thought process itself. In this and the next phase as well, the child exhibits a sense of the literal.

In the third of Piaget's four phases, genuine logic begins to emerge. This phase, called the period of concrete operational thought (see Inhelder and Piaget 1964), extends from five or six up to about ten to twelve years of age. This is very much the phase of Freud's secondary process thinking, defined as ordinary, conscious thinking that is primarily verbal and follows the usual laws of syntax and logic. However, the logical thought that emerges at this time has critical limitations. It lacks generality, and it is tied to the concrete world of actual or fantasized objects and events. The child has logical thinking, but it is logical thinking about particular concrete events and particular concrete fantasies. This logical thought is embedded in a literal context of linear causes and effects. Sullivan's syntactic mode of experience begins to emerge in this phase, but it is concretely anchored in the parataxic mode.

The sensorimotor experience, the thinking of the preoperational phase, and the logical thought of the concrete operational phase are, then, the precursor forms to the organization of thought that emerges in adolescence, in the phase of formal operational thought. What develops, here, in adolescence is a kind of universal metalogic system. That is, the adolescent develops a general system of logic that allows him to think about his ordinary concrete logical thinking systematically (see Inhelder and Piaget 1958).

The emergence of this new level of thought organization can have profound influences on many dimensions of the adolescent's life. However, only a brief sketch of some of these will be presented before we undertake an equally brief consideration of how this organization can play a role in the self-regulation of affect and behavior.

Formal Operational Thought: Consequences

As a preamble to sketching some of the consequences of this new formal level in the organization of thought, we should urge you to think of this acquisition as a tool rather than as an end in itself. Like any tool, once acquired, it can be used or not used (i.e., once it becomes available, it may be accessed or not accessed). Similarly, like any tool, it may be used in some situations and not in others. Finally, like any tool, it can be used for either good or ill. Not having the tool at all, or being delayed in getting it, or perhaps getting it too early, can have negative consequences. Acquiring the tool at the appropriate time, however, still leaves open the question of how it will be used.

A considerable body of contemporary research has demonstrated that formal reasoning undergoes a transformation and a well-defined developmental progression between the ages of approximately ten to eleven and seventeen to eighteen years (Bady 1979; Bucci 1978; Byrnes and Overton 1986, 1988; Moshman 1979; Moshman and Franks 1986; O'Brien and Overton 1980, 1982; Overton, Byrnes, and O'Brien 1985; Overton, Ward, Noveck, Black, and O'Brien 1987; Pollack, Ward, and Overton 1988; Reene and Overton 1989; Ward and Overton 1990). This same body of research—as well as additional studies (Clement and Falmagne 1986; Franco and Overton 1984; Markovits 1986; Overton, Yaure, and Ward 1986)—supports the position that, prior to adolescence, the competence to reason formally is largely unavailable while, by late adolescence, adolescents as a group uniformly demonstrate the availability of this skill. This research shows that formal reasoning competence is a rather universally available tool. It does not argue that this tool must be manifested in all contexts.

We can now turn to some consequences for the adolescent of having this tool available. If formal operational thought is a generalized system of logic or a logic of logic, then it functions to permit the adolescent to stand at a level above his day-to-day syntactic thought. From this new-found reflective vantage point, the everyday thought of secondary process thinking or syntactic thinking can be evaluated in terms of its coherence, consistency, lack of contradictions, and precision. In other words, formal thought permits the individual to reflect on her systems of thought systematically. This freedom psychologically to move beyond the actual world of day-to-day fantasy and commonsense experience opens the door to an array of related experiences.

Once the individual acquires the freedom of reflection, it becomes apparent that this emancipation process need not stop at this level. If, as the person discovers, he can think about his thinking, why not systematically think about his thinking about his thinking. Indeed, why not think about thinking, about thinking, about thinking, and on and on. If this sounds frivolous, consider the obsessive patient. Just as you believe that you have made some experience near contact, off he flies to the next higher level, to reflect on that experience. When you follow, he flies higher yet.

As the adolescent continues the emancipation process, an inversion of the relation between the actual world and the world of the possible takes place. In the past, the actual world led directly, in an empirical inductive fashion, to what would be possible or not possible. Now, the world of possibilities rather than actualities becomes primary. Now, utopian and counterintuitive worlds can be generated in thought, and these thought experiments can be used as standards against which to judge the actual.

The new system of logic itself permits deduction of consequences, moving from the world of possibilities to the world of the actual. Thus, thought can now evince a hypothetical-deductive quality. The adolescent can generate hypotheses and test them in a systematic, logically coherent, deductive manner.

Formal Operational Thought and Self-Regulation

What effect, then, may these consequences have on the self-regulation of affect and behavior? First, consider again the caution that the consequences just sketched do not describe what adolescents who have attained a level of reflective thought actually do. It describes what they become capable of, and what they may do, if they use the tool.

In considering the consequences of formal thought, it should be understood that having this new skill available may be considered a mixed blessing, for there is both an up side and a down side to the use of formal thought. Each of these will be addressed briefly.

With respect to the up side, knowing that early nonformal adolescent behavior tends to be dominated by impulses, it is not surprising that the achievement of a level of formal reflection provides the adolescent with both a method of distancing himself from the impulses and unwanted affect and a structure for their self-containment. Here, Bion's metaphor of the container and the contained is useful. It is only at the level of formal reflection that the individual can truly, herself, operate as a container for the contained impulses and affect. That is, impulses and affect can now be projected onto this level, processed there, and introjected back in a metabolized form by the self as a whole (i.e., this might be thought of as an internalized form of projective identification). It should also be noted that this new level corresponds to what classic psychoanalysis described as the "observing" or "reasonable" ego in contrast with the "experiencing" ego (Greenson 1967) that is characteristic of earlier, lower levels of operation.

The outcome of this process of developing both a distance and a containing structure is both a greater sense of self-control and the further development of self-identity. With respect to self-identity, note that research scientists working in the field of adult attachment (Main, Kaplan, and Cassidy 1985) have proposed that the achievement of formal thinking is a necessary condition for altering the status of the internal working models of relationships. That is—referencing Piaget—these researchers state that such change is possible because "these operations may permit the individual to think about thought itself, that is, to step outside a given relationship system and to see it operating" (p. 77).

If formal reflection is a mechanism for the change of internal working models, then by definition it also establishes the basis for changes of affect regulation. Movement from, for example, an "avoidant/dismissing" type of model to a "secure/free autonomous" model means a change—to quote Kobak and Sceery (1988)—in the "rules that guide individuals' responses to emotionally distressing or challenging situations" (p. 142).

Furthermore, if formal thinking presents a mechanism for the change of internal working models, then by the same logic it suggests a mechanism for the renegotiation of the individual's status within the actual family context. Indeed, we are aware from both the clinical and the research literature that adolescence is a period of renegotiation of status within the family context. The suggestion here is that formal reflective thought can be a critical feature both in the initiation and in the course of that renegotiation.

As a final point concerning change, self-identity, and formal thinking, it seems most probable that the reflective system of formal thought is a necessary component of therapeutic change, at least therapeutic change as understood in any psychodynamic sense. If we conceive of the point of change as the container of the formal level that receives and metabolizes affect and impulse, then psychotherapy involves the joining of therapist and patient at this juncture in the arena that Winnicott called the "playground." Here, the reflective capacities of both the individual and the therapist connect to operate as containers and process dangerous affect and impulse. At the outset, the available conflict-free area of the patient's container is severely restricted, and the therapist serves as primary container. Therapeutic progress entails the progressive transfer of the processing function to the patient's container or to the patient's "reasonable" ego.

This discussion of the up side of formal reflection has, to this point, focused on the way that this capacity entails a vantage point and a system that enables affective and impulse control in a self-regulatory context. It should also be noted that formal thinking gives the adolescent tools that are even more directly related to the regulation of overt behavior. These consist of the ability to make rational decisions and the ability to think ahead or plan in a long-range systematic and coherent fashion.

Further, the very abstractness, universality, and hypothetical quality of the systems of thought made available by movement to the level of formal reflection have a major effect on the way that the adolescent can think about a host of concepts. These include, for example, the way of thinking about personal identity, the nature of society, existence, religion, justice, morality, friendship, and knowledge itself.

As noted earlier, if there is an up side to the use of formal reflection, there is also a down side. The first potentially negative feature of formal reflection is the phenomenon of egocentrism.

Earlier the emancipation process and the freedom of reflection were mentioned. This process can be a very heady experience. In its early phases, it leads the adolescent to the belief that this new experience is special and unique and, thus, because the adolescent is having this experience, that she must also be very special and unique. Here, we have the beginning of what is called adolescent egocentrism.

The quality of uniqueness itself is captured in what Elkind (1967) has called the "personal fable." This is the adolescent's complex of beliefs about his experiences: for example, "only he can suffer with such agonized intensity, or experience such exquisite rapture" (p. 1031); or about his mortality, for example, "I am so unique that I will not die." This last characteristic is particularly implicated in the high degree of risk-taking behaviors found in early adolescence.

The belief in being special also leads—particularly during the early part of this period—to the projection that others see the individual as special. One outcome of this is the adolescent's creation of what has been termed the "imaginary audience." To the extent that the individual is critical or admiring of himself or herself, so too must this projected audience be admiring or critical. As Elkind has said about this phenomenon, "The adolescent's wish for privacy and his reluctance to reveal himself may, to some extent, be a reaction to the feeling of being under the constant critical scrutiny of other people. The notion of an imaginary audience also helps to explain the observation that the affect which most concerns adolescents is not guilt, but shame, that is, the reaction to the audience" (1967, p. 1030). It also helps explain the adolescent's attempts to affect the style and behavior of the anticipated "critical and admiring audience" (see also Elkind 1985).

Another consequence of the use of formal reasoning that has a negative potential is the emergence of skepticism and dogmatism. The emancipation process of becoming capable of thinking about thinking about thinking begins to demonstrate that all knowledge involves the human activity called thinking. This opens the door to the recognition of the relativity of all knowledge (Chandler 1987). As this door opens, the adolescent tends initially to move in the direction of a complete skepticism about the validity of any knowledge or toward a dogmatic appeal to some authority for the correct answers. The formal cynical stance leads the adolescent to behavioral strategies based on "impulsivism (acting without thought), intuitionism (doing what affect demands), conformism (doing the done thing), and indifferentism (tossing a coin or acting on whim)" (p. 151). The dogmatic stance, on the other hand, provides both secular and nonsecular options. For example, the secular option is illustrated in what Elkind (1967) described as the adolescent's endemic search for religious faith. The nonsecular option includes things like a blind faith in the canons of "scientism" or other ideologies. In general, both the skeptical and the dogmatic approaches tend to chase each other during the early adolescent period.

As a final down-side feature of formal thought, it should be noted that this reflective ability can operate to reinforce earlier defensive strategies. That is, formal thinking can operate as a powerful force to be put in the service of whatever defensive structure was developed earlier in life. This is the case regardless of whether the original adaptive structure was primarily externalizing or internalizing in nature. For example, the primitive form of projection becomes the systematized set of projections under the sponsorship of formal reasoning, and the isolation of affect of the obsessional neurotic becomes the intellectualization of the adolescent. In a similar vein, the avoidant regulative style of the infant and the dismissing regulative style of the adolescent, or the ambivalent style of the infant and the preoccupied style of the adolescent, represent the later reinforcement of earlier defensive strategies.

In closing, it should be noted that this combination of up-side and down-side implications of formal reflection makes the task of generating any linear predictions concerning the relation between formal operational thought and developmental psychopathology extremely complicated. We may be able to suggest that all those with disturbances of affect and impulse will show less formal reasoning, and we may be able to make suggestions about certain groups demonstrating early or late formal reasoning availability. However, we are beginning to believe that ultimately the most productive avenue will be to explore the patterning of attachment classifications, family interactions, various diagnostic groups, and formal reasoning more closely in order to arrive at a systematic and clinically useful picture of the self-regulation of affect and impulse.

Measurement of Formal Reasoning and Empirical Evidence

Ward and Overton (1990) present an overview of measurement techniques used to diagnose formal reasoning in this investigation. Essentially, this technique involves a modification of the Wason four-card or selection task. This is a task that requires that the subject test a conditional (if . . . then . . .) rule. The subject does this by selecting the conditions under which he or she would be absolutely certain (i.e., it would be logically necessarily the case) that the rule was being broken.

To this point, we have data on some ninety-one hospitalized adolescents with IQ scores above 75 in our sample. The group is relatively evenly divided into a young adolescence (younger than 14.6 years), a middle adolescence (14.6–16 years), and a late adolescence (older than 16 years) group, with both males and females in each group. Thirty-six subjects have a diagnosis involving substance abuse, and these are distributed across the three age groups.

When the age-level performance for combined diagnostic groups is compared with a control group of nonhospitalized adolescents, it appears that the hospitalized adolescents have only slightly lower scores than the normal control group. When diagnosis is taken into account, the following appears. (a) The young substance abusers and a normal control group perform at identical levels, but other hospitalized subjects perform somewhat more poorly. (b) The middle-adolescent substance abusers and a normal control group also perform at identical levels, but again other hospitalized subjects perform more poorly. (c) At late adolescence, both the hospitalized substance-abusing subject and the hospitalized non-substance-abusing subject perform at identical levels, and this level is poorer than the normal control subject.

When gender is considered, the following begins to emerge. (a) In early adolescence, male substance-abusing patients perform at higher levels than nonabusing patients. (b) In middle adolescence, the same picture holds, but there is some very tentative evidence that female substance-abusing patients perform better than non-substance-abusing patients. (c) In late adolescence, it begins to appear that male substance-abusing patients perform better than male non-substance-abusing patients and female non-substance-abusing patients perform better than female substance-abusing patients.

It should be kept in mind that, given the small sample size, these reported findings are impressionistic and cannot be considered reliable at this time.

REFERENCES

Bady, R. J. 1979. Students' understanding of the logic of hypothesis testing. *Journal of Research in Science Teaching* 16:61–65.

Bucci, W. 1978. The interpretation of universal affirmation propositions. *Cognition* 6:55–77.

Byrnes, J. P., and Overton, W. F. 1986. Reasoning about certainty and uncertainty in concrete, causal, and propositional contexts. *Developmental Psychology* 22:793–799.

Byrnes, J. P., and Overton, W. F. 1988. Reasoning about logical connectives: a developmental analysis. *Journal of Experimental Child Psychology* 22:793–799.

Chandler, M. 1987. The Othello effect: essay on the emergence and eclipse of skeptical doubt. *Human Development* 30:137–159.

Clement, C. A., and Falmagne, R. J. 1986. Logical reasoning, world knowledge, and mental imagery: interconnections in cognitive processes. *Memory and Cognition* 14:299–307.

Elkind, D. 1967. Egocentrism in adolescence. *Child Development* 38:1025–1034.

Elkind, D. 1985. Egocentrism redux. *Developmental Review* 5:201–217.

Erikson, E. 1980. *Identity and the Life Cycle*. New York: Norton.

Franco, R., and Overton, W. F. 1984. Deductive reasoning in young and elderly adults: a competence-moderator-performance approach. Paper presented at the biennial Southeastern Conference on Human Development, Athens, Ga.

Greenson, R. G. 1967. *The Technique and Practice of Psychoanalysis*. New York: International Universities Press.

Inhelder, B., and Piaget, J. 1958. *The Growth of Logical Thinking from Childhood to Adolescence*. New York: Wiley.

Inhelder, B., and Piaget, J. 1964. *The Early Growth of Logic in the Child*. New York: Harper & Row.

Kobak, R. R., and Sceery, A. 1988. Attachment in late adolescence: working models, affect regulation, and representations of self and others. *Child Development* 59:135–146.

Main, M.; Kaplan, N.; and Cassidy, J. 1985. Security in infancy, childhood, and adulthood: a move to the level of representation. In I. Bretherton and E. Waters, eds. *Growing Points of Attachment Theory and Research. Monographs of the Society for Research in Child Development*, vol. 50, nos. 1–2, serial no. 209. Chicago: University of Chicago Press.

Markovits, H. 1986. Familiarity effects in conditional reasoning. *Journal of Educational Psychology* 78:492–494.

Moshman, D. 1979. Development of formal hypothesis-testing ability. *Developmental Psychology* 15:101–112.

Moshman, D., and Franks, B. A. 1986. Development of the concept of inferential validity. *Child Development* 57:153–165.

O'Brien, D., and Overton, W. F. 1980. Conditional reasoning following contradictory evidence: a developmental analysis. *Journal of Experimental Child Psychology* 30:44–60.

O'Brien, D., and Overton, W. F. 1982. Conditional reasoning and the competence-performance issue: a developmental analysis of a training task. *Journal of Experimental Child Psychology* 34:274–290.

Overton, W. F.; Byrnes, J. P.; and O'Brien, D. P. 1985. Developmental and individual differences in conditional reasoning: the role of contradiction training and cognitive style. *Developmental Psychology* 21:692–701.

Overton, W. F.; Ward, S. L.; Noveck, I.; Black, J.; and O'Brien, D. P. 1987. Form and content in the development of deductive reasoning. *Developmental Psychology* 23:22–30.

Overton, W. F.; Yaure, R.; and Ward, S. L. 1986. Deductive reasoning in young and elderly adults. Paper presented to the Conference on Human Development, Nashville.

Piaget, J. 1980. *Recent Studies in Genetic Epistemology*. Geneva: Cahiers Foundation Archives Jean Piaget.

Piaget, J. 1987. *Possibility and Necessity*. Vol. 1, *The Role of Possibility in Cognitive Development*. Vol. 2, *The Role of Necessity in Cognitive Development*. Minneapolis: University of Minnesota Press.

Piaget, J., and Garcia, R. 1986. *Vers une logique de signification*. Geneva: Editions Murionde Pierault Le-Bonniec, 1988.

Pollack, R. D.; Ward, S. L.; and Overton, W. F. 1988. Early adolescence: a transitional time in logical reasoning. Paper presented at the biennial meeting of the Society for Research on Adolescence, Alexandria, Va.

Reene, K. J., and Overton, W. F. 1989. Longitudinal investigation of adolescent deductive reasoning. Paper presented at the biennial meeting of the Society for Research in Child Development, Kansas City, Mo.

Ward, S. H., and Overton, W. F. 1990. Semantic familiarity, relevance, and the development of deductive reasoning. *Developmental Psychology* 26:488–493.

THE AUTHORS

JOHN BAIARDI is a faculty member, the Masterson Institute, New York.

JOHN BOWLBY, although retired, continued his research at the Tavistock Institute of Human Relations, School of Family Psychiatry and Community Mental Health, London, until his death, September 2, 1990, at eighty-three.

DAVID DEAN BROCKMAN is Clinical Professor of Psychiatry, University of Illinois, Chicago; and Training and Supervising Analyst, Chicago Institute for Psychoanalysis.

BARRY S. CARLTON is Associate Professor of Psychiatry, University of Hawaii School of Medicine, Honolulu.

REGINA C. CASPER is Professor of Psychiatry and Director, Eating Disorder Program, Pritzker School of Medicine, University of Chicago.

WILLIAM D. ERICKSON is Medical Director, St. Peter Regional Treatment Center, St. Peter, Minnesota.

SHERMAN C. FEINSTEIN is Clinical Professor of Psychiatry, University of Illinois, Chicago; Acting Director, Child and Adolescent Psychiatry, Humana Hospital–Michael Reese; Consultant, Rancho Park Hospital, San Diego; and Editor in Chief of this volume.

RICHARD FISCHER is a faculty member, the Masterson Institute, New York.

CHARLES P. FISHER is Associate Clinical Professor of Psychiatry, University of California, San Francisco; Director, Adult Psychiatry, Children's Hospital, San Francisco; and Member, San Francisco Psychoanalytic Institute.

BENJAMIN GARBER is Associate Attending Psychiatrist, Humana Hospital–Michael Reese; and Supervising Analyst, Chicago Institute for Psychoanalysis.

HARVEY GOLOMBEK is Associate Professor of Psychiatry, University of Toronto; and Head, Preventive Studies Program, C. M. Hincks Treatment Centre, Toronto, Ontario.

RICHARD M. GOTTLIEB is Assistant Clinical Professor of Psychiatry, Albert Einstein College of Medicine, Bronx, New York; and faculty member, New York University Psychoanalytic Institute.

HARVEY A. HOROWITZ is Clinical Associate Professor of Psychiatry, School of Medicine, University of Pennsylvania; Director, Adolescent Psychiatry Research, Institute of Pennsylvania Hospital; Medical Director, American Day Treatment Center, Bryn Mawr, Pennsylvania; and President (1991–1992) of the American Society for Adolescent Psychiatry.

ALLAN M. JOSEPHSON is Associate Professor of Psychiatry and Director of Training, Child, Adolescent, and Family Psychiatry, Medical College of Georgia, Augusta.

SAUL LEVINE is Professor, Department of Psychiatry, University of Toronto; and Head, Department of Psychiatry, Sunnybrook Hospital, Toronto, Ontario.

AMIA LIEBLICH is a faculty member, Department of Psychology, University of Haifa, Israel.

FELIX F. LOEB, JR., is Clinical Professor of Psychiatry, Oregon Health Sciences University, Portland, Oregon.

516

LORETTA R. LOEB is Clinical Associate Professor of Psychiatry, Oregon Health Sciences University.

RICHARD C. MAROHN is Professor of Clinical Psychiatry, Northwestern University Medical School; Faculty, Chicago Institute for Psychoanalysis; and Past President and Fellow, American Society for Adolescent Psychiatry.

PETER MARTON is Assistant Professor of Psychiatry, University of Toronto; and Head, Research Department, C. M. Hincks Treatment Centre, Toronto, Ontario.

JAMES F. MASTERSON is Adjunct Clinical Professor of Psychiatry, Cornell University Medical College; and Director, the Masterson Institute, New York.

DEREK MILLER is Professor of Psychiatry, Northwestern University Medical School, Chicago, Illinois.

DONNA L. MOREAU is Assistant Professor of Clinical Psychiatry, Columbia University College of Physicians and Surgeons; and Clinical Director, Child Anxiety and Depression Clinic, Presbyterian Hospital, New York.

CANDACE ORCUTT is a faculty member, the Masterson Institute, New York.

WILLIS F. OVERTON is Professor of Psychology, Temple University; and Senior Research Scientist, the Institute of Pennsylvania Hospital.

VIVIAN M. RAKOFF is Professor of Psychiatry, University of Toronto, Clarke Institute of Psychiatry, Toronto, Ontario.

ANA-MARIA RIZZUTO is Training and Supervising Analyst, Psychoanalytic Institute of New England, Boston.

DIANA ROSENSTEIN is Research Psychologist, the Institute of Pennsylvania Hospital.

JOSEPH SANDLER is Freud Memorial Professor and Professor of the Psychoanalysis Unit, University of London; and Training and Supervising Analyst, British Psychoanalytical Society, London, England.

RICHARD M. SARLES is Professor of Psychiatry and Pediatrics, University of Maryland; Vice President, Child and Adolescent Clinical Services, Shepard and Enoch Pratt Hospital, Towson, Maryland; and Past President, American Society for Adolescent Psychiatry.

JOHN L. SCHIMEL is Clinical Professor of Psychiatry, New York University–Bellevue Medical Center; and Associate Director and Training and Supervisory Psychoanalyst, William Alanson White Institute, New York.

STANLEY SCHNEIDER is Professor of Psychology and Social Work, Yeshiva University, New York; and Executive Director, Summit Institute, Jerusalem, Israel.

KIMBERLY A. SCHONERT is a postdoctoral fellow, Clinical Research Training Program in Adolescence, University of Chicago Committee on Human Development.

SCOTT SNYDER is Adjunct Associate Professor, Department of Child and Family Development, University of Georgia, Athens.

JOHN H. STEIDL is Director, Outpatient Clinic; and Director, Family Therapy, Research, and Training, the Institute of Pennsylvania Hospital.

MICHAEL H. STONE is Professor of Clinical Psychiatry, Columbia University College of Physicians and Surgeons, New York; Director of Research, Middletown Psychiatric Center; and Lecturer in Psychiatry, New York State Psychiatric Institute.

MAX SUGAR is Clinical Professor of Psychiatry, Louisiana State University and Tulane University, New Orleans; and Past President, American Society for Adolescent Psychiatry.

HAROLD M. VISOTSKY is Owen L. Coon Professor of Psychiatry and Behavioral Science, Department of Behavioral Science, Northwestern University Medical School.

HADAS WISEMAN is a faculty member, Department of Psychology, University of Haifa, Israel.

518

CONTENTS OF VOLUMES 1–17

529

NAME INDEX

Abbott, M. H., 306, 307, 318
Abend, S., 422, 437
Abraham, K., 349, 358
Achenbach, T., 249, 254
Adams, R., 64
Adatto, C., 133
Adelson, J., 208
Ainsworth, M. D. S., 474, 484, 492
Ajuriaguerra, J. de, 199
Aldershof, A. L., 360
Aleksandrowicz, D., 342
Aleksandrowicz, M., 342
Alexander, J., 215
Allport, G. W., 215
American Psychiatric Association, 147, 465
American Society for Adolescent Psychiatry, 381
Andersen, A. E., 92
Anderson, D., 202
Anthony, J., 357
Anthony, P., 29
Appel, W., 63
Arend, R., 494
Aries, P., 133
Aristotle, 108, 114, 115
Arlow, J., 357
Arnoff, F. N., 381
Arnold, L., 221
Arnstein, R. L., 133, 412
Asgard, U., 299
Avrahami, A., 158

Baars, B., 453
Bachara, G., 343
Bady, R. J., 505
Bahn, A. K., 348
Bailey, G. W., 465, 466
Baker, L., 316
Ballenger, J. C., 348
Bar-El, I., 410

Barraclough, B. M., 299
Bartholomew, A. A., 31
Bateson, G., 119, 121
Baudry, F., 181
Beauvoir, S., 48
Beavers, W. R., 485, 486
Becerra, R. M., 106
Beck, A. T., 299
Beit-Hallahmi, B., 156
Bell, R., 94, 96, 97
Bell, S. M., 492
Benedek, E., 381
Bergman, A., 158, 474
Berkowitz, L., 82, 85
Berman, A. L., 82
Beskind, H., 382
Bettelheim, B., 156, 159, 174
Biven, B. M., 182
Black, D., 29, 119
Black, J., 505
Blasi, J., 156, 158
Blatt, M., 209
Blehar, M. D., 484
Blishen, B. A., 224
Block, J., 216
Blos, P., 136, 138, 140, 149, 159, 182, 186, 193, 213–14, 215, 422, 440, 441, 442
Blumer, H., 78
Bollas, C., 428
Borowitz, G., 228, 239
Bower, E. M., 348
Bowlby, J., xi, 38, 215, 216, 218, 267, 272, 474, 481, 491, 494, 496, 498
Boyd, J. H., 145
Boyd, W. W., 134
Boyle, M., 234, 255
Brandstaetter, L. A., 144
Brandt, J., 306
Brenner, C., 357
Brent, D., 465, 466
Brethreton, I., 216

SUBJECT INDEX

ASAP. *See* American Society for Adolescent Psychiatry

Abandonment and depression, 6

Absorption, 448–59; and self-transcendence, 456

Abstraction principle, 141

Abuse, 481

Academics, 30, 341, 481; and learning disabilities, 324, 325, 344; personality disturbance, 256; self-esteem, 325; and remediation, 326, 345. *See also* Learning disabilities

Achievement and dismissing attachment organization, 497

Acting out, 149, 295, 467; and guilt, 358–59; and manic depressive disorder, 355–57; and personality functioning, 234; and therapist training, substitutes for, 9–10

Actualization and object manipulation, 404

Adaptation: and development, 469; environmental, 259, 264

Adaptive issues, epigenetic, 471

Adjustment, 259, 264, 265, 269; reaction, and manic depressive disorder, 348, 357

Adolescence: biological end of, 134; chronological end of, 132–33; and clinical treatment, 271–73; continuity of stages of, 259; defined, 215, 226, 290, 382; developmental groups, 247–48; and Huntington's Disease, 306–19; identity, 419; length of, 132–33; and personality disturbance, 255–56; phases of, 237, 245–48; and psychodynamic theory, 271; psychological end of, 136–37; stages of, 240, 271; and tribalism, 443–44; turmoil, 268, 269, 270, 273. *See also* Early adolescence; Middle adolescence; Late adolescence

Adolescens, definition, 132

Adolescere, definition, 132

Adoption and identity formation, 136, 413

Adult Attachment Interview, 495

Adulthood: acquiring responsibilities of, 159; and adolescent development, 372; and clothing, 443; and culture, 158; defined, 132, 215; developmental state of, 139; expectations of young, 266; and identity, 450; and late adolescence, 132–33; manic depressive disorder in, 355; transition to, 135, 157

Adultus, definition, 132

Affect, 266, 437, 479, 494; and attachment, 475, 491; and attitudes, 237; attunement, 473, 474; and avoidance, 434; and behavioral exchange, 473; blunted, 296; and bodily interactions, 435; changes in, 316; and clinical assessment, 270; communication of, 469; and comorbidity, 465; contagion of, 488; containment of, 464; continuity of, 241, 248; coordination of with cognition, 474; and defense mechanisms, 434; and developmental sequence, 470; and dismissing attachment organization, 498; disturbed, 267, 268; and early thought, 504; and experience of satisfaction, 433, 434; and exploratory behavior, 475; falsification of, 498; and formal operational thinking, 503, 507, 510; harmony of, 258, 264, 265; and Huntington's Disease, 306, 317, 318–19; and identification, 434; and identity, 434; and identity of experience, 431; and incorporation, 434; in infants, 493; and infant-caregiver dyad, 477; and insecure-avoidant attachment organization, 493; instability, 463, 467, 481; and internalization, 433–34; and intersubjectivity, 473; and introjection, 434; and language, 427; and late adolescence,

561

confusion, 408, 409; and communication, 432; consolidation of, and identity crisis, 448; and creativity, 454; crisis, 419; crisis, defined, 448; crisis, and personal continuity, 448; crisis, and role confusion, 448; crystallization, 218; crystallization, and personality development, 228; and cults, 67, 69; cultural, defined, 408; and culture, 393–94, 407–15, 450; diffusion, 408, 419, 448, 497; diffusion, and culture, 412; diffusion, and parent relationship, 497; disorder, 147; equilibrium, and culture, 409; as ego-syntonic, 437; as entity, 426; first psychic process of, 431–32; flexibility of, 430; vs. growth, 449; as illusion, 451; and infant-caregiver dyad, 432; inner, 412; and inner arrest, 451; internal structure of, defined, 452; and language, 393; and love, 429; maintenance, 219; maintenance, and personality development, 228; and meaning, 156; and perception, 404; as personal myth, 393; and projective identification, 507; and pronouns, 428; as relational narrative, 429; and relationships, 226; and resistance, 393; resistance, and growth, 450; and self-esteem, 394; and self-image, 394; and self-object relations, 405; sexual, and initiation, 443; social, definition of, 449–50; as structural illusion, 454; as subjective experience, 392–93, 412–38; as system, 453; and therapist training, 384; transcendence of, 449–50, 451, 454; vagueness of concept, 437–38

Identity formation, 132, 412–15; and adoption, 136; and communal living, 156–77; and culture, 158; and defense mechanisms, 448–49; defined, 448–49; and friendship, 110; in history, 111; and identification, 448–49; and ideology, 158; and integrating libido, 448–49; and learning disabilities, 342; and military service, 157; and movies, 86; and consistent roles, 449; and social networks, 112; and sublimation, 448–49; and transcendence, 459; as task in late adolescence, 136

Identity of experience: and affect, 431; and communication, 431; and psychic processes, 431–32

Ideological systems and separation from, 177

Ideology: and communal living, 162, 170, 172, 173, 175, 176–77; and formal operational thinking, 510; and identity formation, 158; and movies, 77; sex differences in, 175

Illinois State Psychiatric Institute Adolescent Program, 377

Imaginary audience, 509

Imitation effect and suicide, 82

Immune system and late adolescence, 134

Impulse control, 258, 259, 264, 265; and infant-caregiver dyad, 475; and language, 475

Impulses, containment of, 464

Impulses, regulation of, 507

Impulsivism, 509

Impulsivity, 463; and self-control, 479; behavioral, and comorbidity, 467

Incest, 290, 293, 298; and body image, 444; and borderline personality disorder, 291, 293, 294, 300–301; and boys, 301; and family relationships, 301; and psychosis, 300; and schizophrenia, 301; and sex differences, 301; and suicide, 300, 303

Incestuous wishes of parents toward children, 143

Incoordination and learning disabilities, 326

Incorporation: and affect, 434; and experience of satisfaction, 434; explained representationally, 399; and psychic structure, 392

Independence: and attachment organization, 495; avoidance of, 145; and communal living, 167–68; and late adolescence, 132; psychological, 147

Indifferentism, 509

Individual: psychopathology, isomorphic, 486, 488; psychopathology, and regulation, 464; second, and cathexis, 440–41

Individuality, respect for, 486

Individuation, 136–37, 397; and adulthood, 157; communal context of, 173; and communal living, 156–77; and communal living, 173–74; and control, 163; cultural support for, 142; and girls, 140, 143; and Huntington's Disease, 319; and late adolescence, 137; and parental sup-

Movies and adolescent development, 74–90

Myth: as identity, 454; personal, and identity formation, 451

Narcissism, 7–9, 298, 309; and Huntington's Disease, 317; and learning disabilities, 344; in movie characters, 86–87; primitive, 372; and repressive defense mechanisms, 499; secondary, and superego, 441; treatment of, 318

Narcissistic depression, 60; equilibrium, 23; imbalance, 403; needs, 56, 61; pain, 9; personality disorder, 5, 7–8; personality disorder, abandonment depression, 8; personality disorder, closet, 8; personality disorder, confrontation and, 21; personality disorder, defense mechanisms, primitive, 8; personality disorder, exhibitionistic, 8; phase, injury to, 293; vulnerability, 5, 24

Need satisfaction, 397

Negentropy, 485

Neuropsychology and learning disabilities, 323–24

Neurosis: manic-depressive, and biochemistry, 358; and internal conflict, 414

Noncompliance and self-control, 479

Nonreflectivity, 463, 467, 480

Nonself, 397, 399

Nurturance and depression, 147–48. *See also* Care

Object: choice, 140; idealization, 8; image, and fiction, 456; internal, power of, 441–42; loss, and migration, 414; love, and manic depressive disorder, 357; relating, 503; relations, 372; relations, borderline triad, 6; relations, consolidation of, 148; relations, explained representationally, 403–4; relations, and memory, 427; relations, split, 5; relationships, 3, 26–27, 38, 412; relationships, and fathering, 38; relationships, and group relationships, 27, 30; relationships, and mothering, 38; removal, 138

Object representations, 392, 395, 433, 437, 451; and attitudes, 237; and self-representation, 396–405; substitution

of, 455; use of, 503. *See also* Separation anxiety

Objectification and pronouns, 435

Observing ego, 464

Obsession and manic depressive disorder, 355

Obsessional neurosis and formal operational thinking, 510

Obsessive-compulsive: disorders, 249; thoughts, and movies, 81

Oedipal conflict: and manic depressive disorder, 357, 358; and learning disabilities, 342; and troubled adolescence, 444; psychopathology of, 372

Oedipus complex, 56; and libido, 442; and secondary individuation, 442

Offer Self-Image Questionnaire, 257

Omnipotence, 44

Opportunities and communal life, 164–65, 172, 173

Optimism: defined, 238; and personality development, 240–41; and personality functioning, 243, 246

Oral-anal character traits, and manic depressive disorder, 358

Organization: and development, 469; family, and self-regulation, 481

Other: and affect, 219; and attachment theory, 218; and reality-testing, 219; and self-image, 218; schema, and infant-caregiver dyad, 479

Outpatient treatment, 28

Pain and adolescent females, 144

Planning and formal operational thinking, 508

Pamrih, 449

Parallel processing and the unconscious, 453

Paranoia, 498

Parent-child interaction and laughter, 119

Parent-child ties, 109

Parental control, 143; and anorexia nervosa, 98–99; and cult membership, 72; and friendship, 109–10; and late adolescent development, 136, 137; and late adolescent psychopathology, 147

Parental expectations, 143

Parental support: and autonomy, 143; and individuation, 143

interview, 220; parental, and pronoun acquisition, 435; and personality development, 226; and personality pattern, 220; problems in, 255–56; and psychopathology, 463; and role assumption, 226; and self-esteem, 226; and the unconscious, 430. *See also* Friendship; Social networks

Religion: and formal operational thinking, 510; influence of, 299

Remediation, academic, 326

Reorganization phase, 136

Representation: and experience of satisfaction, 435; and memory, 433; psychic, and affect, 427; psychic, and language, 427; and pronoun acquisition, 428; in psychic structure, 392; through the opposite, 121

Representational thinking and self-awareness, 475

Representational world, 397, 399–400

Repression, 498

Reproduction, 141, 142; and environment, 133–34; and height, 133–34; and therapy, 148

Resentment and communal living, 167

Residential treatment, 28

Resistance: and identity, 393; in late adolescent therapy, 147

Resonance, class differences in, 83

Responsibilities and communal living, 167

Reward and communal living, 165

Rewarding object-relations part unit, 6

Risk factors, interactivity of, 466

Risk taking: and ego-centrism, 509; and formal operational thinking, 509; and self-control, 479

Ritual and persuasion, 67

Ritual, cultic, 67

Role aspirations and personality development, 220

Role assumption: and personality development, 219–20, 229; and relationships, 226

Role: confusion, 409; confusion, and identity crisis, 448; confusion, vs. identity, 408; consistency, and identity formation, 449; cultural, and pseudo-speciation, 451; differentiation, 315, 316; economic, and pseudo-speciation,

451; identity, diffuseness of, 443; integration of, 449; models, father for sons, 314; models, in Huntington's Disease families, 314–15; responsiveness, 404; reversal, 496, 497; taking, and boys, 209; taking, and cognitive development, 207–8; taking, and moral development, 207–8; taking, and moral development, 207–8. *See also* Identification

Sacrifice, fasting as, 96

Sadism, 44, 56

Safety and motivation, 402–3; and object relations, 403–4

Schizoaffective disorder, 290, 296, 297; and comorbidity, 467; sex differences in, 300

Schizophrenia, 249, 273, 290; and incest, 301; and substance abuse, 147

Schizophrenoform disorders, 290

School phobia and manic depressive disorder, 348, 357

Scientism and formal operational thinking, 510

Second individuation and autonomy, 441

Secondary personality distortion, 313

Secondary process thinking, 504

Security: as adolescent/adult, 495; and attachment, 491; and attachment theory, 218; and behavior regulation, 474; and communal living, 162–63; and communal living, 172; and infant-caretaker dyad, 492

SED. *See* Severely emotionally disturbed

Self: actual, 400; affective, structuralization of, 474; coherence of, 480; coping, 259; as developmental organization, 470; familial, 259; fluidity of, 452; fragmented, 8; grandiose, 8; ideal, 400; ideal, and defense mechanisms, 400–401; ideal, and reaction formation, 400; ideal, sources of, 401–2; as inner object, 452; internal working model of, and attachment figure, 496; meaning of, 395–405; as object representation, 267, 405; psychological, 258; psychotherapeutic, 378; sexual, 259; social, 258, 265, 269; stability of, 452; vs. "I," 452. *See also* False self